PRACTICAL EXERCISE THERAPY

Fourth Edition

Edited by

Margaret Hollis

MBE, MSc, FCSP, DipTP
Formerly Principal, Bradford
School of Physiotherapy

and

Phyl Fletcher-Cook

MEd, MCSP, Cert Ed
Senior Lecturer, Huddersfield
University

With contributions by

Sheila S. Kitchen
MSc, MSCP, DipTP
Course Co-ordinator, Physiotherapy Group
King's College, London

Barbara Sanford
DipPE (Lond. Univ.)
Formerly Lecturer in Physical Education
Bradford School of Physiotherapy

The late **Patricia J. Waddington**
BA (Hons), FCSP, DipTP
Formerly Principal, School of Physiotherapy
Manchester Royal Infirmary

Blackwell
Science

© 1976, 1981, 1988, 1999 by
Blackwell Science Ltd
Editorial Offices:
Osney Mead, Oxford OX2 0EL
25 John Street, London WC1N 2BL
23 Ainslie Place, Edinburgh EH3 6AJ
350 Main Street, Malden
  MA 02148 5018, USA
54 University Street, Carlton
  Victoria 3053, Australia
10, rue Casimir Delavigne
  75006 Paris, France

Other Editorial Offices:

Blackwell Wissenschafts-Verlag GmbH
Kurfürstendamm 57
10707 Berlin, Germany

Blackwell Science KK
MG Kodenmacho Building
7-10 Kodenmacho Nihombashi
Chuo-ku, Tokyo 104, Japan

First published 1976
Reprinted 1997
Second edition 1981
Reprinted 1983, 1984, 1985, 1987
Third edition 1989
Reprinted 1990, 1992, 1994, 1997
Fourth Edition 1999

Set in Sabon 10 on 13.5 pt
by Best-set Typesetter Ltd., Hong Kong
Printed and bound in Great Britain at
The Alden Press, Oxford

DISTRIBUTORS

Marston Book Services Ltd
PO Box 269
Abingdon
Oxon OX14 4YN
(*Orders*: Tel: 01235 465500
          Fax: 01235 465555)

USA
Blackwell Science, Inc.
Commerce Place
350 Main Street
Malden, MA 02148 5018
(*Orders*: Tel: 800 759 6102
              781 388 8250
       Fax: 781 388 8255)

Canada
Login Brothers Book Company
324 Saulteaux Crescent
Winnipeg, Manitoba R3J 3T2
(*Orders*: Tel: 204 837-2987
       Fax: 204 837-3116)

Australia
Blackwell Science Pty Ltd
54 University Street
Carlton, Victoria 3053
(*Orders*: Tel: 03 9347 0300
       Fax: 03 9347 5001)

A catalogue record for this title
is available from the British Library

ISBN 0-632-04973-1

Library of Congress
Cataloging-in-Publication Data
Practical exercise therapy/edited by Margaret Hollis
  and Phyl Fletcher-Cook; with contributions by
  Sheila S. Kitchen, Barbara Sanford, the late
  Patricia J. Waddington. —4th ed.
      p.   cm.
    Includes bibliographical references and index.
    ISBN 0-632-04973-1
    1. Exercise therapy.   I. Hollis, Margaret.
  II. Fletcher-Cook, Phyl.
  RM725.P73   1999
  615.8′2—dc21   98-53120
                                           CIP

For further information on
Blackwell Science, visit our website:
www.blackwell-science.com

CONTENTS

PREFACE

In revising this book I have been greatly assisted by my co-editor Phyl Fletcher-Cook who has written new chapters on basic techniques for respiratory care and the neurological basis of movement. Barbara Sanford has checked and revised the chapters on which she worked originally but, sadly, Pat Waddington died in 1997. She gave her blessing to any revision we might make.

We have omitted some sections, notably some of the suspension and spring exercises, as these can now be achieved in the more readily available therapeutic pools, and also the exercises for babies.

Much of the first edition of the book was based on our knowledge gained in practice both with patients and in teaching students, so we have omitted the original bibliography which mostly related to those parts of the book we have not altered. The two totally rewritten chapters each have their own references.

It was not necessary to revise the mechanics chapter as these concepts are eternal truths, as are many of the concepts of movement and muscle action. The first edition became a 'latin primer' as I kept in mind that recovery of movement and re-education of muscle could only be achieved in a limited number of ways. The main principle that all students have to understand is that progression is of the patient, with the physiotherapist constantly adapting techniques to the new needs and demands of the patient. Machines need all the basic principles applied to their use and as more expensive forms of equipment become more freely available in the developed world, there is still great need for the under-developed world to be able to carry out exercise without modern gadgetry.

In this fourth edition we have stuck to the principle of producing a basic teaching book so that in the different educational environments which prevail in some countries, students can still turn to simple explanations

of the 'how' of 'therapeutic exercise'. We hope that
future generations of students of all nationalities will find
this a book from which they can practise physiothera-
peutic skills with the lesser guidance that now prevails.

Mr Peter Harrison AIMBI has again undertaken the
photography and Janice Eccles has also again been able
to type the manuscript. We thank them for their work.

I would like to pay tribute to the contribution the late
Pat Waddington made to the book and to thank Barbara
Sanford for her continued willingness to check and
revise.

The staff at Blackwell Science continue to encourage
me by wanting further editions of my books. I cannot
help feeling there must be a swan song sometime soon
and in finding Phyl Fletcher-Cook I feel I have assisted
with continuity of the idea I first projected, of giving
students a background knowledge based on sound principles of mechanics, anatomy and physiology.

Margaret Hollis
MBE, MSc, FCSP, DipTP
Bradford

and

Phyl Fletcher-Cook
MEd, MCSP, Cert Ed
Bradford

ACKNOWLEDGEMENTS

I am grateful to the following companies who lent photographs.

Days Medical Aids of Bridgend for Figs 10.2, 10.3, 10.5 and 10.6 of their walking aids.

Kirton Designs Ltd of Norwich for Fig. 7.1.

Nomeq of Redditch for provision of their extensive bibliography and articles on isokinetics and for Figs 7.2, 7.3, 7.4, 7.5, 7.6, 7.7, 9.29 and 10.1.

Portabell Keep Fit Systems Ltd for Fig. 9.38B.

Rank Stanley Cox for Fig. 8.3 of the Guthrie Smith suspension frame and Fig. 9.32 of their Variweight boot.

Fig. 9.3 is from the booklet issued by The Hygienic Corporation, to whom we are grateful.

Table 11.2 is modified from Skinner A. T. & Thomson A. M. (1983) *Duffield's Exercise in Water*, 3rd edn, Baillière Tindall, London, with permission.

Our photographers were Mrs V. Cruse of Pudsey, Mr P. Harrison AIMBI of Bradford and Mr R F S Murray AIIP of Manchester to whom we owe our thanks for their patience and their expertise.

> *To our students*
> *who, in learning from us,*
> *teach us so much*

Chapter 1
INTRODUCTION

M. Hollis

The application of therapeutic exercise to a patient is a process which demands an initial examination of the patient's needs and a constant reassessment of the situation in the light of progress or retrogression. It also demands a knowledge of the condition from which the patient suffers, the potential recovery rate and complications which may arise. In addition the therapist must constantly bear in mind the anatomy of the part being treated and of the whole body; the physiological reactions of the body to all exercise and the particular exercise she is applying at the moment; and the underlying mechanical principles associated with the exercise and/or techniques applied.

Therapeutic exercise is also influenced by a psychological reaction in which the patient may or may not wish to get better. If he wishes to improve he may be overeager to please and do too much or perform badly and in haste. If he does not wish to improve it may be because he is afraid. He may be in pain and fear more pain, he may be afraid his illness or accident may recur, or he may have a fundamental fear of the whole field of medicine and hospitals in particular.

This barrier must be overcome and a rapport established between patient and therapist so that the therapist may initiate the proceedings which will eventually lead to the patient achieving his maximum independent potential.

To this end a few simple but important rules should be followed by the therapist. First, each patient should be known by name and greeted and welcomed at each treatment session. Secondly, fear of more pain can be overcome by working and teaching on parts which are not painful. Each action should be taught on the soundest or least painful part, then on the afflicted part gradually working towards the part he most dreads having treated. In this way he will not only be reassured but there will probably be less pain due to facilitation of inhibition. As he relaxes he will relax his protective painful spasm and so have less discomfort.

Thirdly, his activities must always be harnessed to a goal which is within his potential of achievement. This has two uses: it is a goal for which he can strive and a matter for congratulation when achieved. The objective can be reset each day or each week or with no regularity at all, but it is most important that the early goal is remarked upon when achieved as then the patient will gain confidence in his therapist as well as in himself.

It is said that initially patients have a 'love–hate' relationship with their therapists. This may be so as the therapist may have to insist on the patient performing an uncomfortable manoeuvre and he will not be grateful for it until some time has elapsed. Examples of this situation arise when a patient with an ineffective cough must be persuaded to cough more effectively to void his chest secretions in spite of the pain of his abdominal incision; and when patients have to contract the quadriceps muscle group following knee surgery. In both these cases patients freely admit later on that they hated the therapist at the time, but are grateful now that they were persuaded to do their therapeutic exercise.

Therapists who work in this climate become accustomed to this attitude from their patients and learn to use all their manual and psychological skills for the improvement of the patient.

With the patient who has a long-term problem, short-distance goal setting is even more important, and knowledge of the medical history of the patient, his social background and his home and work environment will be necessary to determine the sequence of the goals to be achieved. Personal independence should usually be aimed for initially. This may be toileting, personal care and dressing, feeding or ability to get about. Some go hand in hand. It is no use being able to undress and dress in the toilet if there is no possibility of physically getting there.

It is essential that the therapist gradually withdraws what she does for the patient so that eventually he does every task for himself. If this goal cannot be achieved then it is important to recognize that substitution must occur, e.g. if independent walking is unsafe and not improving, the patient must come to terms with the appropriate walking aid. Recognizing the moment when no further progress is being made is as important as the first assessment of a patient. Failure to recognize this fact leads to false hopes on the part of the patient and his family and a waste of the resources of the therapist, the tools of her work and the patient's time and effort.

Physical definitions of muscle performance

Force

The force output of a muscle, usually called its strength, is that which develops tension in the contracting muscle so that it contracts to produce work.

Work is defined as the action of a force over a specific distance in space. In the human body it refers to the product of muscular force exerted through a specific range of movement.

Power refers to a rate of doing work. In muscle action it is the output of the muscles at specific speeds of contraction.

Endurance is the capacity to contract muscles at a specific rate (power) for a specific interval of time.

Muscles require to be able to do work at varying tempos and to maintain the work for a period of time; failure to be able to produce satisfactory strength of muscle leads to weakness in one or more of the roles in which muscles play their part in normal activities. The roles of muscles are dealt with later in this chapter. Any failure of strength can lead to joint malfunction as well as functional incapacity in any of the daily activities to which the human body is subject during normal living.

Types of muscle work

There are two main ways in which a muscle may work naturally. It may contract and produce no movement, called isometric contraction, or it may produce movement during contraction, called isotonic contraction. Both these types of contraction may be used therapeutically, but a third type of muscle action may be applied to muscles to strengthen them. This uses *isokinetic* or *accommodative* resistance to achieve isotonic contractions (see Chapter 9).

Isotonic contraction

When a muscle works isotonically it contracts and the part of the body to which it is attached will move. There are two types of isotonic contraction.

Isotonic shortening

When a muscle performs a contraction and its two attachments are approximating to one another, the contraction is known as an isotonic shortening, e.g. when the arm is raised from the side and the abductors of the shoulder contract, the contraction is one of isotonic shortening.

Isotonic lengthening

When the attachments of a muscle move slowly away from one another and the muscle allows this movement to occur in a controlled manner, the muscle action is one of isotonic lengthening, e.g. when the body is in the upright position and the arm is lowered from abduction to adduction, the abductors of the shoulder will control the movement and these abductors will be acting in isotonic lengthening.

Isotonic shortening can take place under any circumstances, i.e. whenever movement takes place in which the attachments of a muscle approximate, the muscle work will be isotonic shortening. Isotonic lengthening, however, may only be brought about if an outside force is applied to the component which is to be moved and the body part is slowly moved so that the attachments of the muscle are moved away from one another.

Gravity may be the outside force which pulls body components towards the earth as in lowering the arm from the abducted position to the side, or in sitting on the edge of a table lowering the outstretched leg to a right angle at the knee. However, under many other circumstances, in order to work a muscle in isotonic lengthening it is necessary for the therapist to be the outside force. The command given is '*resist slightly whilst I move your leg*', or arm as the case may be, to a new position. The patient offers slight resistance, the therapist applies pressure which is greater than the resistance offered by the patient and is on the surface which is on the same aspect as the muscles which are required to be worked in isotonic lengthening. For example, if a patient is in side lying and the quadriceps are to be worked, the leg will be arranged straight at the knee, one hand will be placed as a stabilizing hand on the thigh and to palpate the quadriceps. The other hand will be placed on the anterior aspect of the leg and the command will be given '*resist slightly while I bend your leg*'. The patient resists, the therapist bends the leg and the quadriceps will be worked in isotonic lengthening.

Many other examples of isotonic shortening and isotonic lengthening can be found and therapists should attempt to work out the single movements of each of the joints of the body with and without resistance so that they are able to identify isotonic shortening and isotonic lengthening. When therapists can identify these two types of muscle work they should then try to apply the range of muscle work as described below.

Isometric contraction

When a muscle works isometrically it shortens its muscular length and slightly lengthens its non-contractile components and in doing so no movement occurs at any of the joints over which that muscle passes. It is easiest and in fact usual for an induced isometric contraction to be performed when a muscle is resting at the innermost part of its range, i.e. with the muscle attachments approximated, but with practice the skill can be developed so that it is possible isometrically to contract a muscle or muscle group at any part of the range. Isometric contraction can be taught to a muscle by the application of a manual resistance which is exactly equal to the contraction which the muscle produces. The command which the therapist will give will be '*don't let me push or pull that body component about*', e.g. '*don't let me push you forwards*' with pressure on the back of the shoulders will initially cause contraction of the extensor muscles. '*Don't let me pull you back*' will cause contraction of the flexor muscles. '*Don't let me push your foot up*' will cause contraction of the plantarflexors of the foot. '*Don't let me push your foot down*' will cause contraction of the dorsiflexors of the foot.

When isometric contractions are done to one group of muscles only, they are usually taught in order that the patient might practise these contractions alone without the therapist. Indeed isometric contractions are the only contractions which are possible when the patient is wearing a support such as a plaster or a fixation splint. This is the type of muscle work which is used when the joint is so inflamed that movement would be both painful and inadvisable. The strength and tone of the muscles working over that joint may be maintained by teaching the patient isometric contractions. When a patient is initially incapable of performing an isometric contraction on a damaged part, the technique may be taught on the opposite limb or may be taught on any part of the patient, and if this is completely impossible the contraction *per se* may be taught with the use of a faradic type current

applied in such a manner that it merely teaches the patient what to do and is immediately followed by patient participation. In other words the current is used for re-education of contraction.

Range
The word range may be used in two senses. First, it may refer to the amount of movement which occurs in a joint. Secondly, it may refer to the amount of shortening or lengthening of a muscle as it acts to produce or control movement.

Range of movement at a joint   This is the total quantity of movement when a joint is moved to its full extent. The names of the movements are those anatomical names which are normally applied (see Chapter 3) and the method of recording range is well laid down in the book *Joint Motion* published by the American Orthopaedic Association.

One may measure and record the amount of range of movement in a certain direction, e.g. the range of abduction of the shoulder joint is 90°. The range of adduction of the shoulder joint is 90°. This is normal range. If, however, the range is limited the available range can be recorded when a zero starting point is necessary and the recording could be from 10° of abduction to 80° of abduction, i.e. the first 10° and last 10° of movement are absent and the available range is 70°.

Muscle
When a muscle contracts and performs a movement it is said to have acted through a certain range. When a muscle is fully stretched and contracts to the limit of its normal capacity it is described as having contracted and produced a movement in *full range*. For purposes of description full range is broken down into three components which overlap (Fig. 1.1).

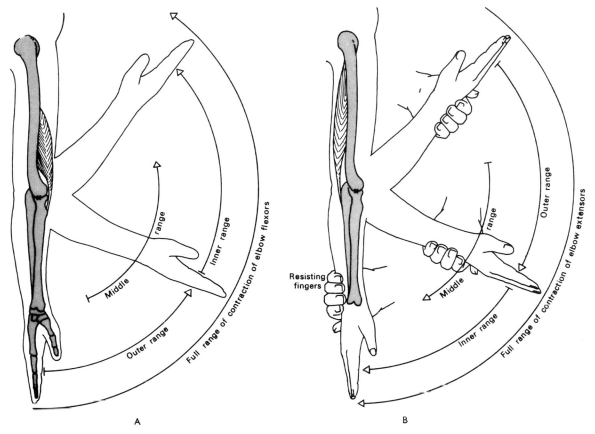

Fig. 1.1 A, The range of movement produced by contraction of brachialis. Gravity resisting; B, The range of movement produced by contraction of triceps. Manually resisted.

Outer range of contraction is from full stretch of the muscle to mid point of the full range. Inner range of contraction is from the above-mentioned mid point to full contraction. Middle range of contraction is any distance between the middle of the outer range and the middle of the inner range. Middle range of contraction is that in which many muscles work most of the time when they are producing movement.

Extreme inner range is more difficult to perform because it requires a contraction of a greater number of motor units of which a muscle is composed and usually also the muscle is pulling with an adverse angle of pull which diverts some of the effort to distracting the two joint surfaces.

Extreme outer range is also difficult because usually the angle of pull is adverse and some of the effort is diverted to compressing the two joint surfaces and, in addition, the muscle may have to overcome inertia and be working against a long or heavy weight arm. It is possible when some movements occur that in moving from full outer to full inner range, with the body in certain positions, gravity may resist the movement when outer range is performed and assist the movement when inner range is performed. When this occurs the same muscles will not be working througout

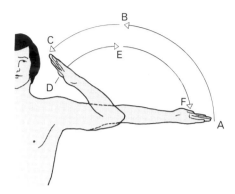

Fig. 1.2 In the movement from A–B the elbow flexors are working in isotonic lengthening in outer range (pulled by gravity). In the movement from D–E the elbow extensors are working in isotonic shortening in outer range (resisted by gravity); from B–C the elbow extensors are working in isotonic lengthening in outer range (pulled by gravity). In the movement from D–E the elbow extensors are working in isotonic shortening in outer range (resisted by gravity); from E–F the elbow flexors are working in isotonic lengthening in outer range (pulled by gravity).

the range of movement. The last part of the range of movement (gravity assisted) will be controlled by the antagonists working in their outer range but working in isotonic lengthening. It is thus possible to describe muscle work by mode of action, i.e. type of muscle activity (isotonic shortening or lengthening or isometric) and, in the former case, to describe the range of the muscle work (Fig. 1.2).

Group action of muscles

Muscles do not work in isolation. They must, for smooth co-ordinated movement to occur, operate in one of the following roles.

Prime movers or agonists
In this case they are those muscles which initiate and perform movement.

Antagonists
These can produce the opposite movement to that produced by the agonists. When the agonists work the antagonists must relax reciprocally, i.e. exactly an equal amount. The tension of the agonist contraction is equalled by the relaxation of the opposing muscles in order to allow smooth movement to occur.

Synergists
These are muscles which contract in order to bring about a joint position to make the action of the agonists stronger. They most frequently may be observed in action when the agonists are bi- or multi-axial muscles, e.g. the wrist extensors. Synergists also contract to prevent extra or additional movements that the agonists might otherwise perform. They operate from unconscious levels.

Fixators
These muscles also operate from unconscious level to fix the attachments of the agonists, antagonists and synergists. This does not mean that they fix a component of the body and keep it there throughout the whole of one particular muscle action; rather their role is dynamic as is that of the synergists. Fixator muscle work probably constitutes about 75% of normal daily muscle action. Their role is not isometric except for very short periods; it becomes isotonic in alternating patterns so that movement is smooth. In the example quoted above the fixator muscle work would be those around the elbow to fix the forearm and hand, the shoulder to fix the arm and shoulder girdle and of the remainder of the body to fix such parts as are not totally supported.

The fixator muscle work of an action such as threading a needle will be very different from that in throwing a heavy ball, both in quantity and quality. In the former case the starting position may be sitting and therefore the fixator work will be confined to those muscles which maintain the sitting position and the shoulder girdle and arm muscles involved in a fine pincer grasp and approximation of thread to needle. In the case of throwing a heavy ball, the fixator work will change rapidly as the body prepares for and carries out the throw followed by a braking action to prevent loss of position or balance.

Types of movement

Movement takes place at joints and is brought about by either the patient's muscular efforts or by the application of an external force.

Movements may be classified as passive or active.

Passive

Passive movements are those brought about by an external force which in the absence of muscle power in the part may be mechanical or via the therapist:

(1) Mechanical – the pull of gravity causing 'flopping'.
(2) The therapist performing movements. The therapist may produce accessory or anatomical movement at joints.

Accessory movements occur when resistance to active movement is encountered and fall into two types. The first type is seen when the metacarpophalangeal joints, which do not normally do so, rotate when grasping an object such as a hard ball. The rotatory movement is not possible unless resistance is encountered.

The second type of accessory movement can only be produced passively. It is produced when the muscles acting on the joint are relaxed and cannot be performed actively in the absence of resistance. An example is distraction of the glenohumeral joint when the fingers are hooked under a heavy piece of furniture and the body is pulled upwards.

Anatomical movements are those which the patient could perform if his muscles worked to produce that movement. These are dealt with in detail in Chapter 5 but can be subdivided into relaxed, forced and stretching.

Active

These are performed by the patient either freely, assisted or resisted.

(1) Freely – in which case mechanical factors will play a part offering either resistance or assistance.
(2) Assisted – when the therapist adopts the grips as for passive movements and assists the patient to perform the movement. The disadvantage of assisted active movements is that it is impossible for either party to detect how much work is being performed by each of them.
(3) Resisted – when mechanical or manual resistance is applied. The mechanical resistance may be in the form of weights, springs, water, auto loading or the mode of performance of the activity.

All these types of movement are described in the following chapters but it must be remembered that the human being is subject to most of the laws of mechanics and to physiological factors which make it able to react to stimuli in accordance with the state of development of the neuromuscular system and with the integrity of both the mechanical and neuromuscular systems of the body. A broken bone, a torn ligament, a ruptured muscle or damage to the nervous system will each have their detrimental effect on the normal activity of the body.

In some of these cases rest may be an essential prerequisite to recovery with the consequent deterioration in muscle power; in others the muscles will react in an abnormal manner due to the abnormal impulses impinging on the central nervous system.

It is not the intention of this book to outline all the rapidly advancing frontiers of knowledge of the present day in respect of the neuro-muscular system nor of the well understood mechanics of normal motion, but a fundamental study of anatomy, physiology and mechanics must proceed at the same time as this text is being used.

Chapter 2
BIOMECHANICS

M. Hollis & S.S. Kitchen

Some understanding of the action of forces on bodies and of the reactions of the human body to the application of forces is essential if the therapist is to comprehend the various factors which affect human motion. Mechanics is the study of forces and their effects upon a body; biomechanics is the study of those forces applied to the human body. A good working knowledge of mechanics will often help to isolate the therapeutic problems and suggest a solution.

This chapter will consider the various aspects of mechanics which the therapist will need in order to study the working of the body.

The main areas considered are:

(1) Force and motion
(2) Newton's Laws and their relationship to force and motion
(3) Force analysis
(4) Moments
(5) Friction
(6) Equilibrium and stability
(7) Work, power and energy
(8) Machines based on the principles of moments
(9) The behaviour of materials under stress
(10) Fluid mechanics.

Force and motion

It is difficult to separate force from motion; motion may be considered to be continuing change in position while force is that which generates or modifies motion.

Force

The study of force may be divided into two areas:

(1) *Statics*: the study of the effect of forces on a body in equilibrium, i.e. at rest or in constant motion. No change in the state of motion is produced.
(2) *Dynamics*: the study of forces not in equilibrium. Unbalanced forces produce some change in the state of motion of a body.

In order to study this subject, mass, force and weight should be defined.

Mass
Mass is the quantity of material a body contains. Units of mass: kg.

Force
Force is a push or pull, measured by its effect on a body. A force can:

(a) change or tend to change the shape or size of a body
(b) cause or tend to cause movement of a stationary body
(c) change or tend to change the movement of a body in motion.

Force is expressed as

Force = mass × acceleration

$$F = m \, a$$

The unit of force is the newton (N). A newton is defined as 'a force which, when applied to a body of one kilogram, gives it an acceleration of one metre per second squared'.

A force may be described as having:

(a)   Magnitude
(b)   Point of application
(c)   Line of action (Fig. 2.1A).

It is therefore known as a *vector quantity* and may be represented by an arrow of specific length, proportional to the magnitude of the force, pointing in the direction of the force (Fig. 2.1B).

Weight

Weight is a specific type of force and is the effect of the earth's gravitational force on a body.

$$W = m \, g$$

where W is the weight, m is the mass and g is the gravitational constant ($9.8 \, \text{m/s}^2$). The gravitational constant (or gravity) represents the *acceleration* of the body towards the earth in free fall.

Compare:

$$F = m \, a$$

and

$$W = m \, g.$$

Motion

Motion involves a change in the position or place of a body. Motion depends on the application of forces. In order to initiate movement, speed it up or slow it down, unbalanced forces

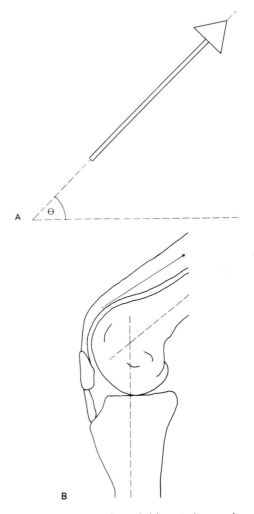

Fig. 2.1 A, A vector: the solid line indicates the magnitude, the arrow tip the direction, angle θ the orientation and the base of the arrow the point of application of the force; B, The force vector applied by the quadriceps muscle to the patella with the knee joint at 50° of flexion.

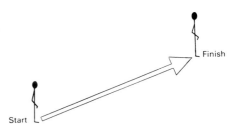

Fig. 2.2 Linear motion.

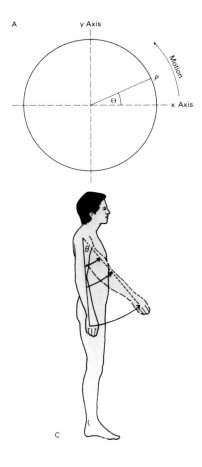

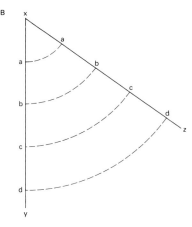

Fig. 2.3 A, Angular motion: angle θ represents the angular displacement between the 'x' axis and position *P*; B, The distance between lines XY and XZ lengthens with an increase in the radius of the arc; C, Angular motion occurring at the shoulder joint.

(1) *Displacement* (*s*): how far the object moves: the amount of movement. Units: metres.
(2) *Velocity* (*v*): how fast the object moves: the rate of change of displacement in time. Units: metres/second.
(3) *Acceleration* (*a*): any alteration in speed: the rate of change of velocity in time. Units: metres/second^2.

must be applied. If a body is to remain at rest or in constant motion balanced forces must prevail.

Types of motion
(1) *Linear motion*: linear motion occurs when an object or part moves in one direction only (Fig. 2.2).
(2) *Angular motion*: angular motion occurs when an object describes a circle or arc of motion about a fixed point (Fig. 2.3A–C).
(3) *Curvilinear motion*: a combination of the two is possible and is termed curvilinear motion. This is most often seen in the flight path of a projectile (Fig. 2.4).

Motion is described in the following terms:

Angular motion and velocity
It should be noted that at a given rate of displacement the velocity of motion of any point along the course of a part moving through an arc will be constant for that point only. The velocity of movement of the point depends on the radius of the arc and corresponding distance to be covered (Fig. 2.3B). Thus (Fig. 2.3C) during flexion of the arm, the hand will be seen to move at a greater velocity than the elbow. Both parts take the same length of time to reach their destination; the hand, however, has to describe a greater distance. This effect would be

increased by the placing of a tennis racket or golf club in the hand. The head of each will move with increased speed.

Natural speed

Therapists may speak of *natural speed* by which is meant the optimum velocity at which an individual can perform an exercise with maximum muscular efficiency. This velocity will vary with different patients of different physical builds and ability.

Newton's Laws of Motion

The study of the behaviour of forces in the production of motion is based on Newton's three laws:

Newton's First Law of Motion

Every object will remain at rest or continue to move with uniform velocity unless acted upon by an unbalanced force.

No alteration in condition can occur without the action of a further force.

Inertia

Newton's first law is often referred to as the *Law of Inertia*. Inertia may be defined as the reluctance of a body of mass 'x' to start moving. The greater the mass of a body the greater the inertia.

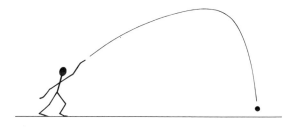

Fig. 2.4 Curvilinear motion.

When muscles are extremely weak, they may not be able to generate enough force to overcome the initial inertia of the part and so initiate a movement. They may, however, be able to continue that movement once begun. Under these circumstances the therapist will need to initiate the movement and the weak muscles will be encouraged to continue it.

Momentum

Similarly, a moving body shows reluctance to alter its velocity in any way. This property is known as the *momentum* of the body. Momentum is dependent on:

- The mass of the body
- The velocity at which it is travelling.

Hence the difference between catching a tossed games ball and a hurled medicine ball! The therapist may make use of momentum when using pendular swinging exercises for the shoulder joint (see Chapter 12) or when mobilizing the limbs in suspension.

Newton's Second Law of Motion

When a force acts on an object the change in motion experienced by the object takes place in the direction of the force and is proportional to the size of the force and the duration for which the force acts.

Any change in motion is due to the application of an unbalanced force. The application of such a force may:

(1)   Initiate movement
(2)   Increase the velocity of movement
(3)   Decrease the velocity of movement
(4)   Change the direction of movement.

All forces capable of achieving these changes are contact forces; that is, the object must be touched by the force. The exception to the rule is the one great attraction force of gravity.

Any change in the velocity of a moving body is called *acceleration*. An increase in velocity represents positive acceleration; a decrease in velocity is termed negative acceleration. The latter may be termed deceleration.

The above may be re-phrased as *Law of Acceleration*. 'The acceleration experienced by an object when acted upon by a force is directly proportional to the size of the force, inversely proportional to the mass of the object and takes place in the direction of the force.'

All alterations in the movements of the human body obey this law. Acceleration of movement occurs following the application of greater muscle force in the existing direction of movement. Deceleration may occur following the application of a breaking force, provided by an opposing group of muscles. Deceleration may also occur as the result of a loss of force in the primary muscle group as a result of fatigue or reduced neurological stimulation.

Newton's Third Law of Motion

To every action there is an equal and opposite re-action.

Whenever a force is applied to an object, as when the weight of the body is applied to the floor in standing, an equal reaction force is returned by the floor to the foot. This is demonstrated in Fig. 2.12, showing the phases of gait.

Force analysis

Forces often have to be analysed before their full implications can be seen. They may be:

(1) *summated*: added together and represented by a single force
(2) *resolved*: divided into component parts.

A free body diagram is used in force analysis; it consists of a diagrammatic sketch having all forces imposed on it in vectoral form (Fig. 2.5A and B).

Summation of forces

Forces rarely present singly. Often, more than one force will affect a part and it will be necessary to summate them in order to appreciate

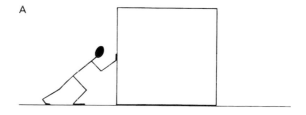

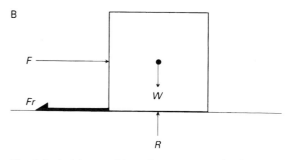

Fig. 2.5 A, Man pushing object; B, Free body diagram to show forces present in (A) in vectoral form. *F* – force applied by man. *W* – weight of box. *R* – reaction force. *F_r* – frictional resistance.

what is happening. The single force which can reproduce the action of the group of forces is known as the *resultant*. A group of forces acting together is called a system.

There are two ways of summating forces:

(1) Graphical
(2) Mathematical.

Summation of linear force systems

Graphical solution (Fig. 2.6A and B)
A free body diagram is drawn. In order to find the resultant, the vectors are redrawn, the head of the first being joined to the tail of the next. The resultant is found by drawing a single vector which will represent the total length of the constituent forces. Both negative and positive forces may be considered.

Mathematical solution
$$R = F1 + F2 + F3 + [-F4] \ldots$$
$$R = \sum F$$

where R is the resultant, F is the vectoral force, and $\sum$ is the sum of.

Forces directed towards the right – positive;
Forces directed towares the left – negative.

Complex systems are often regarded as linear in order to simplify the mathematics.

Summation of co-incident, co-planar force systems

Co-incident forces originate or terminate at a single point. Co-planar forces act within a single plane.

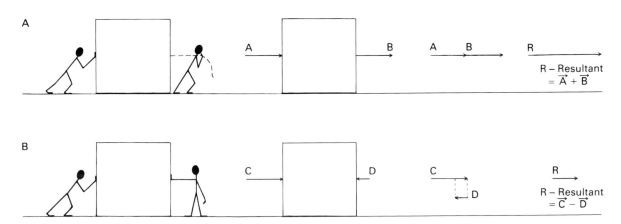

Fig. 2.6 Graphical summation of forces. A, Summation of two forces acting in the same direction; B, Summation of two forces acting in opposite directions.

Forces acting both in a single plane and through one point may be summated either graphically or mathematically.

Graphical solution

There are two types of summating graphically.

Parallelogram of forces

This method may be used for two forces.

A free body diagram is drawn (Fig. 2.7A). A parallelogram of forces is then constructed as in Fig. 2.7B. The resultant may then be imposed as in the diagram. This method is satisfactory for use with many muscular examples. Figures 2.7C and 2.7D show its application to the sternal and clavicular fibres of pectoralis major. Other examples would be the anterior and posterior fibres of deltoid, the two heads of gastrocnemius and both sets of oblique abdominal muscles.

Use of coordinates

This method may be used for two or more forces.

A free body diagram is drawn. The forces are numbered progressing in a clockwise direction (Fig. 2.8A). A set of coordinates may then be superimposed on the free body diagram. The position of F_1 is noted. The coordinates and forces are then redrawn, the forces being reproduced head to tail and in numerical order. Finally, the tail of the first vector is linked to the head of the last. This vector represents the resultant force (Fig. 2.8B).

Fig. 2.9A–C shows the same procedure being used for a more complex problem.

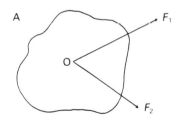

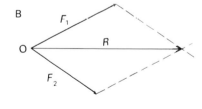

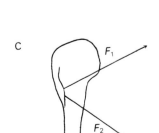

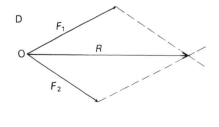

Fig. 2.7 Graphical summation of forces. A, Free body diagram; B, Parallelogram of forces: *R* – resultant force; C, Anatomical example: pectoralis major; D, Parallelogram of forces – pectoralis major. F_1 – clavicular fibres. F_2 – sternal fibres. The resultant gives rise to adduction of the upper limb.

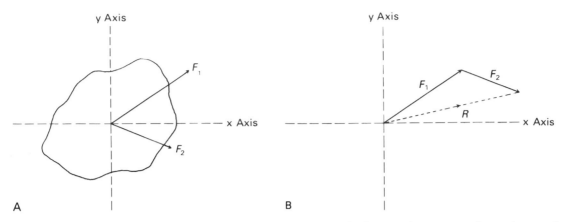

Fig. 2.8 Use of coordinates in the summation of forces. A, Free body diagram, having coordinates imposed; B, Summation of forces, showing resultant.

Mathematical solution

Equation: $R = (Fv_1 + Fh_1) + (Fv_2 + Fh_2) + \dots$

or

$$R = \sqrt{\left(\sum Fv\right)^2 + \left(\sum Fh\right)^2}$$

where R is the resultant, $\sqrt{}$ is the square root and $\sum$ is the sum of.

Fv – force: vertical component (see resolution of forces).
Fh – force: horizontal component (see resolution of forces).

Resolution of forces

It is possible to divide any single force into a number of components; two are normally adequate. These are the vertical and horizontal components of the original force (Fig. 2.10A).

In order to ascertain the values of Fv and Fh a right angle triangle is constructed as in Fig. 2.10B. The values of the component forces may then be calculated by means of the following equations:

$Fv = F\sin - \theta$
$Fh = F\cos - \theta$

The following examples will show the importance of component forces.

(1) A force of 10 newtons (10 N) is applied by the therapist to the leg of the patient at an angle of 60° (Fig. 2.11A). The component forces are calculated (Fig. 2.11B and C):

$Fv = F\sin\theta$	$Fh = \cos\theta$
$= 10 \times \sin 60$	$= F\cos 60$
$= 10 \times 0.87$	$= 10 \times 0.50$
$= 8.7\,\text{N}$	$= 5.0\,\text{N}$

Fv is the effective force for resisting the upward movement of the thigh; Fh is wasted effort on the part of the therapist. Therefore, all resistance should be applied at an angle of 90° to the part in order to be most effective and eliminate wasted effort.

(2) Both vertical and horizontal components may be important, as in gait (Fig. 2.12A–C).

In all phases of gait the vertical component is responsible for providing ground support. In the phase of restraint (or heel strike), it is the horizontal force

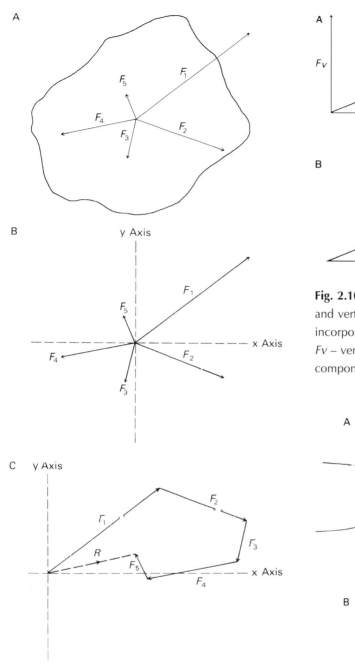

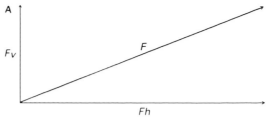

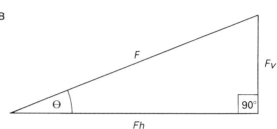

Fig. 2.10 A, Resolution of forces into horizontal and vertical components; B, A right angle triangle incorporating the two component forces. *F* – force. *Fv* – vertical component. *Fh* – horizontal component.

Fig. 2.9 A, Free body diagram; B, Forces superimposed on coordinates; C, Forces joined head to tail to give resultant. F_{1-5} – Forces. *R* – resultant.

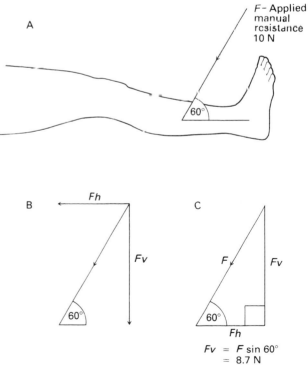

Fig. 2.11 A, Application of force to the lower limb; B and C, Vectoral diagrams to show that only *Fv* resists the upward movement of the limb. *F* – force. *Fv* – vertical component. *Fh* – horizontal components.

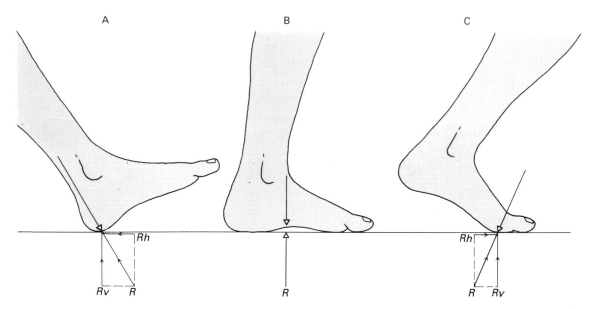

Fig. 2.12 Analysis of forces in walking. A, Heel strike; B, Stance; C, Toe-off. *R* – reaction force. *Rv* – vertical component of reaction force. *Rh* – horizontal component of reaction force.

which prevents the foot from sliding forward and checks the momentum of the body. In the propulsive (or toe off) phase, the horizontal force is responsible for allowing the driving force which propels the body forward.

Moments

A moment may be defined as the turning force resulting from the application of a force some distance away from the fulcrum of movement.

Figure 2.13A show a typical moment; Fig. 2.13B shows the same moment when applied to a cylinder, causing twisting. This presentation is often termed a *torque*. The effective value of the applied force is magnified as a result of being placed at a distance from the centre of motion:

Moment = Force × Distance

$$M = Fd$$

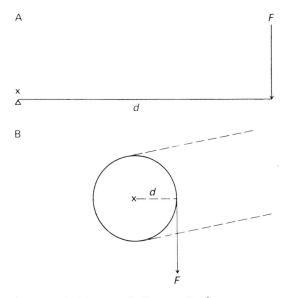

Fig. 2.13 A, Moment; B, Torque. *F* – force. *d* – distance. *x* – fulcrum.

The *moment arm* is the perpendicular distance from the axis of motion (fulcrum) to the applied force.

The *action arm* is the actual distance from

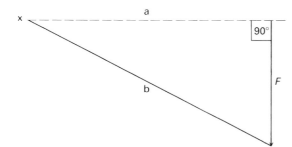

Fig. 2.14 The moment arm and the action arm may not be the same. x – fulcrum. *F* – force. a – moment arm. b – action arm.

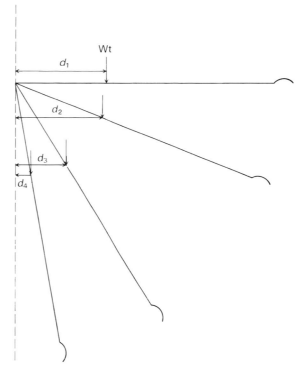

Fig. 2.15 Moments taken about the shoulder joint with the arm in varying degrees of abduction. d_{1-4} – distance, moment arm. Wt – weight.

the axis of motion to the point of application of the force along the bar, limb or lever.

The moment arm and action arm are frequently not the same (see Fig. 2.14). Figure 2.15 shows the upper limb being abducted. The length of the action arm will remain the same throughout a movement; the distance from the shoulder joint to the centre of gravity of the limb will remain constant. The length of the moment arm will change according to the degree of movement

The following are examples of moments as encountered by the therapist.

(1) Moments of force are very common in the human body. The axis of motion, or fulcrum, occurs at a joint. The action arm is the limb or trunk segment and the force is supplied by body weight or muscular work. The example seen in Fig. 2.16 is that of the upper limb being taken into abduction. The shoulder joint acts as the fulcrum, the limb acts as the action arm, and the weight of the part acts as the force. This force acts through a point about one third of the way along the arm.

The moment arm varies with the degree of abduction, for

$$M_1 = F \times d_1 \ldots \text{through to:}$$
$$M_4 = F \times d_4$$

Greater effort is seen to be necessary to hold the arm in a position of 90° abduction. This is important in the planning of progressed exercises. The amount of effort may also be reduced by altering the length of the action arm and consequently the length of the moment arm (Fig. 2.16).

(2) A second example of the effect of moments is seen in the design of the re-education board as used by therapists (balance boards).

Re-education boards are primarily used to re-educate balance and increase the strength of the muscles of the lower leg. They consist of a platform, which may

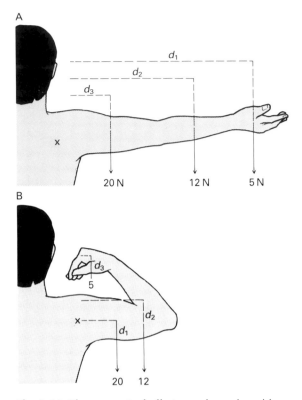

Fig. 2.16 The amount of effort may be reduced by shortening the length of the moment arm.

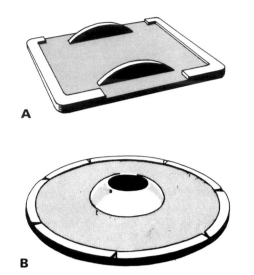

Fig. 2.17 A, A square re-education (wobble) board; B, A round re-education (wobble) board.

be either rectangular or circular, resting on curved supports (Fig. 2.17A and B). The aim of the exercise is that the subject should learn to balance on the board, holding the central position. Re-education boards are based on the principle of moments, as can be seen in Fig. 2.18. The moment F_1d_1 will equal F_2d_2 when the weight of the body is evenly balanced relative to the moments created. The position of the foot on the board will affect the moments as the distances either side of the axis alter.

Force couple

Two forces of equal magnitude acting together in opposite directions and displaced from

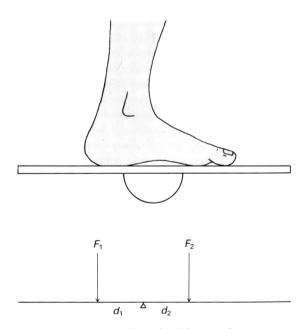

Fig. 2.18 Moments about the fulcrum of a re-education board. When the weight is balanced $F_1d_1 = F_2d_2$. F – force. d – distance.

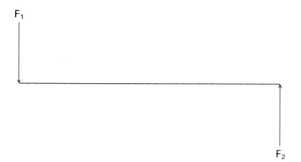

Fig. 2.19 A force couple. $F_1 = F_2$. F – force.

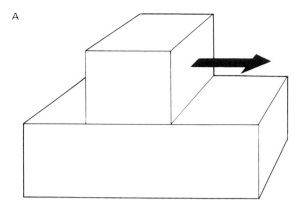

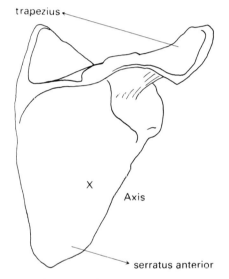

Fig. 2.20 A force couple producing lateral rotation of the scapula.

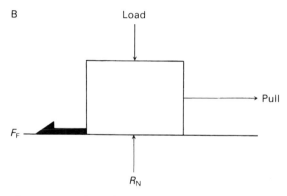

Fig. 2.21 A, Shear force occurring as two bodies slide relative to one another. B, Free body diagram of forces occurring in (A). R_N – reaction normal. F_F – friction force.

one another are called a force couple (Fig. 2.19). A force couple may be regarded as a pair of moments acting at an axis of rotation which may be placed at any point along the length.

Couples, composed of a muscle force and a joint reaction force, are present during limb movements.

The forces acting on the scapula in order to bring about the lateral rotation necessary for full abduction of the upper limb constitute a force couple and are shown in Fig. 2.20. The axis of motion falls through the body of the scapula and the forces are provided by serratus anterior inferiorly and trapezius superiorly.

Friction

Friction occurs when one body slides in relation to another (Fig. 2.21A and B); the frictional force (F_F) is a shear force occurring between two adjacent surfaces which are in contact. As the pulling force is applied to the body, the frictional force will match its value (Newton's Third Law – 'to every action there is an equal and opposite reaction') prior to movement; once movement occurs the frictional force will be of a constant value, determined by:

(1) The nature of the materials involved
(2) The value of the normal load pressing the two surfaces together.

Any difference in force value between the pulling force and F_F will be available to produce movement.

Static friction is the term used for the frictional force occurring prior to movement of the body taking place.

Dynamic friction is the level of frictional force observed during movement.

The value occurring at the transition from static to dynamic friction is termed the limiting value.

Types of friction

(1) *Dry*: the surfaces of the materials are dry and clean.
(2) *Boundary*: the surfaces of the material are coated with contaminants, e.g. grease, dust and other debris.
(3) *Viscous* (fluid): fluid is present between the surfaces.

The principles considered above are for dry friction; those for boundary and viscous friction are basically the same except that the additional material will modify the surfaces and therefore the frictional values.

Rolling friction

When a body rolls, no frictional resistance will occur as point contact only is made. In order for 'rolling friction' to occur, deformation of either the body or the surface must take place,

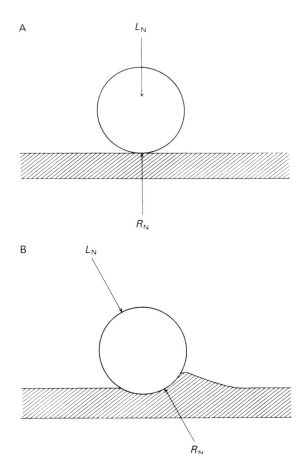

Fig. 2.22 Rolling friction. A, Point contact – no shear force occurs; B, Surface deformation resulting in increased surface contact and therefore shear.

as shown in Fig. 2.22. Under these circumstances, sliding between the two deformed surface areas will take place and friction will occur. This friction may be of any of the above types.

Friction can be of great value to the therapist. Shoes should always have soles of a material which will not slip easily; ferrules on crutches and sticks should be in good condition and the brakes on most wheelchairs depend on friction for their effect. Conversely, friction can be damaging to skin if the part is dragged over rough surfaces such as bedclothes and the edges of wheelchairs.

Lubrication

Friction is important in the prevention of slipping. However, there are times when the therapist wishes to reduce its value in order to facilitate an action. Lubrication is the use of an additional material to separate surfaces. Much shear resistance is due to the uneven nature of the surfaces of materials and the consequent tearing resulting during motion. Lubricants, therefore, act to even out the surfaces. Lubricants should consist of materials having a relatively low intermolecular co-efficient of friction. This will reduce the intrinsic resistance of the lubricant.

Lubricants come in many forms; for example, talcum powder to lubricate the skin as it slides over re-education boards, fabric for use in blanket pulls across the gym floor and oil in massage.

Equilibrium and stability

In order to discuss the concepts of equilibrium and stability the line of gravity, centre of gravity and base of support need to be defined.

Line of gravity

A human body consists of a number of segments, each of which contributes a percentage weight to that of the whole. Each segmental weight may be represented by a resultant force acting through a single point (Fig. 2.23). These segmental resultants may be summed in order to give the resultant force exerted by the weight of the whole body. This resultant is known as the line of gravity (Fig. 2.24).

Centre of gravity

The point through which this line would pass with the body orientated in any direction is

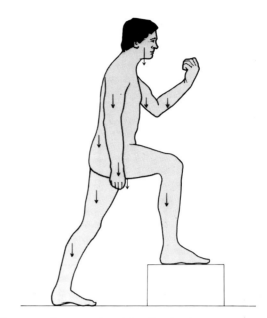

Fig. 2.23 Segmental weight distribution.

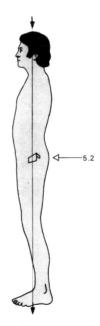

Fig. 2.24 Centre and line of gravity. The centre of gravity of the standing human is at the level of the second sacral vertebra. The line of gravity falls from the vertex, through the centre of gravity, in front of the ankles and within the base.

called the centre of gravity (Fig. 2.24). In the standing position, this lies at approximately the level of the second sacral vertebra. The body segment diagram (Fig. 2.25) is designed to show the position of the centres of gravity of the parts and the whole. The position of the centre of gravity and consequently the line of gravity will vary with body posture (Fig. 2.26A–G). Raising the weight distribution will raise the centre of gravity whilst moving it sideways will laterally displace both the centre of gravity and the line of gravity.

A body always behaves as though all its weight is acting through its centre of gravity; for example, a body rests on a surface (Fig. 2.27A and B), only falling when the line of gravity falls beyond the edge of the supporting surface (Fig. 2.27C).

Base of support

The base of support refers to the supporting area beneath a body. It includes both the parts of the body in direct contact with the surface and the area enclosed by the contact points. For the therapist, the points of contact in question will be such areas as the feet in standing, buttocks in sitting, and the heels, calves and back in lying. Additional supports such as sticks and walking frames also function as points of contact enclosing an enlarged base.

Equilibrium

When a body is at rest in equilibrium there is:

(1) No tendency to move in any direction, i.e. resultant force = 0
(2) No tendency to rotate in any direction, i.e. resultant moment = 0.

A body may be defined as being in equilibrium but its hold on its position may be more or less

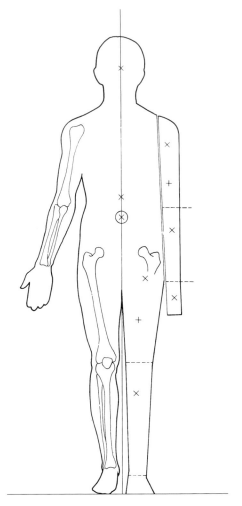

Fig. 2.25 Body segment diagram showing centres of gravity. ⊗ – of whole body. + – of limb. × – of segment.

precarious. This is referred to as its degree of stability.

Types of equilibrium

Stable equilibrium

The body returns to its original starting position following the application of a displacing force. The centre of the body is usually low and considerable effort is required in order to raise

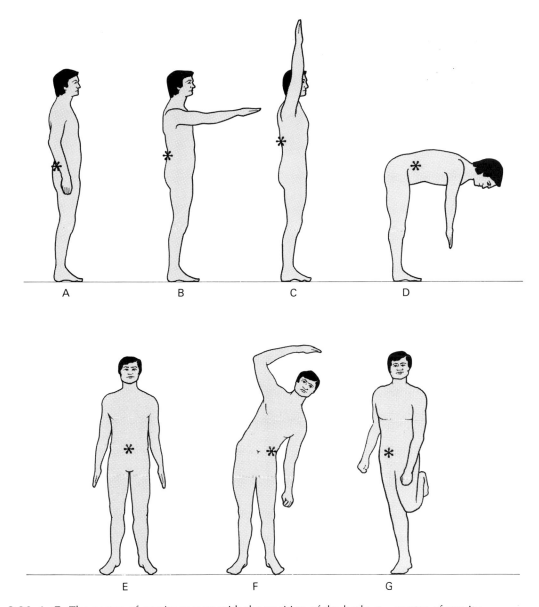

Fig. 2.26 A–G, The centre of gravity moves with the position of the body. * – centre of gravity.

it sufficiently to displace the body (Fig. 2.28A). The base is usually large, allowing the line of gravity to fall easily within it.

Unstable equilibrium
The body continues in the line of the displacing force leading to overturning. The centre of gravity tends to be high initially and the base small; the line of gravity falls easily out of the base. Overturning leads to a lowering of the centre of gravity (Fig. 2.28B).

Neutral equilibrium
The height and position of the centre of gravity remains the same despite displacement; rolling is the prime example.

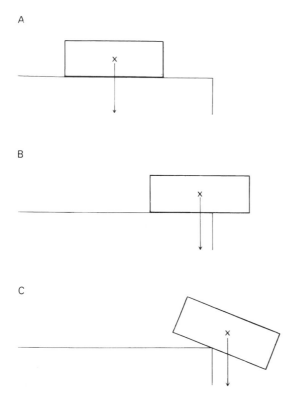

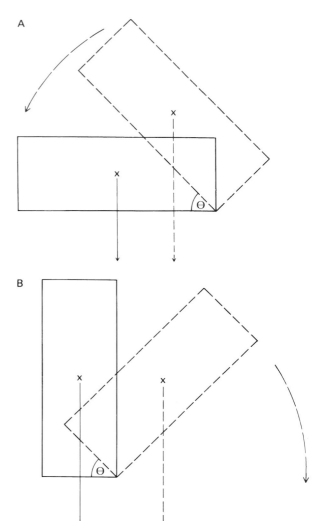

Fig. 2.27 A, Body fully supported; B, Body partially supported – the centre of gravity is over the supporting base; C, Body falls – as the centre of gravity is no longer over the base. X – centre of gravity.

Fig. 2.28 A, Stable equilibrium – the body passes through angle θ, but falls back; B, Unstable equilibrium – the body passes through angle θ and falls over. X – centre of gravity. ↓ – line of gravity.

The stability of a body

When a body rests on a surface its line of action must pass through its base of support. When tilted the body will fall onto the face intersected by the line of action. Thus in Fig. 2.29A, when the cube is only raised slightly, the line of action will continue to fall through the face bounded by AB. However a greater angle of raise will cause the line of action to fall through the face BC. The body will therefore fall onto this face – the structure 'falls over' (Fig. 2.29B).

The degree of stability of a body depends on two factors: base, and height of centre of gravity.

Base

A larger base allows greater displacement of the body without overturning.

This factor is very important when dealing with the human body. Walk standing and stride standing (Fig. 2.30A and B) increase the stability of the body in the upright position; both toddlers and the elderly spontaneously increase

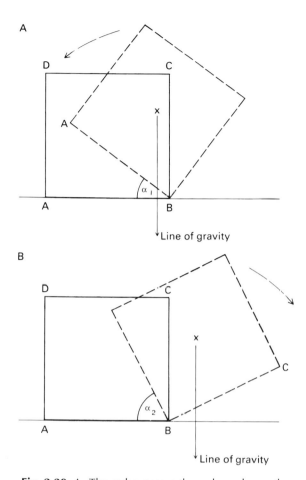

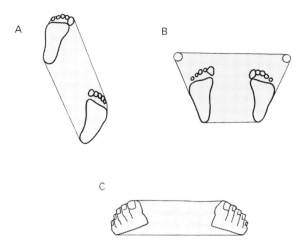

Fig. 2.30 Bases. A, Walk standing; B, Stride standing with walking aid; C, Toe standing.

Fig. 2.29 A, The cube passes through angle α_1; the line of gravity remains through the base and the body returns to its original position; B, The cube passes through angle α_2; the line of gravity passes out of the original base and the body falls over.

their base size by widening the space between their feet and out-toeing. Walking aids such as sticks and frames have a similar effect (Fig. 2.30B). The converse is true in that a reduction in stability arises from close standing, standing on one leg and ultimately from standing on the toes (Fig. 2.30C).

Height of centre of gravity
The line of action passes through the centre of gravity. The higher this point is, the less stable

the body tends to be (compare Figs 2.28A and B). The height of the centre of gravity will depend on the size and shape of the body as well as the material type and distribution. A body with most of its weight distributed towards the top will be less stable than one which has its centre of weight at a lower point. Thus standing is much less stable than sitting and lying gives ultimate stability to the human body.

A consideration of base and height of centre of gravity are of great importance when devising and progressing exercises. Raising the centre of gravity of the part and decreasing the base size will increase the difficulty of an exercise by decreasing the stability of the body and thus increasing the muscle work and co-ordination required to perform satisfactorily.

Centre of gravity and motion

It is essential for the weight of the body and thus the line of gravity to pass through the base, in order that the body weight may

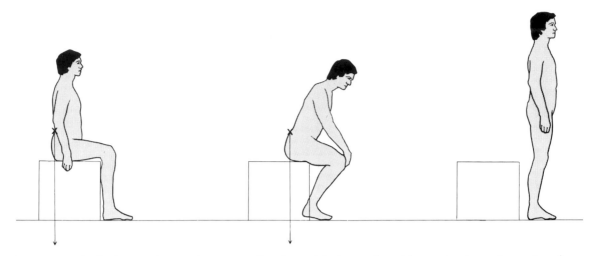

Fig. 2.31 As the body rises from sitting to standing the weight is transferred forward to keep the centre of gravity over the base. X – centre of gravity. ↓ – line of gravity.

be supported by that base. Thus it is essential for weight to be transferred over the supporting structures upon change of position. It is, for example, impossible to stand up from a chair or to climb stairs without first transferring the weight over the supporting part (Fig. 2.31). More complex movements, such as running, skipping, jumping and even cartwheels can be performed provided that control of movement of the weight of the body is achieved. Thus dynamic equilibrium is achieved.

Work: power: energy

Work

Mechanical work is done when a load is moved through a distance. The biceps brachii muscle performs work when it contracts in order to raise a load in the hand.

Power

Power is the rate at which work is done.

Energy

Energy is the capacity to do work; it is manifested in two forms: potential energy and kinetic energy.

Potential energy (PE)

Potential energy refers to the capacity of a body to do work as a result of stored energy. This stored energy may be the result of deformation of the body or the result of the position of the body. A spring held in extension is an example of potential energy resulting from deformation. An arm raised in flexion has the potential to fall under the influence of gravity and is an example of potential energy due to position.

Kinetic energy (KE)

Kinetic energy is the work performed by a body as a result of motion. Thus releasing the spring will allow work to be performed, as will allowing the arm to fall towards the floor.

The illustration in Fig. 2.32 shows the interrelationship of kinetic and potential energy during swinging. Greatest potential energy is stored at the maximum excursion of the pen-

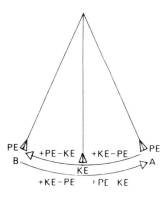

Fig. 2.32 A pendulum demonstrating kinetic (KE) and potential (PE) energy.

dulum in either direction and released during fall as kinetic energy. Thus in Fig. 2.32, when the weight on the end of the cord is lifted to position A, and whilst it is held there, it has potential energy. When it is released and begins to fall, it gains kinetic energy and loses potential energy. As it passes through the lowest point of its arc of motion, the energy is entirely kinetic. As it rises towards point B, it loses kinetic and gains potential energy until, at point B, the energy is entirely potential. The pendulum will continue to oscillate in this way until the energy originally imparted to it as a result of the work done in lifting the weight has been used up in frictional losses.

Machines

A machine is a mechanical device which does work. Those used by therapists are based on the principles of moments.

All machines are able to produce a mechanical advantage (MA), which may be either positive or negative. A mechanical advantage is a 'trade off' between effort and distance. The total force *in* must equal the total force *out* in all machines. The relative lengths of the moment arms and forces may, however, vary whilst achieving this equality.

The mechanical advantage is the ratio of *load arm* : *effort arm*:

$$MA = \frac{\text{length of effort arm}}{\text{length of resistance arm}}$$

When the two lengths are the same, the mechanical advantage is equal to 1.

When the MA is greater than 1 the machine is regarded as being efficient and has a positive mechanical advantage. This means that the effort required to shift a given resistance is less than the value of that resistance. This is possible because the total force is equal to $F \times d$. When the MA is less than 1, the machine is less efficient and exhibits a mechanical disadvantage. This means that the effort required to shift a resistance is greater than the value of the actual resistance.

Two types of machines, both based on the principles of moments, are used by the therapist – levers and pulleys.

Levers

A lever is a rigid bar which rotates about a fixed point, known as the fulcrum or axis of motion. A force is applied to the bar allowing work to be performed at some other point. Figure 2.33 represents the parts of a lever. The varying relationships between the constituent parts result in the three orders of levers.

Classification of levers

First order levers
The fulcrum is placed between the effort and the resistance (Fig. 2.34A).

When the two arms are of equal length the mechanical advantage is 1; Fig. 2.34B shows that the MA may be more than 1; Fig. 2.34C shows that the MA may be less than 1.

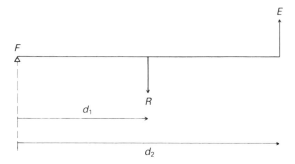

Fig. 2.33 The parts of a lever. *F* – fulcrum. *R* – resistance. *E* – effort. $d_1(F-R)$ – resistance arm. $d_2(F-E)$ – effort arm.

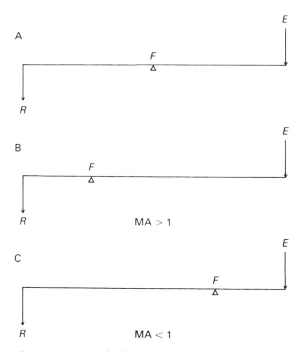

Fig. 2.34 First order lever. A, in balance – MA = 1; B, MA is greater than 1; C, MA is less than 1.

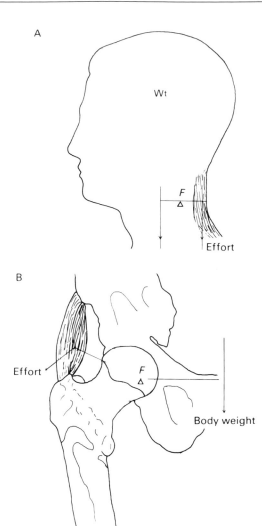

Fig. 2.35 First order levers in the human body. A, the neck extensors balancing the weight of the head; B, the hip abductors balancing the weight of the body when standing on one leg.

When the fulcrum is close to the resistance, a force advantage is gained. When the fulcrum is close to the effort, a force disadvantage prevails.

For example:

(1) The action of the neck extensors balancing the weight of the head in the standing position, the atlanto-occipital joint being the fulcrum (Fig. 2.35A).

(2) The action of the hip abductors about the fulcrum of the hip joint in preventing dropping of the pelvis to the unsupported side when standing on one leg. Failure of

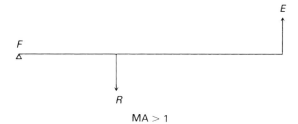

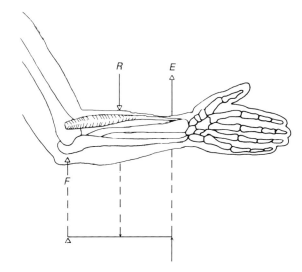

Fig. 2.36 Second order lever – the MA is greater than 1.

Fig. 2.37 Second order lever in the human body. Brachioradialis provides the effort, the segment weight provides the resistance and the elbow joint is the fulcrum.

this mechanism leads to a Trendelenberg Sign (Fig. 2.35B).

Second order levers

The resistance lies between the fulcrum and the effort (Fig. 2.36).

The mechanical advantage is always greater than 1; a force advantage is gained. A small amount of effort can shift a large resistance.

There are few examples in the human body; the action of the muscle brachioradialis when acting as a flexor of the forearm is one example (Fig. 2.37).

Third order levers

The effort lies between the fulcrum and the resistance (Fig. 2.38).

The mechanical advantage is always less than 1; a greater amount of effort is required to shift a resistance.

Most levers in the human body are of this type:

(1) Biceps brachii acting to raise the weight of the forearm about the fulcrum of the elbow joint is one of many examples (Fig. 2.39).
(2) The hamstrings act about the knee joint, flexing the lower leg.

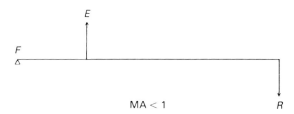

Fig. 2.38 Third order lever – the MA is less than 1.

(3) Deltoid acts about the shoulder joint in order to raise the arm.

Pulleys

A pulley consists of a grooved wheel having a rope running over it. Figure 2.40 shows an example of a pulley used by therapists in suspension therapy. A pulley may be used in order to:

(1) Change the direction of a force
(2) Obtain a mechanical advantage.

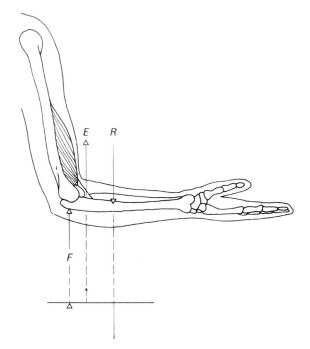

Fig. 2.39 Third order lever in the human body. Brachialis provides the effort, the segment weight provides the resistance and the elbow joint is the fulcrum.

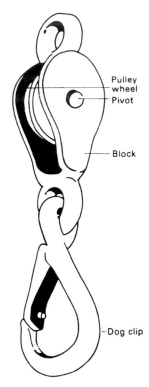

Fig. 2.40 A pulley.

A pulley may be either fixed or moveable. A fixed pulley will only change the direction of a force; a moveable pulley can also obtain a mechanical advantage.

A single fixed pulley has a mechanical advantage of one as the load on the pulley wheel requires an equivalent force to allow it to be balanced. Such a pulley serves to change the direction of the force which must be applied in order to move the load (Fig. 2.41A). Use is made of this simple device in the reciprocal pulley circuits described in Chapter 9 and also in the rope and pulley circuits which allow combined oblique and rotary movements.

A multiple pulley circuit offers a greater mechanical advantage than a single pulley. This is demonstrated if a pulley with a weight attached is inverted and hung from a hook in

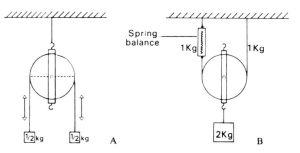

Fig. 2.41 A, A pulley demonstrating that it serves to change the direction of the force; B, A pulley suspended to show how the load is distributed at the suspended points.

the ceiling by a cord, and a spring balance is inserted into the cord circuit to measure the force (Fig. 2.41B). Each side of the cord takes half the weight and therefore the mechanical advantage of the circuit will be two.

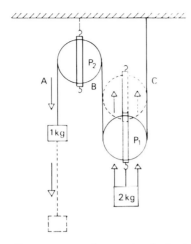

Fig. 2.42 Demonstrates the mechanical advantage offered by inserting more than one pulley in a circuit.

If a second pulley is inserted into the circuit so that a downward pull can be applied to the cord, the mechanical advantage is unchanged. The ceiling still takes half the weight at each suspension point, but the rope can now be moved. As it moves, the loaded pulley will move upwards, but the rope will travel twice the distance that the load will move. In Figure 2.42 the rope C remains stationary but shortens, and rope B moves up and over pulley P_2. Rope A lengthens by the distance pulley, P_1 travels up the rope A and the distance rope B travels over pulley P_2. The load of 1 kg on pulley P_2 balances the load of 2 kg on pulley P_1.

For example:

(1) The tendon of peroneus longus passes around the fixed pulley provided by the lateral malleolus. The direction of pull of the muscle is altered. The tendon of extensor pollicis longus also passes around a fixed pulley, the dorsal tubercle of the radius, in order to change its direction. Neither alters their force value.

(2) The weight and pulley system seen in Fig. 9.29A both alters the direction of the force exerted by the weights and reduces by half the effective force experienced by the patient. That in Fig. 9.30A and B only alters the direction of the applied force.

The behaviour of materials

When a force is applied to a material it will suffer varying degrees of deformation. The internal stress will equal the external load.

Stress

Stress is the intensity of internal force per unit area and may be expressed as:

Stress = force/area

Units: newtons per metre squared (N/m^2).
 Stress may be:

(1) Compressive (negative, −ve).
(2) Tensile (positive, +ve).

(Fig. 2.43A and B)

Strain

All materials under load experience a change in shape or length:

$$\text{Strain } (\varepsilon) = \frac{\text{change in length}}{\text{original length}} \frac{(x)}{(L)}$$

(Fig. 2.44A and B).
 Strain associated with tension is considered positive; that associated with compression, negative.

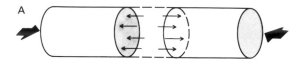

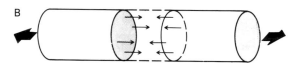

Fig. 2.43 Stress forces. A, Compressive; B, Tensile. ➤ – applied force. → – stress.

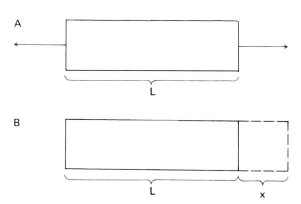

Fig. 2.44 Strain. A, Unloaded beam; B, Loaded beam. L – original length. x – deformation.

The above discussion refers to linear stress and strain; both shear and torsional stress and strain may occur and are frequent in the human body which is subject to complex force systems.

Hooke's Law

Hooke's Law states that: *Strain is directly proportional to the applied stress.*

Stress/strain = constant *E*.

This constant is known as Young's modulus, or the modulus of elasticity (Fig. 2.45).

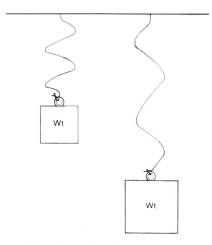

Fig. 2.45 The relationship between stress and strain – the greater the load on the spring the greater the deformation.

Stress–strain curve

The graphical relationship between stress and strain is shown in Fig. 2.46. The behaviour of the material alters as the extension strain increases.

(1) *Elastic behaviour of material*: When a material is stressed within its elastic phase the strain or deformation which occurs is reversible. The material will return to its original length and shape, thus obeying Hooke's Law. This is the region in which it is safe to stress most materials without damage occurring.

(2) The yield point occurs when the material stretches for a period without the addition of any further force.

(3) *Plastic behaviour of material*: Permanent deformation of material arises following the application of stress loads into this phase. Hooke's Law is no longer operational.

(4) The period following the plastic phase leads directly to the point of fracture of

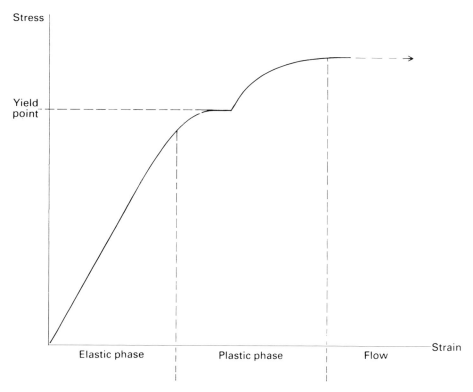

Fig. 2.46 Graph of stress–strain curve.

the material under stress. It consists of a period of localized thinning preceding breakage.

Internal stress patterns

Forces may be applied to a body in a variety of ways and will result in a variety of internal stress patterns. A knowledge of these is useful in determining the way in which a structure will behave under load. For example, it is useful to know how a plaster of Paris splint will behave under direct compression forces and bending forces.

Apart from the previously mentioned direct tensile and compressive forces which may be applied to a body, bending, shear and torsion forces often arise.

Tensile force (Fig. 2.43B)
When a tensile force is applied to a body, opposing patterns of stress arise. The body will resist being pulled apart.

Compressive force (Fig. 2.43A)
When a compressive force is applied to a body, opposing patterns of stress will arise as the body resists being squashed.

Bending force (Fig. 2.47A, B and C)
When a force applied to a body results in bending, tension and compression stresses develop on the convex and concave portions respectively (Fig. 2.47A and B). Greatest stress develops at the periphery of the structure; the neutral axis occurs centrally and is the point at which the stresses change from tensile to

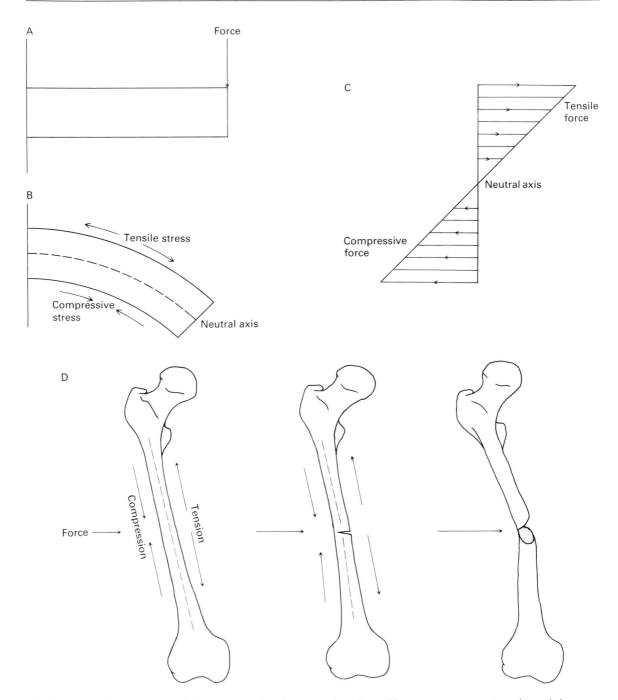

Fig. 2.47 Bending moments. A, force applied to beam; B, bending of beam; C, cross-section through beam showing stress distribution; D, bending of the femur; fracture occurs due to tensile stress.

compressive. This neutral surface is neither stretched nor compressed (Fig. 2.47C).

Figure 2.47D shows the application of bending forces to the femur upon application of a lateral force. It is interesting to note that the cortical bone of the long bones of the body is distributed in such a manner as maximally to resist bending forces. It is placed around the periphery where forces are greatest. The central region contains marrow and corresponds to the central, neutral axis.

Shear force (Fig. 2.48A and B)

When a force applied to a body results in shear, stress forces arise which tend to oppose the shearing motion. Shear forces frequently arise at the same time as bending moments, when one end of the body is fixed. Fractures which occur in the lower limb when weight bearing sustain both types of stress.

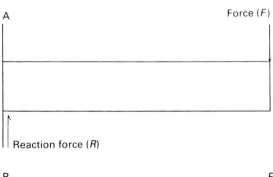

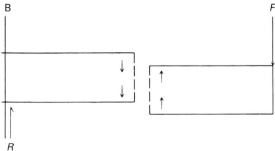

Fig. 2.48 Shear force. A, force applied to beam; B, shear stress occurring in the beam.

Torsion force (Fig. 2.49A–C)

When a twisting force is applied to a body, torsion stresses will arise. These will occur maximally about the periphery of the object. Long bones are ideally suited to resist torsion stress as the material of the bone is primarily distributed around the periphery.

Behaviour under stress

Materials vary considerably in their behaviour when stressed. Some, such as rubber and skin, show great elasticity. Others, such as ligaments, show little elasticity and permanently deform following stress injuries. Still other materials show very little elasticity or plasticity and fracture easily.

The internal structure, shape and orientation of a material affects its behaviour when stressed.

Bone is particularly well adapted to its various functions and the stress applied to it. Its internal structure is modified into two main forms: cortical bone, which is dense, and cancellous bone, which is much lighter though still strong. Cortical bone is present in the shafts of long bones which are relatively slender; cancellous bone is found in the expanded extremities. The latter allows for strength but avoids undue heaviness of the expanded portion. The osteons in both types of bone are orientated along the lines of force, facilitating their transmission through the bone. The trabeculae of the cancellous bone serve the same purpose (Fig. 2.50A). As forces vary in their impact on a bone, the alignment of the osteons and trabeculae can be modified to suit newly arising situations.

The gross shape of the bone is important with regard to its ability to withstand stress. A hollow tube is stronger than a solid cylinder of similar size; a large area allows force to be dissipated and results in less stress per unit area. These two points are seen respectively in the

A

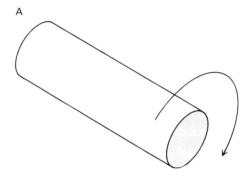

B

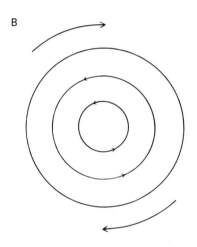

C

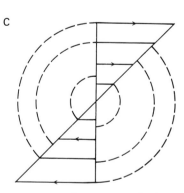

Fig. 2.49 Torsion force. A, applied torque; B, internal stress pattern; C, cross-section through cylinder showing stress pattern.

shaft and extremities of long bones. Bones do not exhibit sudden change in shape which would result in concentration of forces and consequent weak points. Where changes in shape or size do occur, bones will be more susceptible to damage; thus the tibia tends to fracture at the junction between its middle and lower thirds. It is at this point that it is at its thinnest and exhibits a noticeably triangular cross-sectional view (Fig. 2.50B).

Bone has to withstand varying stress patterns; it is strongest in compression and weakest in shear. Tension is reasonably well tolerated. This arrangement suits the stress patterns to which bone is subjected, most of which are compressive.

Collagen, present in ligaments and tendons, is also subject to varying stresses. Its orientation is very important in relation to its response to force. It is unable to resist compressive forces, but is strong in tension; thus ligaments and tendons tend to have their fibres orientated in the direction of greatest force (Fig. 2.51A). Collagen has, however, a very limited elastic phase, and as a result, when stressed, rapidly reaches its full degree of extensibility. This extensibility is primarily due to the 'straightening out' of the relaxed collagen fibres (Fig. 2.51B). This is rather like the straightening that can occur when tension is applied to a piece of string. Any further force will result in plastic behaviour of the material and permanent deformation occurring. Thus, once a ligament has been overstretched, it will not return to its original length, and laxity of the joint will result. This may be seen following inversion injuries to the ankle.

Collagen is also present in skin. Skin, however, exhibits a greater degree of elasticity. This is due to the fact that the fibres do not lie in parallel bundles, but comprise a supportive network. This allows for a greater degree of stretch to be applied to the tissue before the

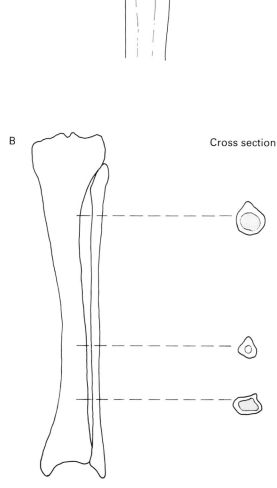

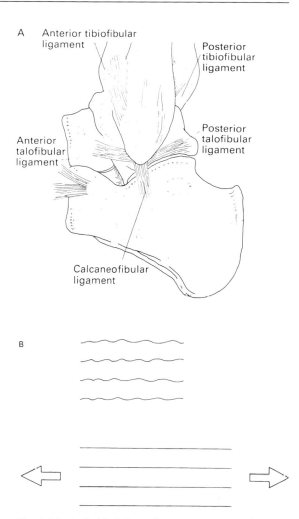

Fig. 2.50 A, Head of femur, showing how trabeculae transmit force from the expanded head to the walls of the shaft; B, Tibia, showing variations in cross-sectional area.

Fig. 2.51 A, Ankle joint – ligaments arranged around the lateral aspect of the joint in such a way as to control any unwanted movements, B, Collagen in its relaxed and tensioned phases.

collagen fibres will become orientated along the applied lines of force.

Non-biological materials are also subject to stress and strain. A spring is a therapeutic example of a structure which is designed to withstand stress and is used to resist muscle work and so strengthen the muscles involved. The wire of which the spring is made may be arranged in a variety of different ways; the spirally wound spring is the most common. Other types include both compression and torsion springs (see Chapter 9). In each case the intention is to allow a controlled amount of elastic deformation to occur upon the application of stress. Thereafter, plastic deformation will occur. Therapeutic springs will tolerate a range of between $1/2$ and 25 kg of force without permanent deformation.

The tolerance of a spring to stress varies with the following:

(1)   The nature of the material
(2)   The diameter of the wire
(3)   The total diameter of the configuration

All therapeutic springs have an inbuilt mechanism to prevent overstretch. The spiral spring has a cord running through its length which will indicate the limit of its elastic extensibility; the compression spring simply cannot be further opposed. The torsion spring is designed for use in a single hand which does not have the range of movement available to overstress the equipment.

Fluid mechanics

A fluid is a substance which will deform continuously under the action of shear stress and may be either a gas or a liquid.

A *gas* completely fills the space in which it is contained and is easily compressed.

A *liquid* usually has a free surface and is compressed with difficulty.

Hydrostatics

Hydrostatics is the study of force and pressure in a fluid at rest.

Mass
Mass is the quantity of material present in a body.

Volume
Volume is the area occupied by a certain mass of material.

Density
Density is the relationship between the mass and the volume of a substance:

Density = mass/volume

Relative density
Relative density is the ratio of the density of a substance to the density of pure water. The relative density of pure water is one. Other examples of densities are wood – 0.57, iron – 7.7 and the human body – 0.95. Objects with a relative density of more than 1 sink; those with a value of less than 1 float. The average human body will just float. Fat and lung tissue containing air are the primary factors which allow the body to float. When the body is allowed to float freely it will do so in the prone position, the rib cage often just showing above the water (Fig. 2.52A). This position has its limitations in therapy! Some effort is required in order to float in the supine position; the head needs to be slightly extended and the arms abducted. Despite such effort, some people will find that their legs will tend to sink and a few others will float in the vertical position (Fig. 2.52B)! Therapists will note that a significant number of patients will need pelvic and/or leg floats when required to exercise in the floating position.

Buoyancy and Archimedes' principle
Archimedes' principle states that any body which is wholly or partially immersed will experience an upward thrust equal to the weight of fluid displaced. This upward thrust is termed the *force of buoyancy*; it acts through a point called the *centre of buoyancy*. This

A

Water

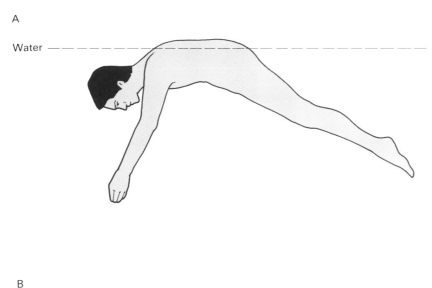

B

Water

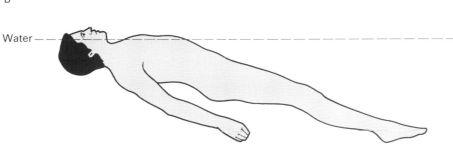

Fig. 2.52 Floating body. A, Prone; B, Supine.

centre need not coincide with the centre of gravity.

The human body will seem 'lighter' when wholly or partially submerged. The therapist can make use of this in the hydrotherapy pool. It both allows the patient to be easily manoeuvred by the therapist and facilitates their movements and postures. It is, for example, easier for a very weak patient to stand upright and maintain the position in the pool.

Moment of buoyancy

If a floating body is to remain in a position of equilibrium, the centres of buoyancy and gravity must lie in the same vertical line (Fig.

2.53). When they are not in line a turning force or couple is produced, the body moving toward a position of equilibrium. This turning force is known as the moment of buoyancy (Fig. 2.54). The effect of the moment of buoyancy can be seen quite clearly in the hydrotherapy pool when treating patients. Figures 2.55A and B show the force being used to advantage when asking the patient to move from the standing to lying position and vice versa. Taking the head backwards will produce a moment which will lead to lying; bending the head forwards will allow the patient to stand again. Figure 2.56 shows the same rotation occurring with the patient in sitting; this follows a backward

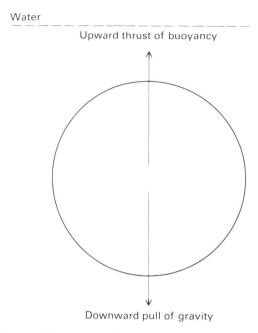

Fig. 2.53 The centres of gravity and buoyancy are in line – no turning occurs.

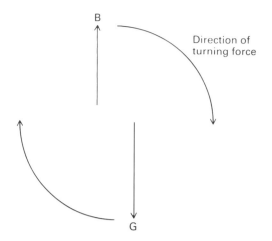

Fig. 2.54 Moment of buoyancy producing a turning force. B – buoyancy. G – gravity.

movement of the head or extension of the lower leg. When the patient is required to sit in the pool and exercise the lower leg it is advisable to counter the natural rotation caused by leg extension by suggesting that they bend the head forwards.

Pressure

Pressure is experienced by a fluid when a force is applied to that fluid when contained in a confined space (Fig. 2.57):

Pressure = force/area

Pressure within a fluid is also the result of the force applied by the weight of the fluid above a given point. The greater the height of the column of fluid in question the greater the pressure. Figure 2.58 shows how pressure increases with depth. To this fluid pressure should be added the value of the atmospheric pressure; this is usually about $101.3\,kN/m^2$.

Pressure in fluid has two important features:

(1) The pressure at a single point is the same in all directions
(2) The pressure exerted at a point on any surface is normal to that surface (Fig. 2.59).

It is very unlikely that the pressure exerted by the water in a hydrotherapy pool will have much effect upon oedema of the tissues as has been claimed in the past. Any reduction of swelling is more likely to be the result of an increase in temperature improving the circulation and the effect of the exercises. However, it has been noted that patients suffering from respiratory distress may have increased problems due to the pressure of the water on their chests when submerged.

Hydrodynamics

Hydrodynamics is the study of fluid in motion. Two types of flow pattern occur as a result of this motion:

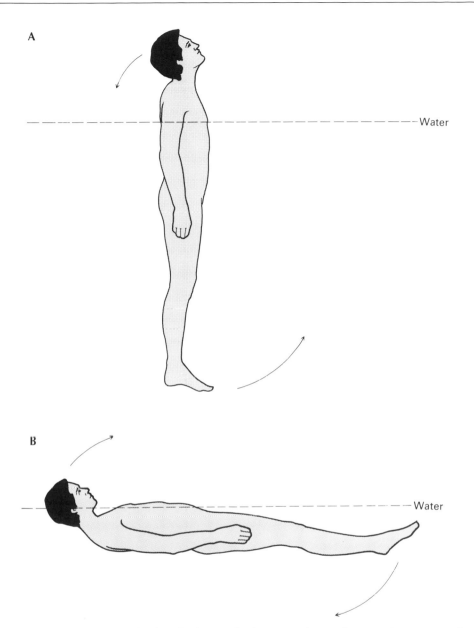

Fig. 2.55 Moment of buoyancy applied to the human body. A, standing to lying; B, lying to standing.

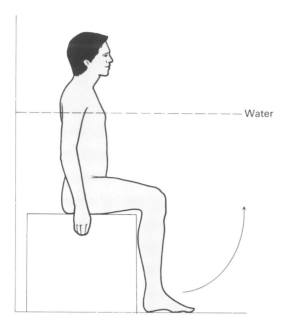

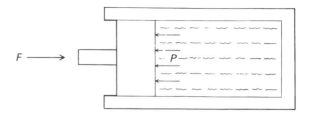

Fig. 2.57 Pressure in a fluid in a confined space. *F* – force applied. *P* – pressure of fluid against piston.

Fig. 2.56 Moment of buoyancy causing rotation of the body in sitting due to extension of the lower leg.

(1) *Velocity of flow.* The velocity of flow of a fluid is the speed at which it moves.
(2) *Viscosity of the fluid.* Viscosity is the internal resistance of a fluid to any change. It is due to the friction occurring between the individual molecules of the liquid.
(3) *Shape.* The shape of the container through which the fluid moves will affect its flow pattern. The shape of objects moving through water will also affect the flow in the fluid lying to the rear of the body.

(1)   Laminar (Fig. 2.60)
(2)   Turbulent (Fig. 2.61).

The type of flow pattern developed in a fluid depends on three major factors:

Laminar flow (Fig. 2.60)
Water molecules move from a point of higher pressure to one of lower pressure. In laminar flow these molecules form layers which slide over one another in a streamlined manner. The

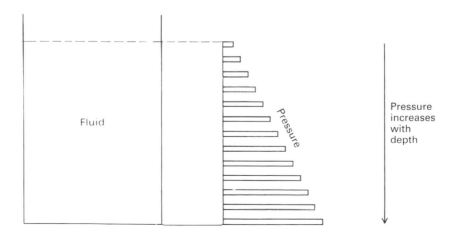

Fig. 2.58 Pressure in a fluid increases with depth.

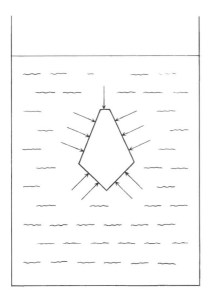

Fig. 2.59 The pressure exerted on a minute body is equal and normal to that body in all directions.

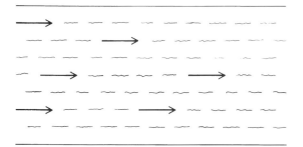

Fig. 2.60 Laminar flow – arrows indicate direction of flow.

path of the molecule is in the same line as that of the general flow. Viscous friction occurs between these adjacent layers, impeding the flow of the fluid. The greater the viscosity of the fluid the greater will be the impediment and thus the slower the flow. Laminar flow only occurs with low velocity fluid movement and it will therefore be seen that fluids of higher viscosity have a greater tendency towards laminar flow.

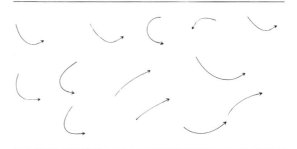

Fig. 2.61 Turbulent flow – arrows indicate motion of fluid.

Turbulent flow (Fig. 2.61)

With an increase in flow rate the laminar pattern will break up and turbulence will occur. The molecules no longer travel in layers but take on an irregular pattern of motion.

Eddy formation

An eddy, or back current, is an exaggerated turbulent pattern which can arise in either laminar or turbulent flow. Its onset is hastened by the presence of initial turbulent flow and increased speed of fluid motion. Eddies arise at points of change in shape in containers or follow the movement of a body through fluid. An area of reduced pressure forms downstream of the irregularity and back currents flow into these areas forming eddies (Fig. 2.62A and B and Fig. 2.63A and B).

Such eddies following a moving body may be termed a wake. A wake will give rise to a drag force which will impede the movement of the object. This effect can be reduced by streamlining the shape of the body (Fig. 2.63B).

The therapist makes considerable use of these factors when treating patients in water. Slow movement of the patient through the medium facilitates laminar flow of the water and consequently there is less resistance to movement.

Further reduction in eddy formation may be

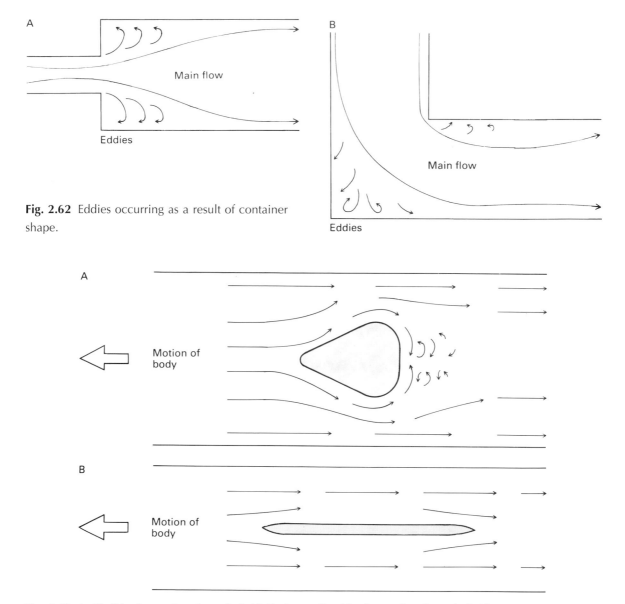

Fig. 2.62 Eddies occurring as a result of container shape.

Fig. 2.63 A, Bluff body moving through fluid; B, Streamlined body moving through fluid.

achieved by presenting the most streamlined aspect of the body to the water. Thus it will be found that walking sideways (slowly) through the water is much easier than walking forward (quickly). Use may be made of the resistance offered by the water; bats are sometimes used in order to present large surface areas to the fluid, encouraging the formation of a wake.

Chapter 3
FUNDAMENTAL AND DERIVED POSITIONS

M. Hollis

There are five fundamental positions which are usually described along with their derivatives as the starting positions from which exercises start or in which they may be given.

Muscle work is deliberately not described as it is dependent upon the way in which the body components relate to one another. It must be recognized that maintenance of position is dependent on the integration of interplay of isotonic muscle action and of some isometric muscle work, but once a position has been assumed the body will reduce its muscle work to the minimum necessary to maintain that position. The abbreviations for each word are also provided.

Lying (Ly) or Supine (Sup.)
The body is supine with the arms by the sides and legs straight. This is the position in which the body is most supported, with a large base and low centre of gravity.

Sitting (Sitt.)
The body is erect, arms by the sides, the thighs are fully supported and together. Right angles are maintained at the hips, knees and ankles. The centre of gravity is low but near to the rear edge of the base which is the area between both the legs of the seat and the feet.

Kneeling (Kn.)
The body is upright from the knees which are held at a right angle. The arms are by the sides. The base consists only of the legs, the centre of gravity is high and the line of gravity falls close to the edge of the base, making the position unstable and difficult to maintain.

Standing (St.)
The body is erect with arms by the sides. The feet are slightly apart at the toes. The base is small and the centre of gravity is high. Providing the lower limbs are strong this position is easier to maintain than kneeling.

Hanging (Hg.)
The body hangs from a beam or overhead support. The arms are wide apart (more than shoulder width) and should be braced so that there is no undue traction on the shoulders. This position should only be used for very strong people as the base consists of the hands grasping the beam and supporting the full body weight.

Positions derived from lying

Side lying (S. Ly.)

This position is rarely used as turning onto the side with the under arm by the side and legs straight is very difficult both to perform and to maintain. The base is small and rounded and the position is one through which the body passes in turning movements or is modified by bending the under arm and leg forwards while the upper arm and leg either rest in the straight position or are flexed slightly. This position is then called the right lateral position (lying on the right side) (R. Lat.) or left lateral position (lying on the left side) (L. Lat.).

Prone lying (Pr. Ly.) or Prone (Pr.)

The body is face down with arms by the side and legs straight. In order to rest comfortably two pillows should be crossed (Fig. 3.1) to support the forehead or the head allowed to turn to the side of the patient's choice.

Quarter turn ($^1/_4$ Tn.)

The body is turned through 45° from either lying, side lying or prone lying and supported by pillows down the raised side of the trunk. The direction of the $^1/_4$ turn is indicated by stating the starting position and direction, e.g. $^1/_4$ Tn.L. from Ly.

Half lying ($^1/_2$ Ly.)

The body is bent at the hips and the trunk is raised from lying to any angle up to 90°. This is the standard position in which most sick people are propped up in bed (Fig. 6.1). More comfortably the legs may be slightly raised or lowered from the horizontal and the knees bent. This modified position is achieved by using ergonomically designed beds or by placing a pillow under the knees.

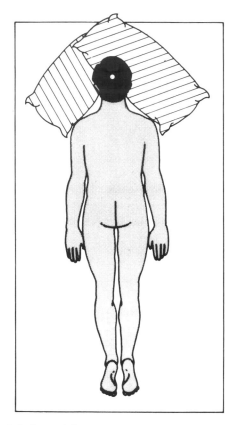

Fig. 3.1 Prone lying.

Side half lying (S. $^1/_2$ Ly.)

The trunk and head are turned to one side so that the patient rests on one buttock and leg and that side of the trunk (Fig. 6.13).

Positions derived from sitting

Forward lean sitting (Fwd. Ln. Sitt.)

The trunk is inclined forwards and the head is supported on pillows on a table at the front (Fig. 6.2).

Half sitting ($^1/_2$ Sitt.)

Sitting on the side of a seat so that only one buttock is supported. The leg on the side of the unsupported buttock is usually bent at the knee as this position is used when the hip is stiff

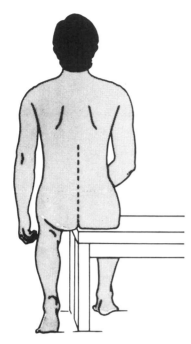

Fig. 3.2 Half sitting.

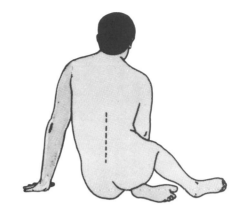

Fig. 3.3 Side sitting.

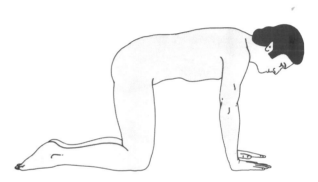

Fig. 3.4 Prone kneeling.

in extension or for lower limb above-knee amputees to allow exercise of the stump (Fig. 3.2).

Long sitting (Long Sitt.)
The legs are stretched out in front, knees straight. The trunk is upright and this position is an uncomfortable one to maintain.

Positions derived from kneeling

Kneel sitting (Kn. Sitt.)
From kneeling to sitting back on the heels. A stable position and much used for retraining balance and by children at play.

Side sitting (Side Sitt.)
From kneel sitting the buttocks are moved sideways so that one or both buttocks rest on the floor beside the feet (Fig. 3.3).

Half kneeling ($^1\!/_2$ Kn.)
From kneeling, one leg is taken forward to be bent at right angles at the hip, knee and ankle. A stage in rising from kneeling to standing or transferring from floor to stool.

Prone kneeling (Pr. Kn.)
Kneeling supported by all four limbs. The arms should be straight and the hands in line below the shoulders. Right angles should be maintained at the hip and knee and the ankles may be plantarflexed or dorsiflexed (Fig. 3.4).

Positions derived from standing

High standing (High St.)
Standing on a platform or stool of any height. Normally used when one leg is to be moved

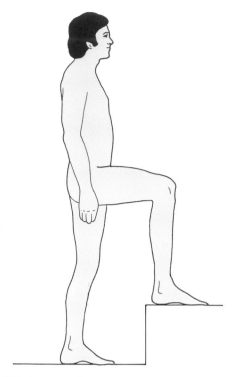

Fig. 3.5 Step standing.

and allows the patient to be more accessible to the therapist. The position is usually stabilized by allowing the patient to grasp a support.

Step standing (Step. St.)
Standing with one foot on a higher level than the other. Used for teaching weight transference before walking upstairs (Fig. 3.5).

Half standing (¹/₂ St.)
Standing on one leg, i.e. one hip is hitched up or one leg is bent at the hip and knee.

Close standing (Cl. St.)
The feet are together and parallel. Harder to maintain than standing, not only because the base is slightly smaller but because the axes of the ankle joints are no longer at an angle to

each other, but together form a single long axis which results in increased interplay of muscles in front of and behind the joints.

Toe standing (T. St.)
The body is raised onto the toes. The smallest possible base is now in use.

Positions derived from hanging

Arch hanging (Arch Hang.)
The starting position for forward and backward swinging of the trunk or for bar somersaults.

Half hanging (¹/₂ Hang.)
Hanging by one arm. The position achieved during lateral travel on the beam.

Positions derived by moving the arms (*A*)

Any of these may be incorporated into the fundamental positions or into those derived from them.

Half (¹/₂)
One arm.

Stretch (Str.)
The arms are held straight above the head in the position of elevation (flexed and laterally rotated) at the shoulder, i.e. palms facing inwards.

Yard (Yd.)
The arms are held straight out from the side of the body, palms facing downwards (Fig. 9.8A).

Reach (Rch.)
The arms are held straight in front of the body palms facing inwards (Fig. 9.9).

Head rest (H. Rst.)
The hands rest on the head, more usually on the occiput, and the position is usually used to gain upper trunk extension.

Bend (Bd.)
The elbow is bent and the hands lie adjacent to the shoulders. A starting position usually used for thrusts upwards, forwards, downwards and backwards.

Wing (Wg.)
The hands rest on the hips. Little used except in rotatory movements of the trunk when the arms are fixed and the quantity of trunk movement is therefore limited.

Heave (Hve.)
Usually used with a grasp. The arms lie abducted at the shoulder, the elbows bent upwards at a right angle so that a grasp may be taken of the edges of the bed or plinth. Used to fix the upper half of the body (Fig. 3.6). Alternatively may be used as heave hanging.

Grasp (Gr.)
The hands grasp a convenient support. May be used with stretch, yard, reach or heave (Figs 8.18 and 9.9).

Low Grasp (Low Gr.)
The hands grasp when they are by the sides.

Forehead support (F. head Supp.)
The forehead rests on the hands placed either palm down or with loosely grasping thumb and forefinger (Fig. 3.7). Used in forward lean positions.

Arm lean (A. Ln.)
The forearms and the hands palms down are placed on a support in front of the body, the head may rest on them or they may rest on and

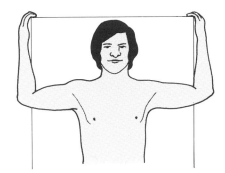

Fig. 3.6 Heave grasp.

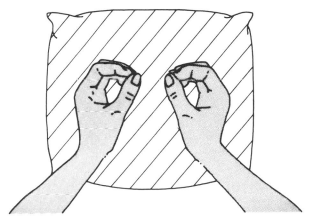

Fig. 3.7 The loosely grasping thumb and forefinger resting on a pillow ready to receive the forehead for forehead support.

be covered by a pillow on which the head rests. Used in forward lean positions (Fig. 6.2).

Forward propping (Fwd. Prop.)
The hands rest flat on the seat and in front of the trunk.

Backward propping (Bwd. Prop.)
The hands rest flat on the seat, fingers pointing backwards and behind the trunk (Fig. 9.30).

Reverse propping (Rev. Prop.)
The hands rest as above but the fingers point forwards. All three propping positions are used

for thrusting actions in which the arm is braced in extension and the trunk may be balanced and/or moved on the arm/s.

Positions derived by moving the legs (*Lg*)

Stride (Std.)

The feet are a sideways pace apart and the base is therefore wide from side to side giving good lateral stability.

Walk (Wk.)

The feet are a forward pace apart and the base wide from front to back, giving good antero-posterior stability.

Oblique stride (Obl. Std.)

The feet are a pace apart part way between walk and stride. This position allows oblique transfer of weight.

Lunge (Lge.)

The feet are well apart and at right angles to each other. If the rear leg is bent, the weight is in a back lunge position. If the front leg is bent, the weight is in a forward lunge position. This position allows transfer of body weight from one leg to the other, with maximum stability for working in this position.

Step

One foot is supported on a stool of any height. The weight may be on either the rear or the stepping foot.

Crook (Ck.)

The knees and hips may be bent slightly by using one pillow under the knees or, in the extremely flexed position, the soles of the feet will be flat on the support (Fig. 3.8).

Cross leg (X Leg)

The legs are crossed at the ankles. The knees are flexed and the hips flexed, abducted and lat-

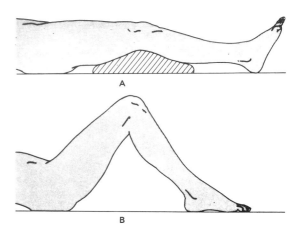

Fig. 3.8 A, Crook lying using a pillow for flexing the knees; B, Crook lying with the knees so flexed that the feet are fully supported.

erally rotated. This position is taken up on the floor or on a high mat.

Cross ankle (X Ankle)

The legs may be crossed at the ankles when the body is in the lying, sitting, kneeling or standing positions.

Positions derived by moving the trunk (*Tr*)

Stoop (Stp.)

The body is bent forwards at the hips with erect back and head.

Relaxed or Slack Stoop (Lax Stp.)

The head and trunk are flexed.

Arch

The head and trunk are extended.

Turn (Tn.)

The trunk is rotated through any degree less than 90° either by moving the shoulder girdle or the pelvis or both depending on the fundamental position (Fig. 8.21).

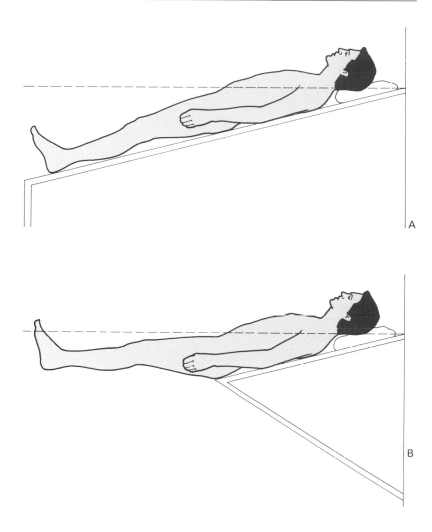

Fig. 3.9 A, Support lying;
B, Half support lying.

Positions in water

The fundamental positions of lying, sitting and standing, used on land, are suitable but, because of the properties of the medium when the patient is immersed, he will need supporting on a plinth or half plinth if his position is to be fixed. The word support (Sup.) is added before the fundamental position when the patient is supported either on a plinth, e.g. support lying (Sup.Ly.) or on a half plinth, e.g. half support lying ($\frac{1}{2}$ Sup.Ly.) (Fig. 3.9A and B).

The further adjective Float (Fl) is added first when the support is by such a facility, e.g. float support lying (Fl.Sup.Ly.). When the plinth is greatly inclined, this word may be the appropriate prefix, e.g. inclined support lying (Incl.Sup.Ly.).

The patient may be fixed by the use of straps or may hold the side rail by:

either grasping with his arms in stretch or heave positions
or by tucking his toes under the side rail.

Greater use is made in a therapeutic pool of inclined postures whereby the patient leans:

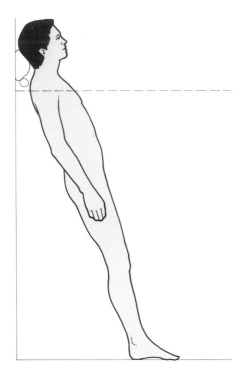

Fig. 3.10 Inclined standing.

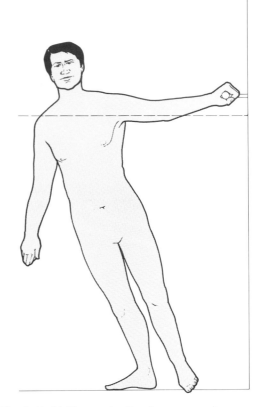

Fig. 3.11 Half grasp inclined away standing.

either forward towards the rail, which he grasps – grasp inclined prone standing (Gr.Incl.Pr.St.)

or backwards to a head support on the pool side – inclined standing (Incl.St.) (Fig. 3.10)

or sideways towards – half grasp inclined towards side standing ($^1/_2$ Gr.Incl. tow. S.St.)

or sideways away from – half grasp inclined away side standing ($^1/_2$ Gr.Incl. aw. S.St.) – the pool side and rail (Fig. 3.11). Sitting on a weighted stool allows arm and trunk movements to be performed with more facility in shallower pools and fixes the legs for ankle exercises.

To describe a position

First consider which parts of the body are not in the normal relationships as in the fundamental position. Then name their position in the following order – head, arm, trunk, leg and fundamental position, e.g. head support arm lean forward stride sitting; $^1/_2$ low grasp $^1/_2$ high standing.

Descriptions of movements

Flexion (Flex.)
An angular movement. A forward movement in which joints are bent. Usually the approximation of two ventral surfaces. Takes place about a transverse axis and in the median or sagittal plane.

Extension (Ext.)

An angular movement, the opposite of the above. A backward movement in which joints are straightened. The opposite of flexion with the same axis and plane.

Abduction (Abd.)

An angular movement. Movement away from the mid-line of the body occurs round an anteroposterior, i.e. sagittal axis and in the coronal or frontal plane. The exceptions are the shoulder joint and the carpometacarpal joint of the thumb.

Adduction (Add.)

An angular movement, the opposite of the above. Movements towards the mid-line of the body.

Circumduction ○

A combination of the above four angular movements so that each position is adopted in turn and in sequence. The moving bone(s) circumscribe a conical space.

Rotation (Rot.)

A turning movement, about a vertical axis and in a horizontal plane, of limbs, head or trunk in which case the direction in which the anterior surface is turning is first indicated.

Medial rotation (M. Rot.)

Occurs round a vertical axis. The anterior aspect of the limb turns towards the mid-line.

Lateral rotation (L. Rot.)

The opposite of the above, though the axis is the same.

Side flexion (S. Flex.)

An angular movement. Movements of the head or trunk away from the mid-line in a lateral direction.

Inversion (Inv.)

Applies to the foot and is a movement of adduction and inward rotation of the forefoot of which the sole faces inwards.

Eversion (Ev.)

Applies to the foot and is the opposite of the above.

Supination (Sup.)

Applies to the forearm. The palm of the hand is turned forwards so that the thumb is lying laterally.

Pronation (Pron.)

The opposite of the above. The movement is limited to the radio-ulnar joints and is best observed when the elbow is flexed. (Neither of the above should be confused with medial and lateral rotation of the arm.)

Symbols, apparatus and counts

⊙ *Circling* may be a movement of a part involving all four angular movements and rotation and the term may also be used to describe an action by a group of people.

○ *Circumduction* consists of a composite of the four angular movements with no intention to rotate.

- ⌢R.L.⌢ *Rolling* in direction of arrow.
- → Movement in that direction, i.e. ↑ up, ↓ down, → R. to the right, L. ← to the left, ⤢ obliquely.
- (Form) (Stool) etc. placed in the exercise name after the fundamental position.
- 4× repeated four times.
- 1–4 to a count of 4, may be followed by an indication of tempo 1–4 (slowly).
- Reb. with a rebound.
- ·/. repeat.

To describe an activity

First name the starting position (see above) then the part to be moved in the activity or movement, e.g. T. turn or jump on spot.

Next name the direction, e.g. T. turn R. and L.

The apparatus to be used is named in brackets after the starting position, e.g. Std. Sitt. (Stool).

The repetition number and count is named after the action and is followed by the tempo description if needed, e.g. Std. Sitt. (Stool); T. turn alt. R. and L. (4×); *or* Std. Sitt. (Stool); T. turn alt. R. and L. (1–4) slowly (5–8) quickly; *or* Std. St. T. turn alt. R. and L. with reb. (1–4) and T. drop fwd. (5) T. Str. up. (6–8).

To analyse muscle work of an exercise

Watch the whole performance and observe which are the moving body parts. Then decide the joints which are moving and the direction of movement at each joint. Remember that direction may be conditioned by movement of the body part either proximal or distal to the joint, e.g. there is rotation of the cervical spine in the action of walking but the head does not move; the rotation is of the vertebral column *below* the head. Next decide on a starting point in the analysis. Most actions are both repetitive and cyclical and thus a starting point is needed so that a decision can be made about the exact part of muscle range being used at any one time. For convenience repetitive actions are often divided into phases described by what is being done at the time, e.g. in walking each leg repeats stance, toe or push-off, swing-through and heel-strike phases, with one leg doing stance while the other performs the movement sequence. In throwing a ball the phases are conditioned by the starting position and the vigour of the throw as well as the size and weight

of the ball; they may be swing back, swing forward and release for the throwing arm, while the other arm may swing in opposite directions to assist balance and the rest of the body may be doing weight on back leg, weight transfer forwards, weight on forward leg with the upper trunk rotating with the throwing arm against a lower trunk rotated with the weight transfer.

The next decision that has to be made is: which are the working muscles over each joint in a sequence? The same sequence should be used to name and describe the different phases of the activity. Thus the muscle groups working over the foot, ankle, knee and hip should always be described in that order if that is the order used for the first part of the analysis and description.

Each time a muscle group is named the type of muscle work it is performing and the range of muscle work should be stated, e.g. the muscle work of the swing phase of the leg in walking may be described in two ways:

either the dorsiflexors of the foot isotonic shortening in full range; the extensors of the knee isotonic shortening in inner range; the flexors of the hip isotonic shortening in outer range;

or because the phrase 'isotonic shortening' applies to all groups mentioned, this phrase can be used at the end of the sentence thus: the dorsiflexors of the foot in full range, the extensors of the knee in inner range and the flexors of the hip in outer range, all in isotonic shortening.

Recognize that at the same time another part of the body may simultaneously be doing something else and that action should be analysed next and recorded so that a synchronous picture and analysis is built up.

It must be remembered that in analysing free

movement the effect of gravity will be important in determining the muscle work and will be varied mainly by the mode of performance in speed and weight. Thus trunk bending slowly forward to pick up a ball will be initiated by a momentary contraction of the flexor muscles in isotonic shortening in the middle range and brought about by the trunk extensors in isotonic lengthening in their outer range along with the hip extensors in isotonic lengthening if the hip joint is moved. In other words, in this case the *movement* is of flexion, but the muscle *action* is of the extensors.

Now if the movement is a swift and hard push into flexion, the flexors will perform the action until the speed and weight of the action is reduced, when the extensors will take over.

Chapter 4
RELAXATION

M. Hollis

The tension of muscles can be affected by conscious effort and thought and can be relieved by the application of conscious thought and/or muscular effort on the part of the patient. The difference between tension and relaxation may be observed, for example, in the difference in posture of an athlete at the beginning of a sprint start and that at the end of the race when the line has been crossed; or in the learner driver who sits tensed and hunched over the steering wheel as opposed to the relaxation of the accustomed and experienced driver.

Relaxation can be taught to patients so that a regime can be practised alone, or active resisted techniques may be used for which the presence of the therapist is necessary. Relaxation may be general or local, i.e. the whole body may be taught to relax or only a small part, as required. Relaxation can be practised in any convenient posture, but is more usually taught in lying, half lying, side half lying, modified side lying and right or left lateral positions, prone lying or in an armchair supported with a high back.

There are two physical methods, contrast method and reciprocal method, which the patient may be taught to practise alone.

Contrast method

The physiology of the contrast method is that a strong contraction of a muscle is followed by an equal relaxation of the same muscle, or

Excitation = Inhibition

The technique consists of a sequence of contractions of muscles performed, usually, in a distal to proximal sequence in each limb or pair of limbs in turn, followed by letting go or relaxation for an equal or longer period of time. Then the contractions for each limb part are usually added to one another so that tension in the limb is total and the relaxation should be controlled in reverse sequence.

The sequence of commands is as follows (alternative or explanatory commands are in brackets):

For the arm
'*Make a fist and let go.*'
'*Tighten your wrist and let go*' (pull your hand back or forwards).
'*Tighten your elbow and let go*' (bend or straighten).
'*Tighten your shoulder and let go*' (pull your arm into your side).

For the leg
'*Point your foot down or pull your foot up and let go*' (the patient chooses whichever is least likely to give him cramp).
'*Tighten your knee and let go*' (straighten your knees).

'*Tighten your hips and let go*' (tighten the buttocks). When the above sequences are added together the commands will be:

For the arm
'*Tighten your fist, wrist, elbow and shoulder and let go shoulder, elbow, wrist and hand*' (stiffen the whole arm, and let go).

For the leg
'*Tighten or point your feet, knees and hips and let go your hips, knees and feet*' (stiffen the whole leg, and let go).
The commands for both pairs of limbs may be added together as follows:
'*Tighten the feet and hands, knees and elbows, hips and shoulders and let go*' in reverse order (stiffen your arms and legs and let go).

For the trunk and head
'*Press your head against your support and let go.*'
'*Press your shoulders against your support and let go.*'
Deep breathing may be practised with relaxation of any part of the body. It is more usual to breathe in while tensing the muscles and to breathe out on letting go.

It is also possible to add the contractions for the trunk on to those for the limbs so that the patient is in whole body tension, but this should not be taught to a patient with high blood pressure, or one who tends to have respiratory incapacity. The value of this technique is that it can be used for a limited part of the body, for example for relaxation of the hand or of the shoulder girdle or the hip adductors and lateral rotators.

Reciprocal method

The physiology of this method is that the antagonist groups of muscles always relax reciprocally and equally to the contraction of the agonist groups of muscles. Tension will be relieved by contraction of the antagonistic muscles. In this technique, the muscles which will take the patient out of the tense posture are those which are required to contract with the consequent diminution in tension in the muscles that are maintaining the tense posture.

The patient is allowed initially to remain in his tense posture, and may lie or sit if he prefers, but specially comfortable positioning should not necessarily be offered; better positions will be achieved as the relaxation proceeds. For success with this technique it is important that the patient learns to recognize his own tension at any time and learns what to do to relieve it without necessarily changing his main working position.

The sequence used is more usually proximal to distal, and each part of the body is given three commands as follows:

(1) To move so that the tense '*infolded*' position of the body is opened up.
(2) To stop moving.
(3) To let the brain appreciate the new posture making the patient think about the new position in which his body component is now resting. Time should be allowed for this and the patient should not be hurried.

The commands are given as follows:

For the shoulders
'*Push your shoulders towards your feet.*'

For the arms
'*Lift your arms outwards and slightly straighten your elbows.*'

For the hands
'*Make the whole palms of the hands and your fingers be fully supported.*'

For the hips
'*Separate the thighs.*'

For the knees
'*Straighten your legs slightly.*'

For the feet
'*Point your feet away from you.*'

For the head
'*Press your head into the support or backwards.*'

For the upper trunk
'*Press your back into the support or backwards.*'

For the jaw
'*Without necessarily opening your lips push the lower jaw away from the upper jaw or towards your feet.*'

Breathing for this technique is usually achieved at greater depth by asking the patient '*to sigh*' and to appreciate what is happening to the waist. To be aware that the waist is becoming smaller, and even that the '*ribs are folding down like a bird's wing*'.

In fact in both these methods asking the patient to sigh as though at the end of a heavy day is the best method of gaining deep breathing because if a good breath out is taken the amount of air that is subsequently taken into the lungs will be slightly increased. Note that in these two techniques the word *relax* is never used and only in the contrast method is the patient asked to *let go*. The positions which may be used for the reciprocal method are the same as those for the contrast method and in neither of these methods is it important that the patient should be in a particularly quiet atmosphere. It is, in fact, much better to teach the reciprocal method against a normal back-ground noise and not to create a soothing hypnotic atmosphere round the patient.

Suggestion method

A third method which may be used for some patients and which is entirely for those who may not perform much muscle work is the suggestion method. In this technique the therapist provides comfortable relaxing conditions for the patient:

(a)   A warm well-ventilated room
(b)   A comfortable support
(c)   Light covering.

Then, by using quiet, hypnotic, mellow tones, suggest that the thoughts be directed to personally enjoyable but repetitive noises or scenes. The patient is told to think about each part of the body in turn. To think that it is '*very heavy*' and the suggestion is repeated several times until the limb gives the appearance of relaxation, e.g. until the lower limb is rolled out. The patient may be invited to try to raise the limb, while the suggestion is made that it will be impossible to do so and that it may feel as though it is floating. The patient is then instructed to direct attention to the other leg and to each arm in turn and then to the whole body. Deep, sighing type of breathing may be practised for a few breaths and the 'suggestible' patients will be found at the end of quite a short treatment session, to have gone to sleep.

Pendular swinging

This is used for relaxation of the limbs. The arm(s) or leg(s) may be swung back and forth until they feel numb. The sensory receptors have accommodated to the constant movement. This type of swinging may be aided by adding a $\frac{1}{2}$ to 1 kg weight to the limb keeping it within the length of the limb, i.e. grasped in the hand or fastened to the ankle. This type of swinging is of particular value to reduce the rigidity of Parkinsonism, but is also used for shorter periods to mobilize joints by patient activity. It is most suitable for the shoulder, hip, knee and lumbar spine.

Active resisted techniques for local relaxation

Hold relax

This technique is described more fully in Chapter 23 on neuromuscular facilitation. Briefly it consists of offering resistance to a muscle group which is in tension. The patient is commanded to '*hold*' the limb in position while the therapist applies resistance to the patient's contraction, which produces isometric contraction of the tense muscles. No movement should occur. When the therapist feels that the patient has reached the limit of his potential contraction, she should grasp the limb firmly, but comfortably, and at the same time tell the patient to '*relax*' or '*let go*' and allow a time to elapse which is at least as long as, or perhaps longer than, the time taken to build up the maximum contraction. This technique is of special use when a patient has no movement because of pain-spasm.

Contract relax

This technique may be used when a patient has a small range of movement and then is prevented from moving further by the spasm of the muscles which are antagonist to the movement. The therapist places her hands on the limb on the same side as the antagonist muscles which are in spasm and asks the patient to make a small strongly resisted contraction back to the original position of rest. At the end of the movement the part is grasped firmly, but comfortably, and the patient is told to '*relax*'. Again the period of relaxation should be an adequate length of time. Then the original movement should again be attempted either passively or actively. A gain in range may be found and a further contract–relax should now allow a small range movement which should not return the limb to the original resting position, but should be less than the total range, i.e. the patient should not return each time to the original position in which the limb was resting. This technique is described more fully in Chapter 23.

Chapter 5
PASSIVE MOVEMENTS

M. Hollis

Anatomical movements which are performed by the therapist for the patient are passive movements. They may be performed at single joints or at several joints in sequence covering any or all of the joint movements and maintaining muscle length. They may also be performed to several joints simultaneously as in many natural and functional movements.

Basic rules

The following must be observed:

(1) Those parts not to be moved should be adequately supported.
(2) The part(s) to be moved should be comfortably grasped.
(3) The sequence of motion should be decided – distal to proximal or proximal to distal. Each have their place, e.g. for giving passive movements to neurological patients a proximal to distal sequence is used. The reverse, a distal to proximal sequence, is more commonly used to aid venous and lymphatic return.
(4) At the extremities of the ranges, the grasp on the stretched skin side should be eased to prevent dragging.
(5) The grasp should be as near the joint to be moved as possible.

(6) As the movement is performed the joint may be given slight traction, but compression should be exerted at the extremities of the range.
(7) The motion should be smooth and rhythmical and the repetition rate maintained at even tempo.
(8) Changes in grasp should be smooth and positioning of the hands arranged so that minimal changes are necessary.

Movements of the right upper limb

Patient's position lying (or side lying)
The therapist stands so that she can see the patient's face and in walk standing with the outer leg (L) forwards. She grasps as follows.

Proximal to distal sequence

Shoulder girdle
There are two different grasps, for:

(1) Elevation and depression – the left hand above the shoulder, the right hand under the bent elbow (Fig. 5.1).
(2) Protraction and retraction – the left hand grasps over deltoid and rolls the arm and, therefore, the shoulder girdle, forwards and backwards (Fig. 5.2).

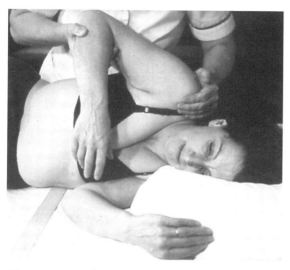

Fig. 5.1 Grasp for elevation and depression of the shoulder girdle.

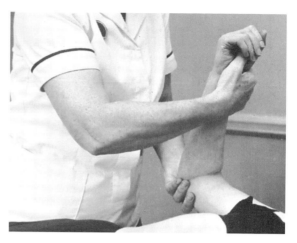

Fig. 5.3 The grasps used for glenohumeral joint movement when the joint is not stiff showing abduction. The same grasp is used for elbow joint movement.

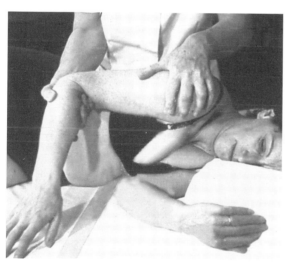

Fig. 5.2 Grasp for protraction and retraction (lateral and medial rotation of the scapula).

Glenohumeral joint

There are two possible grasps:

(1) The left hand at the elbow to grasp as in Fig. 5.3 and to give slight traction; the right hand takes a palm-to-palm thumb grasp which fixes the wrist joint in slight

extension. The starting position of the arm is in neutral abduction. Movements towards the body are done first: adduction and abduction (Fig. 5.3) then remaining in abduction (Fig. 5.4A) flexion through abduction and extension to the limit of the support/joint; medial and lateral rotation (Fig. 5.4B) follow again from neutral abduction. Full elevation follows (flexion/abduction/lateral rotation) (Fig. 5.5).

(2) If the glenohumeral joint is stiff it may be necessary to fix the shoulder girdle, in which case the left hand remains above the shoulder to do so. The right forearm supports the patient's arm with the therapist's hand grasping the elbow (Fig. 5.6). The movements may be performed as above, but flexion through abduction may involve foot movement on the part of the therapist.

To complete the movements of the shoulder joint the patient should be turned into side lying when full extension can be performed (Fig. 5.7).

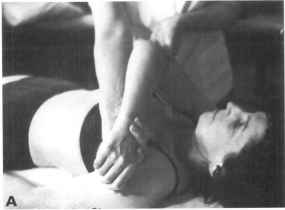

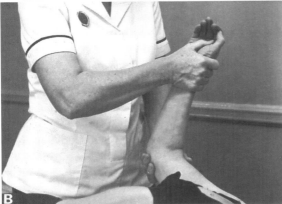

Fig. 5.4 A, Flexion through abduction at the glenohumeral joint; B, The grasp used for medial and lateral rotation at the glenohumeral joint.

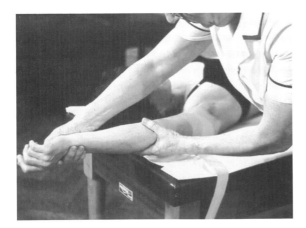

Fig. 5.5 The grasp used to obtain full range movement into elevation of the arm (flexion/abduction/lateral rotation).

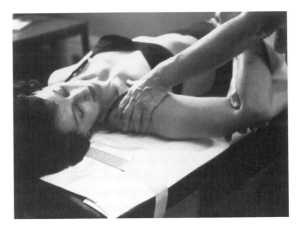

Fig. 5.6 The grasps used to isolate the movement to the glenohumeral joint.

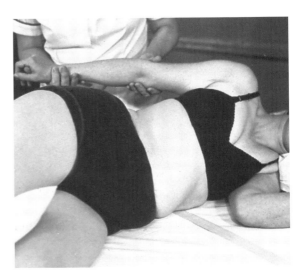

Fig. 5.7 Side lying grasp for full range extension of the glenohumeral joint.

Elbow joint

The left hand grasps behind the elbow and the right hand maintains a palm-to-palm thumb grasp. Flexion is performed first, finishing with slight overpressure, and extension is performed last finishing with slight traction (Fig. 5.8).

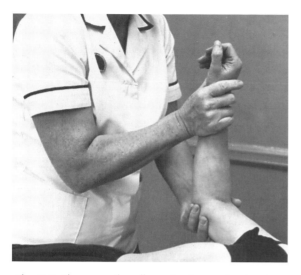

Fig. 5.8 The grasp for elbow flexion and extension.

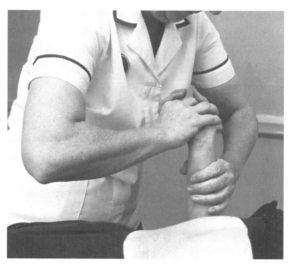

Fig. 5.9 The grasp for wrist flexion and extension.

Radio-ulnar joints

The movements of pronation and supination may be performed using the same grasp as for the elbow, but to confine the movement to the radio-ulnar joint the elbow should be semi-flexed (Fig. 5.8) and kept in this position throughout the movements which follow.

Wrist joint

The right hand grasps the palm and the left hand grasps proximal to the wrist (Fig. 5.9). Flexion is performed first, being careful that the thumb on the dorsum of the hand does not drag on the skin, then extension is performed, followed by ulnar then radial deviation with the wrist in the neutral position, i.e. straight.

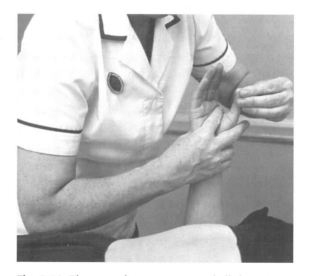

Fig. 5.10 The grasp for movements of all the joints of the thumb.

Thumb movements

The therapist's right hand grasps the palm and the left hand grasps the thumb tip on each side (Fig. 5.10). The movements of full flexion of the carpometacarpal, metacarpophalangeal and interphalangeal joints may be performed together followed by extension, then adduction and abduction of the metacarpophalangeal and carpometacarpal joints, followed by opposition and extension of the carpometacarpal joint. Alternatively, with the arm laid on the supporting pillow the movements of flexion and extension of the individual joints may be performed separately by holding the distal and proximal bone on each side and near the joint to be moved.

Metacarpophalangeal joints of the fingers

The therapist grasps the palm with her right hand and the fingers with her left hand so that she keeps the interphalangeal joints straight (Fig. 5.11). The movements of flexion, extension, abduction and adduction are then performed for all four joints simultaneously, or with the arm laid on the supporting pillow each joint may be moved separately.

Interphalangeal joints

The same grasp is maintained on the palm with the right hand, and the tips of the fingers are grasped with the left hand (Fig. 5.12A). The fingers are bent into the palm (Fig. 5.12B), overpressure is given and, as the fingers are unrolled into extension, they are regrasped at the tips so that slight traction may be given, or, again with the arm laid on the supporting pillow, each interphalangeal joint may be moved separately by holding adjacent to the joint on the sides of the bones.

Combined movements of the upper limb

(1) Elbow flexion with supination and extension with pronation is done to maintain the passive length of biceps brachii and the normal pattern of these two movements.

(2) Elbow extension with pronation and extension/abduction/medial rotation of the shoulder and its opposite elbow flexion and/or extension with supination

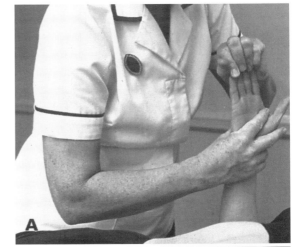

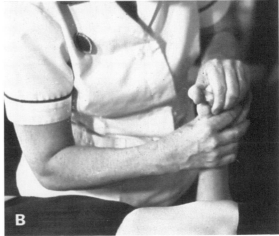

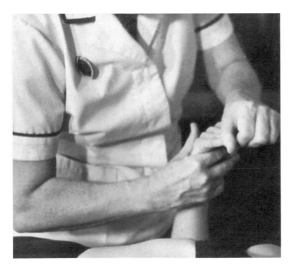

Fig. 5.11 The grasp for movements of metacarpophalangeal joints of the fingers.

Fig. 5.12 The grasp for A, Extension; B, Flexion of the interphalangeal joints of the fingers.

and flexion/adduction/lateral rotation of the shoulder (elevation).

(3) Extension and abduction of fingers, thumb and wrist with supination and elbow extension and its opposite flexion/adduction of fingers, thumb and wrist with pronation and elbow flexion to maintain the passive length of the muscles in the anterior and posterior aspects of the forearm and working over the above joints.

Movements of the right lower limb

Patient's position lying (or side lying)
Hip movements
It should be recognized that full range movement of extension of the hip especially in the male cannot be achieved in lying, and it may be necessary to turn the patient to side lying or prone (Fig. 5.13).

Medial and lateral rotation
The therapist places one hand on the front of the lower tibial region and one on the front of the lower thigh and rolls the leg first in then out (Fig. 5.14) or the leg may be flexed to 80° (approx.) by grasping with the left hand under the lower thigh and with the right hand under the lower leg (Fig. 5.15). The lower leg is then moved outwards to obtain medial rotation and inwards to obtain lateral rotation. The supporting left hand maintains the flexion and allows the limb to pivot at the hip.

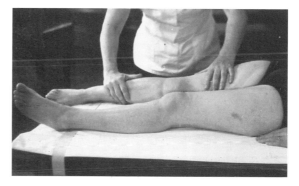

Fig. 5.14 Grasp for medial and lateral rotation of the hip in extension.

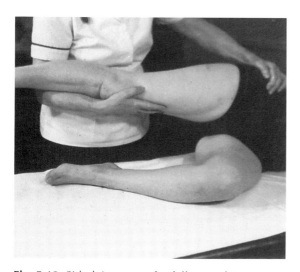

Fig. 5.13 Side lying grasp for full range hip extension.

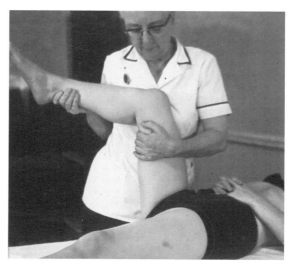

Fig. 5.15 Grasp for medial and lateral rotation of the hip in flexion.

Adduction and abduction

The therapist holds under the lower thigh with her left hand and the ankle area with her right hand with the knee slightly flexed (Fig. 5.16A). To permit full adduction the other leg should be abducted or the moving leg may have to be raised to slight flexion to cross in front of the opposite leg. Abduction should be carried out second and, if the opposite leg is not abducted, the therapist must be careful to note when the limit of abduction is reached and the pelvis starts to tilt laterally, or the therapist holds the leg from the medial side by sliding her right hand under the knee and supports the slightly flexed leg on her forearm whilst her left hand palpates on the anterior superior iliac spine for the onset of pelvic tilting (Fig. 5.16B).

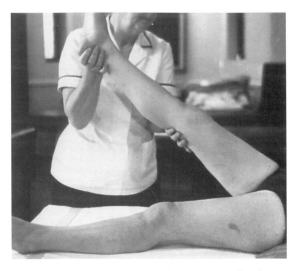

Fig. 5.17 The grasp used for flexion of the hip by performing a straight leg raise.

Flexion and extension

With the patient in lying this may be done in two ways:

(1)   As a straight leg raise by grasping over or under the ankle with the right hand and under the knee with the left hand. The amount of hip joint flexion will be limited by the passive insufficiency of the hamstrings (Fig. 5.17).
(2)   With the knee flexed, when the right hand may hold under the heel and the forearm may support the foot and the left hand holds under the lower thigh and flexion of both hip and knee joints is carried out simultaneously. To obtain full flexion with overpressure it may be necessary to move the left hand to the front of the upper tibial region as the movement passes mid-range, and return it as extension starts (Fig. 5.18A and B).

Knee flexion and extension

This can only be carried out as above if the patient is in lying, but can be carried out alone

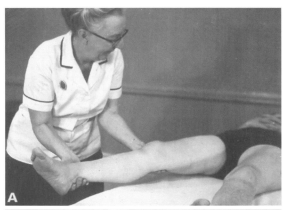

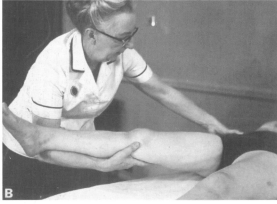

Fig. 5.16 Alternative grasps (A and B) for adduction and abduction of the hip.

if the patient is in side lying. The hip should be kept extended so that full knee extension is possible. With the patient in left side lying the therapist's right hand holds under the medial side of the ankle and the left hand under the medial side of the lower thigh. It may be necessary to allow slight hip flexion in order to carry out full knee flexion because of the stretch on rectus femoris (Fig. 5.19).

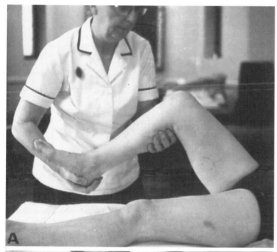

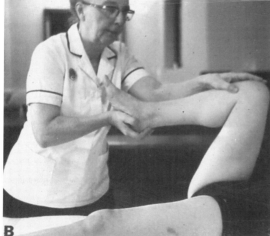

Fig. 5.18 Hip and knee flexion and extension. A, The grasp to start and finish the movements; B, The grasp for the middle stages, i.e. full flexion and the beginning of extension.

Ankle movements
There are several possible grasps; in each case a pillow may be used under the calf to raise the heel off the bed.

(1) One hand on the dorsal and one on the plantar aspect of the mid-foot with the hands crossing the foot, fingers on the medial side. Plantarflexion should be performed first (Fig. 5.20A).

(2) The right hand takes an under heel grasp with the forearm under the foot and the left hand across the dorsum of the foot (Fig. 5.20B). The disadvantage of this grasp is that pressure is exerted on the metatarsal heads which may, in some diseases, cause the onset of ankle clonus. Care should be taken that the toes are not extended with unintentional vigour at the metatarsophalangeal joints.

Mid-tarsal joints
Inversion and eversion can be performed by using grasp (1) described for ankle movements by sliding the hands more distally on the foot, or the foot may be grasped from the outside with the right hand, and the left hand used across the ankle and on to the medial side of

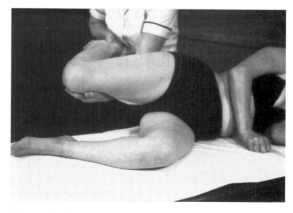

Fig. 5.19 Side lying. The grasp used for knee flexion and extension.

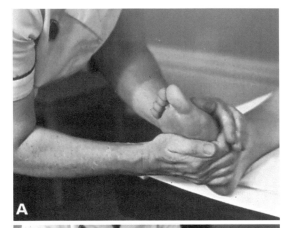

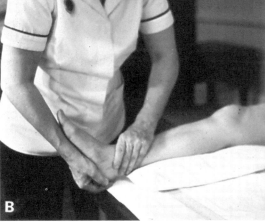

Fig. 5.20 A, The grasp for both plantar- and dorsi-flexion of the ankle and for in- and eversion of the foot; B, An alternative grasp must be used to obtain a passive stretch on a shortened tendocalcaneous.

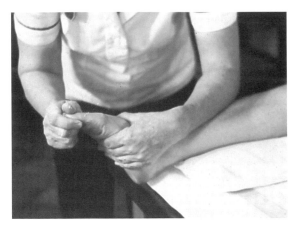

Fig. 5.21 The grasp for all movements of the metatarsophalangeal joints.

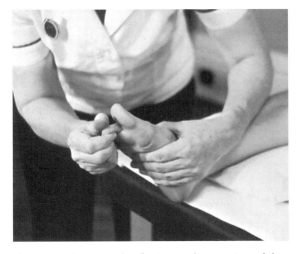

Fig. 5.22 The grasp for flexion and extension of the interphalangeal joints of the lateral four toes.

the calcaneum to stablilize the leg and proximal tarsal bones.

Metatarsophalangeal joints
Flexion, extension, abduction and adduction can be carried out on five joints simultaneously by using the left hand to grasp the metatarsals from the inside of the foot while the right hand grasps the toes (Fig. 5.21).

Interphalangeal joints
Flexion and extension may be performed by sliding the right hand grip on the toes to the tips (Fig. 5.22), but it is easier to deal with the lateral four toes together and the big toe separately. The grasp for the big toe is with both hands reaching over the foot to grasp adjacent to the joint and on the dorsal and plantar aspects (Fig. 5.23).

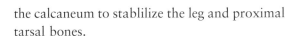

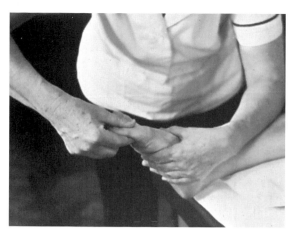

Fig. 5.23 The grasp for movements of the metatarsophalangeal and interphalangeal joints of the big toe.

Individual interphalangeal joints of the toes may be flexed and extended by grasping on the proximal bone at the sides and the distal bone either at the sides or on the dorsal and plantar aspects.

Combined movements of the lower limb

Flexion/adduction and lateral rotation of the hip may be alternated with extension/abduction and medial rotation and flexion/abduction and medial rotation with extension/adduction and lateral rotation. In each oblique pattern of such movements the limb should be supported just about the level of the knee and under the foot and ankle.

The above movements can be combined with knee and ankle movements, those of flexion of the hip combining more usually with flexion of the knee and dorsiflexion of the ankle. Under some circumstances it is necessary to perform an extension pattern of the hip with knee flexion, especially prior to retraining a walking pattern for the 'lift off' phase of the movement.

Foot and ankle movements often combine – dorsiflexion with inversion and plantarflexion with eversion, or dorsiflexion with eversion and plantarflexion with inversion.

Movements of the head

Head movements may be performed with the patient in lying with the head over the edge of the plinth and supported in the therapist's hands.

Flexion and extension
There are three alternative grasps:

(1)   One hand under the occiput, the other hand under the chin. The posterior hand performs the movements and gives traction. The hand on the chin keeps it 'tucked in' and controls any tendency of the head to wobble (Fig. 5.24A).
(2)   Both hands supporting the back of the head. The disadvantage of this grasp is that on full extension of the head there may be inadequate control (Fig. 5.24B).
(3)   The head is supported on the crossed pronated forearms and the finger tips rest on the front of the outer part of the patient's shoulders (Fig. 5.24C).

Side flexion
Grasps (1) and (2) above may be used. If the former grasp is used it may be necessary to change hands so that the head is supported at the back by the hand on the side towards which side flexion occurs.

Rotation
One hand crosses obliquely behind the head from above one ear to below the opposite ear, the other hand, at right angles to it, grasps the jaw line from in front with the fingers cupped round the chin. The head is rotated *away* from

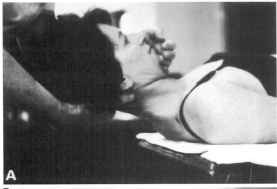

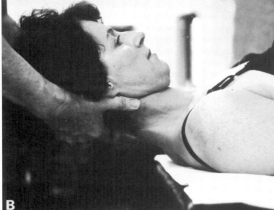

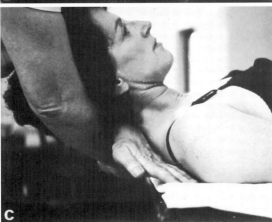

Fig. 5.24 For movements of the head. A, The occiput and chin grasp; B, The double-handed grasp on the occiput; C, The crossed forearm support.

the front hand. To rotate the opposite way the hands should be changed over, moving first the front hand to support at the back and then the back hand to the jaw line.

Movements of the trunk

Passive movements of the trunk are most easily given if half the body is suspended. The unsuspended part of the trunk is further fixed by the therapist who half kneels behind the patient, leans across and places her arm across the front of the trunk. She braces her standing leg and uses her free arm to swing the trunk into flexion, extension or side flexion as the case may be.

If suspension is not available then the patient should be on a high mat or plinth.

To move the lower trunk
Flexion

The patient is in lying with knees fully bent and pressure is applied on the area of the tibial tuberosity with one forearm while the other hand, placed under the sacrum, lifts the lumbar spine into full flexion (Fig. 5.25).

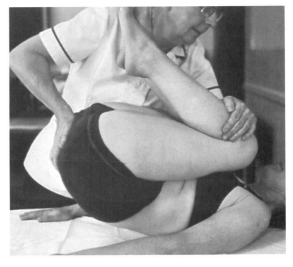

Fig. 5.25 The grasp for lumbar flexion.

Side flexion

The patient is in crook lying. The therapist hooks one arm under the knees, lifts slightly and, counter-pressing on the waist, lifts the patient into side flexion.

Rotation

The patient is in crook lying, the therapist grasps both knees and flexing at the same time presses the knees towards first one shoulder and then to the other (Fig. 5.26A). Alternatively the therapist may press the bent knees to one side away from her while holding the shoulder of the opposite side still (Fig. 5.26B).

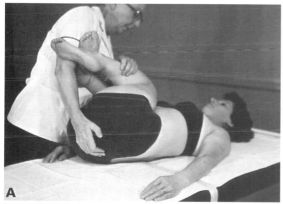
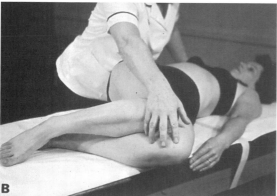

Fig. 5.26 Alternative grasps (A and B) for trunk rotation.

Extension

The patient may be in prone lying and the therapist places one arm under the thighs and the other hand on the lumbar spine and lifts the thighs backwards (Fig. 5.27). Alternatively the patient may be in side lying and the same manoeuvre may be performed by half kneeling behind the patient and carrying the thighs backwards, supporting with one hand across the front and under the lower thigh.

To move the upper trunk

The patient may be in stride sitting with his arms grasped behind his neck.

Rotation

The therapist stands behind and placing one hand in front of and one hand behind the shoulders, she applies opposing pressures. The thigh and pelvis should be supported at the back to prevent unwanted movements.

Flexion

A hand is placed on the occiput and the head, neck and upper trunk are flexed.

Extension

One hand is placed on the forehead and the other in mid-thoracic region and pressure is applied to the forehead while the lower hand

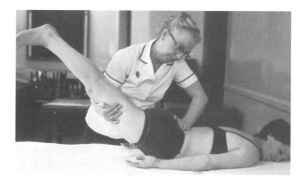

Fig. 5.27 The grasp for lumbar extension.

exerts counter pressure and also acts as the pivot.

Side flexion

The therapist stands at the back of the patient, hooks her arms from in front through his bent elbows and by levering on his grasped arms moves him from side to side.

Assisted active movements

Movements in which the patient participates but is helped by the therapist are assisted active movements. The disadvantage of such movements is that the amount of work being done by the patient is an unknown quantity and may vary considerably in the course of several repetitions or even in different parts of the range of movement.

However, in some circumstances it may be necessary to perform assisted active movements by:

(1) Asking the patient to join in and perform some muscle action.
(2) Initiating and completing the movement for the patient while allowing him to produce all the muscle effort he can for the easier middle range.

The grips for assisted active movement in which the patient is joining in are those for the passive movements as described earlier in this chapter.

For the second type of assisted active movement, i.e. help at the beginning and end, the same grips may be used, but for the middle range the therapist removes that half of her hand which would be the 'helping' part. Thus, the grip is maintained in the direction of the movement and sensory stimulation is only applied to the 'leading' surface.

Forced passive movements

A movement which is taken beyond the easily available range is a forced movement and there must be differentiation between over-pressure and forcing.

A forced movement to lengthen tight articular structures may be performed when the patient is anaesthetized and should only be done by a doctor who has already explored all other avenues of regaining joint range. Following this manipulative procedure the therapist may be required to maintain the required range and will have to do so in spite of the limitations of pain. The 'slow reversal hold relax' technique should be used until maximum active range has been gained and then at the limit of the present range a firm but quick extra pressure is given to regain the lost range. All the rules for giving passive movements must be obeyed in performing this technique.

Gradual stretching is another form of passive movement usually performed on either:

(1) Babies with congenital deformity when the basic rules for grasp and support are obeyed and the corrected position of the deformed part is achieved three times in succession followed by attempted active muscle work by reflex skin stimulation or
(2) Those with shortened structures due to adaptive shortening. Taking the joint to the limit and applying constant over-pressure will result in some lengthening under some circumstances and if associated with the application of appropriate serial plasters or splints.
(3) Passive stretching. Those aspiring to greater length of muscular structures to facilitate movement. These are usually athletes who require greater length of

their muscular components to give a larger range of joint movement. It is most important to stress that length without power is very dangerous and under no circumstances should stretching be performed without the essential follow-up of increase in power by exercise of those muscles which maintain and control the range of new movement.

Passive stretching in itself is not a warm-up procedure prior to intense muscular activity. It is wiser to warm up the muscles to be stretched *either* by passive means – warm water, hot wet or dry packs, massage, dry (radiant heat), *or* by small range gentle swinging exercises. The passive stretching can then be performed on the desired muscle groups *either* by the therapist *or* by the patient/athlete himself. In either case the following rules apply:

(a) First stretch the muscle with gentle force
(b) Then apply greater stretch for a shorter duration
(c) Increase the duration of the stretch before increasing the stretch

(d) Remember the anatomy so that:
  • uni-axial muscles are stretched over the one joint over which they operate;
  • bi-axial muscles are stretched over each joint in turn over which they operate before being stretched over both joints simultaneously. It is better to achieve full length over one joint and apply stretch over the second joint only at any one time (e.g. hamstrings, quadriceps).
(e) Check to ensure that if the patient is doing self stretching he is aware of the above rules and that he knows exactly how to take up and maintain a correct position to attain his own needs.

Finally do not encourage hypermobility – it sometimes produces joints prone to accidental damage (accident prone joints).

It is also important to be aware of the range of movement needed for efficient performance of the sport or activity. Some activities demand small range but greater power while others require the exact opposite. Only pentathletes need both!

Chapter 6
RESPIRATORY CARE – BASIC EXERCISES

Phyl Fletcher-Cook

In health, quiet respiration comprises two phases: the inspiratory phase which is actively brought about by inspiratory muscular effort, and the expiratory phase which is passive, occurring when the inspiratory muscles relax allowing the chest wall to return to its original dimensions and the lungs to recoil. The timing of the two phases is unequal, the inspiratory phase lasting about one third of the time for the expiratory phase.

Respiratory volumes and capacities

The respiratory volumes include the following (Marieb 1995):

- Tidal volume is the amount of air inspired and expired with each breath in quiet breathing and is about 500 ml.
- The inspiratory reserve volume is the amount of air which can be inspired above the tidal volume and is about 3100 ml.
- The expiratory reserve volume is the amount of air which can be forcefully expired after normal tidal volume and is about 1200 ml.
- The residual volume is the amount of air which remains in the lungs after a forced expiration and is about 1200 ml.

The respiratory capacities include the following (Marieb 1995):

- The total lung capacity is the amount of air in the lungs after a full inspiration and is about 6000 ml.
- Vital capacity is the maximum amount of air which can be expired after a maximal inspiration and is about 4800 ml.
- The inspiratory capacity is the amount of air which can be inspired after a normal expiration and is about 3600 ml.
- The functional residual capacity is the amount of air left in the lungs after a tidal volume expiration and is about 2400 ml.

In disease states, these volumes and capacities may be altered, e.g. the residual volume will be increased in chronic obstructive airways disease. Thus, these normal volumes and capacities must be borne in mind to assist in the assessment of patients' respiratory problems.

Breathing exercises

A range of commonly used techniques will be considered in this chapter. The techniques may be listed according to their effects as follows:

Control of breathlessness:
—breathing control
—positioning

Secretion mobilization and clearance:
—thoracic expansion exercises
—forced expiration technique
—active cycle of breathing

Decreasing the work of breathing:
—breathing control

Breathing control

In sitting, with the shoulders, arms and upper chest relaxed, the patient is encouraged to breathe at tidal volume, at his own rate and using the lower chest. On inspiration the upper abdomen and lower chest should be seen to expand and rise slightly (the active phase), and to sink down again on expiration (the passive phase) (Webber & Pryor 1993). At no point should the breathing be forced.

To guide the patient initially, the physiotherapist or patient may place one hand on the upper abdomen (Fig. 6.1) just below the xiphisternum, and should see it rise and fall with the patient's breathing pattern (Webber & Pryor 1993).

The length of time for which the technique is performed will vary depending on the patient's presentation. Those with severe breathlessness and wheeze will require longer treatment time, the aim being to promote a slower respiratory rate with an accompanying increase in tidal volume (Tucker & Jenkins 1996). Such patients may also need to adopt an alternative position such as supported forward lean (Fig. 6.2) while performing the technique (Tucker & Jenkins 1996), as this has been shown to increase diaphragmatic recruitment, relax neck and upper chest musculature and decrease dyspnoea (Breslin 1995).

Breathing control using the lower chest is a form of relaxed breathing at tidal volume (Webber 1990; Tucker & Jenkins 1996; Miller *et al*. 1995), known in the past by the inaccurate term 'diaphragmatic breathing'. Breathing control is commonly interspersed between more active techniques which tend to induce bronchospasm. As this technique is aimed at

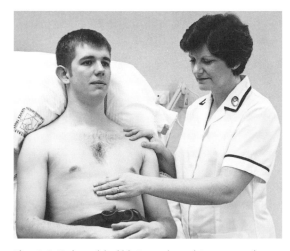

Fig. 6.1 Relaxed half lying – breathing control.

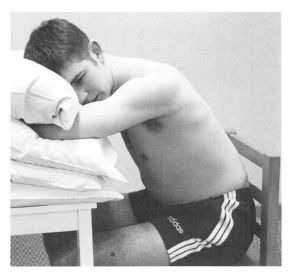

Fig. 6.2 Supported forward lean sitting – breathing control.

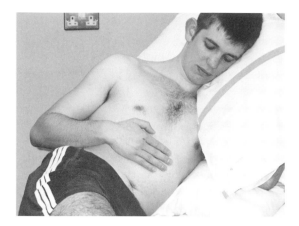

Fig. 6.3 High side lying – breathing control.

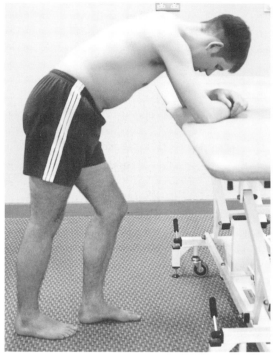

Fig. 6.5 Forward lean standing – breathing control.

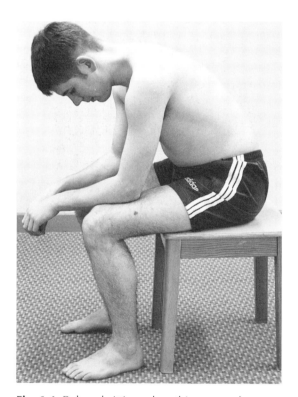

Fig. 6.4 Relaxed sitting – breathing control.

fully supported in sitting or high side lying (Fig. 6.3; Webber & Pryor 1993).

Other positions which may be adopted by patients in their self-management of breathlessness using breathing control include:

- relaxed sitting (Fig. 6.4)
- forward lean standing (Fig. 6.5)
- back lean standing (Fig. 6.6)
- side lean standing (Fig. 6.7) (Webber & Pryor 1993).

Thoracic expansion exercises (TEE)

Thoracic expansion exercises emphasise the inspiratory phase of breathing and are performed from functional residual capacity (FRC) to maximal inspiratory capacity (Tucker & Jenkins 1996).

reducing the work of breathing, and reduction of bronchospasm (Webber 1990), it is usually quietly and gently performed with the patient

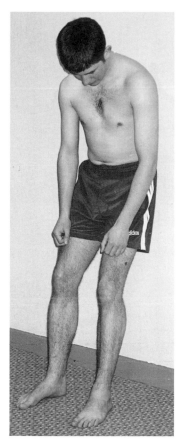

Fig. 6.6 Back lean standing – breathing control.

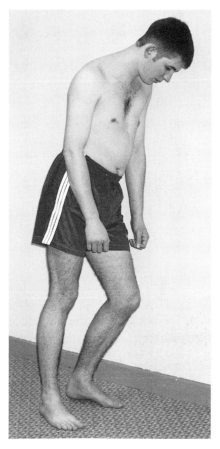

Fig. 6.7 Side lean standing – breathing control.

To perform the technique, the patient is positioned appropriate to the goal of treatment, e.g. if secretion removal and subsequent improved ventilation to a particular lung zone is the goal, then thoracic expansion exercises may be performed in the appropriate postural drainage position (Hollis 1998).

The patient is encouraged to breathe in slowly and as deeply as he can through the nose, followed by a relaxed passive expiration via the mouth. To avoid hyperventilation, this is repeated only three more times (Webber & Pryor 1993), before the patient is allowed to return to his tidal volume breathing. A three-second hold at full inspiration with the

glottis open may be added (Tucker & Jenkins 1996; Webber & Pryor 1993), or alternatively the patient may be instructed to 'sniff' more air in through the nose at the end of the inspiration.

Verbal cues should be given to the patient to encourage maximal inspiration. Tactile stimulation may also be added by the physiotherapist placing her hands over the chest wall where expansion is required (Fig. 6.8). In this position, proprioceptive stimulation may be added by the therapist delivering a quick stretch to the inspiratory muscles (Tucker & Jenkins 1996). This is achieved by quickly squeezing the chest wall between the therapist's hands at the beginning of the inspiration as though trying to produce an expiration. The inspiration is then allowed to continue to its maximum volume.

Once the patient understands what is required of him, additional resistance may be applied via the physiotherapist's hands to max-imize inspiration (Tucker & Jenkins 1996). The resistance should be stronger initially and should decrease as the inspiration progresses, to take into account the changing length–tension relationship of the inspiratory muscles.

Thoracic expansion exercises are thought to prevent atelectasis, to help re-expand collapsed alveoli and to mobilize secretions (Tucker & Jenkins 1996; Webber & Pryor 1993). The increased volume of inspired air promotes flow via collateral channels (Tucker & Jenkins 1996; Webber & Pryor 1993), and this mobilizes mucous plugs and secretions, allowing im-proved ventilation to these peripheral areas (Tucker & Jenkins 1996; Webber & Pryor 1993).

Another mechanism for increasing airflow to these areas is that of interdependence, where the increased volume of inspired air through patent airways expands alveoli which exert pulling forces on adjacent alveoli thus assisting their expansion (Tucker & Jenkins 1996; Mead *et al.* 1970; Webber & Pryor 1993).

Thoracic expansion exercises may be com-bined with other treatment techniques (Tucker & Jenkins 1996), such as postural drainage, chest shaking or vibrations, or as part of the active cycle of breathing technique (Webber 1990). They may be performed unilaterally or bilaterally.

Forced expiration technique (FET)

Forced expiration technique consists of one or two huffs from mid to low lung volume fol-lowed by a period of breathing control to reduce any bronchospasm the huffs may have

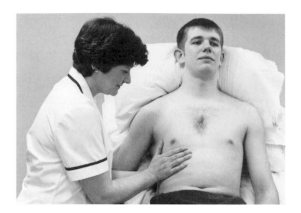

Fig. 6.8 Half lying – tactile stimulation to encourage thoracic expansion.

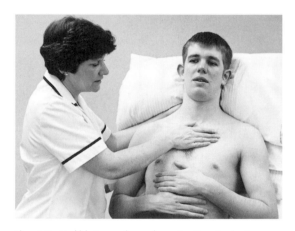

Fig. 6.9 Half lying – forced expiration technique.

engendered (Tannenbaum 1995; Hardy 1994; ACPRC 1996; Webber & Pryor 1993; Webber 1990).

The technique may be performed in postural drainage positions but is commonly performed in sitting or high side lying (Fig. 6.9). The patient is instructed to take a medium sized breath in, followed by a lightly forced expira-tion through an open mouth and glottis (Webber & Pryor 1993). The huff should not be sharply forced or too prolonged as coughing may result. It is usual to perform one or two huffs followed by a period of breathing control to avoid inducement of bronchospasm. The cycle of huffs and breathing control may be repeated until secretions reach the proximal airways when a cough or short huff from high lung volume may remove them (Webber & Pryor 1993).

Forced expiratory technique may also be used as part of the active cycle of breathing technique. In patients with marked instability of the airways, forced expiratory technique is more effective than a cough at removing peripheral secretions, as coughing tends to completely close airways above the equal pressure point (see next section) and therefore obstructs airflow (Hardy 1994).

The purpose of the technique is to mobilize secretions from the more peripheral airways towards the proximal airways in order that they be removed either by a huff from high lung volume or by a cough. The physiological basis of the technique centres around the equal pressure point (EPP) in airways where the pressure within the airway is equal to intrapleural pressure (Tannenbaum 1995; Schoni 1989). Downstream (towards the mouth) of the equal pressure point, the airways are dynamically squeezed and secretions are moved proximally (Tannenbaum 1995; Webber & Pryor 1993). At successively lower lung volumes, the equal pressure point moves more peripherally, mobilizing secretions at lobar and segmental bronchi (Webber & Pryor 1993).

The active cycle of breathing technique (ACBT)

The active cycle of breathing technique is performed to aid clearance of bronchial secretions (Webber & Pryor 1993). It combines thoracic expansion exercises, breathing control and forced expiratory technique in a treatment approach which is flexible to the patient's needs.

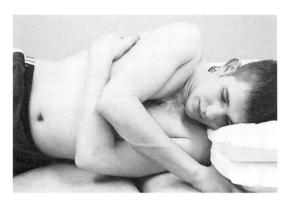

Fig. 6.10 Side lying – self treatment thoracic expansion as part of the active cycle of breathing technique.

A typical active cycle of breathing technique starts with a period of breathing control, the length of which will vary according to the patient's signs of bronchospasm (ACPRC 1996) but may be in the region of one minute or so (Tannenbaum 1995). This is followed by three or four thoracic expansion exercises to mobilize secretions in the smaller bronchi. Forced expiration technique from mid to low lung volume may then move the secretions proximally, and this may stimulate a cough, or alternatively, a huff from high lung volume may remove the secretions. It is vital that breathing control follows immediately after the forced expiratory technique as this helps to reduce induced bronchospasm and minimize patient fatigue (Tannenbaum 1995; Hardy 1994).

It is recommended that the technique be performed in the sitting position if secretions are minimal or it can be combined with postural drainage positions, e.g. alternate side lying (Fig. 6.10) (Tannenbaum 1995). It may also be necessary in those patients with significant bronchospasm to follow the thoracic expansion exercises with a period of breathing control prior to performing forced expiration technique (Webber & Pryor 1993). In cases where mobilization of secretions is slower, two periods of thoracic expansion exercises in the cycle, interspersed with breathing control, may be necessary (Webber & Pryor 1993).

The cycle of techniques is repeated until the huff is unproductive and sounds dry, or earlier than this if the patient becomes fatigued (Webber & Pryor 1993; Hardy 1994). The total treatment time will usually be between 15 and 30 minutes (ACPRC 1996).

Once the patient is conversant with the active cycle of breathing techniques, he can be encouraged to use it as a self-treatment regime (Webber & Pryor 1993), until it becomes habitual and can be used in periods of exacerbation.

References

ACPRC (1996) Clinical Practice Guidelines – Physiotherapy Management of the Spontaneously Breathing, Acutely Breathless Adult Patient – a Problem Solving Approach. Association of Chartered Physiotherapists in Respiratory Care, London.

Breslin, E.H. (1995) Breathing retraining in chronic obstructive pulmonary disease. *Cardiopulmonary Rehabilitation*, **15**, 25–33.

Hardy, K.A. (1994) A review of airway clearance – new techniques, indications and recommendations. *Respiratory Care*, **39**(5), 440–55.

Hollis, M. (1998) *Massage for Therapists*. Blackwell Science, Oxford.

Marieb, E.N. (1995) *Human Anatomy and Physiology*, Ch. 23, 761–2. Benjamin Cummings, Redwood City, California.

Mead, J., Takishima, T. & Leith, D. (1970) Stress distribution in lungs: a model of pulmonary elasticity. *Journal of Applied Physiology*, **28**, 596–608.

Miller, S., Hall, D.O., Clayton, C.B., & Nelson, R. (1995) Chest Physiotherapy in Cystic Fibrosis: A Comparative Study of Autogenic Drainage and the Active Cycle of Breathing Techniques with Postural Drainage. *Thorax*, **50**, 165–9.

Schoni, M.H. (1989) Autogenic drainage: a modern approach to physiotherapy in cystic fibrosis. *Journal of the Royal Society of Medicine*, **82**(16), 32–7.

Tannenbaum, E.L. (1995) Cystic fibrosis – approaches to management. *S.A. Journal Physiotherapy*, **51**(2), 27–9.

Tucker, B. & Jenkins, S. (1996) The effect of breathing exercises with body positioning on regional lung ventilation. *Aust. Journal of Physiotherapy*, **42**(3), 219–27.

Webber, B.A. (1990) The active cycle of breathing techniques. *Cystic Fibrosis News*, Aug/Sept, 10–11.

Webber, B.A. & Pryor, J.A. (1993) *Physiotherapy for Respiratory and Cardiac Problems*. Churchill Livingstone, London.

Chapter 7
APPARATUS: SMALL, SOFT AND LARGE

M. Hollis & B. Sanford

Small apparatus

Small apparatus may be used in as infinite a variety of ways as exist and may be contained within a Physiotherapy Department. Basically three things may be done with any piece of small apparatus. One can 'get rid' of it, 'receive' it or 'hang on' to it. It is the permutations of these three factors with weight and size and material, their relationship to other people or objects, obstructions, distance and direction, that produces the variety of exercise.

Each piece of apparatus will also have two main uses. It may be used as an object to achieve a particular purpose, e.g. threading a needle with cotton, or it may be used for its innate properties. For example, most small pieces of apparatus may be pushed about and therefore may be a load and a means of obtaining the patient's interest to move an object from place to place. According to their innate properties, some pieces of apparatus may be very resistant to being moved, while others may be moved very easily.

In the former case the movement of a heavy weight across a rough surface would form a resistance exercise, while rolling a ball across a smooth surface would give a speedy and there-fore a mobilizing movement. Both would be a means of maintaining the patient's interest.

The properties of any piece of apparatus may also present disadvantages. Any apparatus of compressible material may be squeezed, but it must be the right size for the part which holds it, and if it is inelastic and therefore incapable of returning to its original shape after the squeeze, then further work will be involved in re-arranging the apparatus. A piece of foam rubber if squeezed and released, compresses with the force, stores energy and returns to its original shape; a beanbag or sand inside a bag may be squeezed or pushed into a different shape, but no energy will be stored in this activity and the beans or sand will remain where they have been placed.

A ball may be bounced and will return if aimed properly but is of no use if the patient cannot change balance to catch it. Similarly a rubber quoit may be squeezed and thrown but unlike a ball will not return. A piece of material such as a band or pillowcase can be squeezed with little likelihood of it rolling or sliding away.

Some of the properties of some common pieces of small apparatus are discussed in the following pages.

Whenever small apparatus is used it should have been experimented with by the therapist so that she is aware of the values and limitations which that object may have. Some apparatus is more useful for team games or where two patients are working together.

Experiments will also reveal that the method of use of each piece of apparatus will give a movement line or direction and weight. The weighting of the movement is dependent upon the energy which the patient imparts to the activity he is trying to achieve. All movements are 'loaded' by the quality of the activity and in order to achieve greater or lesser loading by the patient he must be directed exactly as to the manner in which he should use the piece of apparatus. It is not necessary to use a heavy load, e.g. a 5 kg weight, to obtain strong extensor muscle work for the back muscles. Hard bouncing of a light ball against a wall through a long distance, especially a double-handed overhead throw, will work the back extensors very hard in inner range to prepare for the throw and in middle and inner range to catch a high returning ball.

In the same way the line or direction of a movement must be taught to the patient so that he moves the required joints. Whilst the therapist is placing her hands on the moving parts, direction and therefore line will be indicated, but free, objective and interesting movement may not achieve such perfection of line.

Initially perfection of line does not matter. The patient will achieve his objective the best way he can, constructive teaching and encouragement will improve the direction of the movement, and adjustment of the starting position and method of performance will eventually improve the line and method of work.

Careful consideration has to be given at all times to the use of basic principles. The starting position should be selected to limit the movement to a particular part if the object is mainly to strengthen muscles locally or to limit movement to a small number of joints, but if strength and range are to be improved by corporate work of the whole body then a less limiting starting position should be chosen. Much will also depend on other factors and it is important to know if the patient is capable of static balance, and has good dynamic balance, good vision, cutaneous perception and co-ordination.

Safety of the patient using the apparatus and of other patients around should be considered. The load, whether in the form of weights or weighted balls, should be within the patient's capacity. If he fetches equipment himself he will be revealed to be capable of doing this much with it. He should have the minimum equipment near him and apparatus should be moved to a safe place or put away in its storage place after use so that it does not constitute a hazard to other people in the vicinity.

The safety of the use of apparatus is dependent on the correct selection of a suitable piece of equipment for the task in hand. Injured elbows should not be treated by the use of weights or heavy balls; elderly people and small children need yielding pieces of apparatus so that if they miss a catch and are struck no damage is done. More agile patients can work with small, rapidly moving pieces of equipment to which great energy may be imparted.

Finally, it should be observed by personal practice that by using apparatus it is not necessary to direct the patient's efforts all the time to the affected part of the body. Running bouncing a ball is as much an exercise for a weak or stiff foot, knee, hip, back, shoulder, elbow and hand as it is for poise, balance and co-ordination.

Balls

Balls may be used to exercise every part of the body by objective activity, and the infinite variety of their size, weight and materials gives added value to their use.

One of the most important points to be considered before choosing to use a ball for any activity is the ability of the patient to retrieve it. The nature of a ball which is 'lost' by the patient is to continue its motion in the direction of the force last imparted to it and to continue until the energy is consumed or it meets an obstacle. A static patient who needs objective exercise should be given a non-rolling or less mobile object which he can retrieve if he misses or drops it.

If these properties are considered and related to the three principles described above and to the three basic uses of apparatus ('hang on' to it, 'get rid' of it or 'receive' it) then some uses will emerge.

Balls may be solid such as a small ball bearing or marble used for fine intrinsic movements of the fingers, semi-solid such as a medicine ball made of a leather case and packing to a specific weight, or semi-solid but aerated in varying materials from sorbo rubber, the common ball of our youth, or from man-made materials varying in density and aeration from the Supa ball, which is small and needs little energy imparted to it to create bounce, to the polyurethane foam balls which are compressible round soft 'shapes'.

Aeration may be total, i.e. the ball is a case around a permanent supply of air, and the degree of bounce will depend on the air pressure inside the case. These balls need constant attention to their pressure and the larger balls may need to have air pumped into them regularly to make them harder and better bouncers. In time the casing will deteriorate with use and the ball will then need replacement as a bouncer but may still be used for its compressibility.

The size of ball matters in relation to the capacity of the patient as well as to the part to be exercised. Large and brightly coloured balls are best used for the very young and more elderly as the eye and body co-ordination demanded are least with such balls and at their maximum with small, 'fast', balls. (Some balls of artificial material have higher elastic properties and produce 'fast' response to a small force, e.g. Supa balls.)

The part of the body to catch, hold or retrieve the ball will also control the size of ball to be chosen. A hand with small span, i.e. which cannot be opened into full extension, needs a small ball, as a big ball demands full extension of the hand joints if it is to be held or caught. Fine foot movements can be performed using a small ball, but most people need a bigger ball for coarse foot movements or leg movements. On the whole a large ball is easier to control, but may require fuller range movements if it is to be held.

The distance through which a ball is thrown will alter both the joints moved and the muscles worked. Try the following experiment:

Take a small hand-held sorbo rubber ball. Stand near to a wall on to which it can be thrown and have a clear space behind you. Start throwing the ball overarm and one handed at the wall and walk backwards a half pace between each throw. Get a colleague to observe your movements and think about your own muscle work. Near to the wall the head and neck must be extended as well as having the arm elevated and elbow extended to perform the throw. As the distance from the wall increases the head and neck movement is lost and the whole arm is flexed and extended, then the upper trunk is rotated and finally the legs are flexed and extended to impart thrust to the ball.

Repeat the same activities with an underarm throw and then with a double-handed throw, both under- and overarm, and observe which position produces most movement and therefore most muscle work for each part of the body. Some of the positions and types of throw are obviously more mobilizing, i.e., they carry the body component past a potentially blocked point in the range. In the case of other positions and types of throw the effect is more one of strengthening for various muscle groups, i.e., the amount of effort imparted to the ball is greater and therefore the muscles work harder.

Now continue to explore the uses of the different sizes, weights and types of balls, using ball and floor, ball and wall, ball and air space, ball and body relationships in, say, standing, sitting and lying, using the ball with the upper limb(s) for finger and thumb, hand, wrist, radio-ulnar, elbow and shoulder movements; with the lower limb(s) for toe, foot, ankle, knee and hip movements. Consider which, if any, of these involve the trunk and/or head to enhance the movement, increase the muscle effort or ensure co-ordination.

Do not forget that a ball can be kicked, kneed, hipped, shouldered or headed if it is suitable and the action appropriate to the needs of the patient. Also discover that space may control selection of the ball size and weight. To throw a light ball in such a way that movement of the lower thoracic or lumbar spine is produced needs a long space. The same effect will be produced in less than half the space if a 1 kg medicine ball is substituted with no very great increase in effort for the trunk muscles, but considerably more effort for the arm muscles.

The way in which a ball is held in the hand will also produce variations in joints used and muscles worked. The type of grip must be adapted to the size and weight of the ball and so must the manner in which the ball is to be thrown or received, e.g. overarm, underarm, single handed or double handed.

Quoits

Quoits are rings of about 20 cm (8 in) diameter made of either sorbo rubber or rope. If the former they have the property of elasticity, if the latter they will be semi-rigid.

Only the sorbo rubber quoit can be turned inside out involving movement of all the upper limb joints and work of muscles against resistance, but both types offer other similar features. They form a ring round a space and so can be used for all threading activities, whether it be transfer from foot to foot, passing a stick or hand through them or 'aiming' to thread or throw them over a skittle or hand-held pole.

Quoits are a circle of material and can be gripped by foot or hand by one person or by two people and so used for pushing, pulling and twisting exercises, done in standing, sitting or long sitting.

A quoit is also a suitable object to be rolled or thrown, although the rope quoits will roll less well than the rubber quoits and both types are objects which may be pushed over higher structures such as the top of the wall bars, or thrown to a partner over a beam or high rope. A quoit may also be tied on the end of a rope as a weight so that it can be whipped in a circle and jumped over in leg exercises, thus increasing timing ability in eye and leg co-ordination.

A quoit is sometimes substituted for a ball in games such as deck tennis when the space is confined. It is of value in such games because it rolls less if the receiver fails to catch it and therefore requires movement through only short distances in order to retrieve it.

Hoops

Hoops may be made of bamboo or other wood and may be somewhat uneven and brittle, or of plastic and therefore even, but compressible. They are of varying sizes and may be of small enough diameter to be used to pass the body through in 'mock dressing', or of large enough diameter to run through as the hoop bowls along.

Spinning a hoop (hula-hoop) may be done with the whole body or any part of the upper or lower limb and in so doing, very complex movements will be performed in a co-ordinated manner. Alternatively a hoop can be rotated between hand and the ground or a wall, so producing finely co-ordinated finger and thumb movements with the arm in many different relationships to the trunk while dynamic balance is maintained.

A hoop may be used as a fixed outline enclosing a space, enabling many jumping, stepping, bouncing games to be devised, or the outline may be used for co-ordinated leg movements by stepping round the margin of the hoop.

Suspended hoops can form part of an obstacle course and can be held by a partner as a stepping or jumping obstacle.

Ropes

Many activities with a rope involve the use of the hands and arms. Ropes can be of a length of about 2 m for individual use or of any longer length to allow group participation. They should preferably be made of hemp and can vary in diameter from approximately 1.5 cm to many centimetres, when weight will become a feature to be considered. On the whole, lighter weight ropes are usually used for individual work but a heavier texture is more useful and 'whips' and deviates less than the light rope and thus is more useful for group work. Ropes for individual use are more useful if the ends are bound and sealed, and not fixed to handles.

The most obvious use of a rope is for various forms of skipping and jumping exercises performed either slowly or quickly, thus involving arm and leg movement and great co-ordination. But a rope can be used for intrinsic work with the hands, when one or both is inco-ordinate. It may be tied into a malleable circle and used as though dressing and it can be laid on the ground and stepped along in a straight or wriggling path.

The whole length of the rope can be crumpled by hand or feet and if bound together it becomes a non-bouncing object which may be used for target work. With a quoit tied to one end and the therapist or a patient holding the other end the rope may be swung round in circles while the remaining patients forming a ring, jump over it as it passes. If a patient is swinging the rope he can sit or stand according to his ability. He might even be a patient with a disablement of the shoulder or arm and so work with patients who need primarily leg exercises.

A rope may also be used to create shapes on the floor and to be an obstacle to be jumped over, climbed up or pulled as in a tug-of-war.

Bands

Bands are soft webbing or braid in a variety of colours and of a length of approximately 75–100 cm, sewn at the ends to make a circular band. Like a rope their uses are multiple.

First, as they are flat and of moderately rough material they have a high co-efficient of friction and will therefore stay where they are dropped, put down or tucked in. They can, in consequence, be used as markers of all sorts, either as a tail in chasing games, a marker on a rope for tug-of-war, or for distance jumped or hopped over.

The material is just springy enough to be a challenge in pulling the whole length of the band into the hand or under the foot by lumbrical action or by digital flexion, whichever is desired. Since the bands are soft and tend to cling they can be used for dressing and undressing practice before a patient is ready to tackle putting on or taking off actual clothing.

A series of bands looped into one another will make an emergency rope of some length and they can be looped round hoops or quoits as a means of hanging these objects up. A series of experiments on the lines suggested for balls will reveal that they can be used in similar manner but as non-returning objects, and their use need not be limited to marking the members of the red and blue teams.

Beanbags

A beanbag is usually made of cotton twill squares so that a flat bag approximately 20–30 cm square is produced containing enough dried beans to half fill the bag. It should be double stitched at all seams.

This produces a small object of variable shape and with no elastic properties. If thrown it must land and be fetched or be caught and returned. It can thus be used for aiming or target exercises with or without a partner. Without a partner the target can be a bucket, bowl, hoop, rope or band circle and the patient will need quite a pile of beanbags to keep him busy. Additional exercise is provided by the initial positioning of the stock of beanbags. Thus a sitting patient may have to pick up his beanbag from his right with his right hand and so side flex, and/or flex and/or extend according to where on his right the beanbags are

placed. Alternatively, they may be put on his left and he must then rotate and flex or extend and perhaps also extend his left arm for propping purposes. The object of the exercise might then well be to use the left arm for this purpose and recover balance after the target practice.

Many finger and hand exercises can be performed with beanbags as they may be used above or on a table. Each bean may be manipulated across the bag and stereognostic ability increased, or the bag may be flicked with flexion, extension, ulnar or radial deviation of the wrist or with any of the movements of the fingers and thumb. The smaller bags are especially useful for flicking exercises where rapid digital extension must be performed.

As they are a handsized object to grip they can simulate a duster, wash leather or dishcloth for domestic tasks and so be a means of performing unloaded arm, leg and trunk movements in full range and in a functional way.

Poles

Wooden rods of varying lengths and diameters and thus of varying weights provide a means of devising a challenging variety of exercises.

A thin pole such as a broomstick handle is approximately 1250 cm long and 2 cm in diameter, whereas a pole which is the same diameter as a tennis ball, i.e. functional grip size, may be 10–15 cm in diameter and would be very heavy if it were 1250 cm long. However, such a pole would still have its uses in heavy resistance exercise and for those without fine grip.

Most exercises using poles involve the hand and arm directly as grip is usually needed. Exceptions are paired exercises in which a thicker pole is placed on the floor between two people each in crook sitting with their heels on the floor on the far side of the pole from themselves. They try to pull the pole with their heels, thus flexing the hips and knees and working the hamstrings hard. Or the pole may be used as a 'raise' over which to exercise the foot lumbricals or may be rolled (underfoot) in sitting, moving the foot through dorsi- and plantar-flexion and the knee in middle range.

The trunk muscles and leg muscles are mainly exercised by again either using pairs of people to twist, pull up and down or side to side on a suitable pole, or by passing people in a circle round a series of standing poles in a ring – the idea being speedy leg, trunk and arm movement to catch each pole while it is still vertical.

Solo exercises might involve pronation and supination using a grip at the middle of the pole and the long weight arm on each side as the load. Rolling out pastry across a table or rolling a pole up the wall are progressively harder arm exercises, or again the pole may be an object to be jumped over, walked round or stepped over. Its advantage in these cases is its mobility in one

plane by rolling, but this can also be a disadvantage; i.e., if the patient lands on the pole it will roll under his foot and he will initially need the therapist on hand as a 'catcher' until his balance is sound.

Ball pools

A ball pool is a free standing container for small balls (Fig. 7.1). The container walls are of semi-rigid foam covered in plastic. The walls are sectional to form either a square or a multi-sided container. The floor is not usually padded. One side may have a small cut-out section to facilitate entry and exit, and a foam step may be needed to assist access. The walls should maintain their integrity when leaned on by an average adult and sometimes are wide enough for a child to sit on. The balls, bright and multi-coloured, used for filling are themselves air

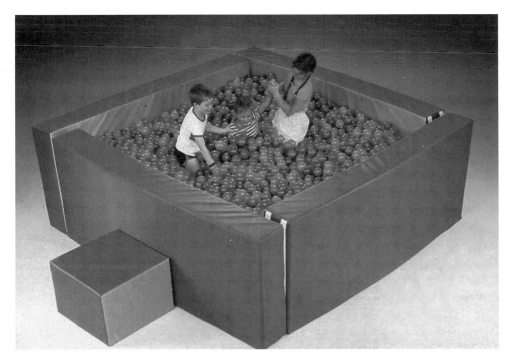

Fig. 7.1 A ball pool.

filled and slightly larger than a tennis ball, having a diameter between 50 mm and 70 mm. They usually fill the container to four-fifths of its capacity but when small children are to use the pool some of the balls should be removed to allow the child to be able to stand on the base and have his head visible. The surplus balls may be used in a non-rigid bag container with which very small children may be happier.

The balls offer a mobile support so that the feeling is of floating, and surface movements may be made over them. In other words they are buoyant in a similar way to water. The resistance they offer to downward movements into their depths is also similar to that offered by water, but the advantages are that the patient does not get wet and that sinking into the pool allows unimpeded breathing. The balls offer the same problem as water, however, in that turning over is difficult due to lack of a fixed point.

The greatest value of a ball pool is in the treatment of children, who can have great fun and enjoyment as they are released from the effects of gravity, and discover hitherto un-known movements and a greater facility of muscular activity. Any movement on the part of the child causes response in displacement of the balls. The resistance offered to movement is very slight, and children seem to explore new movements constantly when left to 'play' rather than practise repetitive actions.

A ball pool may be used as a play facility to encourage an otherwise 'frozen' and immobile physically or mentally handicapped child to move, as it gives tactile feedback and visual stimulation. It can be used as an introduc-tion to therapeutic measures, especially to the hydrotherapy pool as the child can learn to float, to blow into the depths of the balls and to turn upside down and touch the bottom without the hazard that water may present and the fear that may then be induced.

The therapist should introduce the child to the ball pool slowly and carefully and remain close at hand until the child gains confidence.

Soft apparatus

The development of foam with plastic covering and plastic inflatables has given some thera-peutic exercise areas a whole new concept of equipment. Soft apparatus presents no injury hazard to patients. Colour, shapes and sizes allow imaginative use by patient and/or the therapist. The most commonly used shapes in a therapeutic environment are balls, rolls and wedges.

Soft balls

Soft therapy balls are available in many sizes, from the smallest which are about the size of a tennis ball to the largest which have a diameter of 120 cm when fully inflated. In sizes up to a diameter of about 56 cm they are made in two different materials – soft foam or inflatable plastic. Balls larger than 56 cm are only avail-able with a single or double inflatable plastic skin, the size, pliability and rebound capacity of which can be controlled by the amount of air injected into them. The soft foam filling is of varying densities each of which produces a dif-ferent rebound capacity. In this material the 56 cm ball has a rigid core to prevent sagging when it is supporting heavy weights. All the balls are brightly coloured. Because of their texture, pressure is minimized on the areas of body contact.

All soft therapy balls can be bounced, thrown, pushed, kicked, held, squeezed or handed from one person to another in a variety of ways using either one or both upper or lower limbs. They can also be used as a moveable target to be aimed at (see the section on small apparatus at the beginning of this chapter). Larger balls are particularly useful for patients whose problem is spasticity of the upper limbs as they may be used in a variety of ways to facilitate normal movement. Visually handicapped people work with greater confidence when using larger balls. When patients roll larger balls ahead of them these provide minimal aid to walking for those in the later stages of walking re-education.

Larger balls can be used to provide a firm, comfortable support for the whole body when the patient lies over them (Fig. 7.2), whilst the more advanced patients may be able to sit astride them with or without the feet touching the floor as the occasion demands. From both these positions active or passive movements can be performed, e.g. head and upper trunk extension whilst lying over the ball, or arm, shoulder joint and shoulder girdle movements whilst sitting astride the ball.

Balance, co-ordination and body awareness may also be re-educated using the larger balls as a support. The therapist may rock the balls in various directions as the patient tries to maintain his position, or movement of the ball may be initiated by the patient himself making slight shifts in body weight. More advanced patients who are younger may enjoy trying to jump along the floor whilst maintaining their balance sitting astride the ball, but the therapist must ensure that the feet can comfortably reach the floor in case the patient loses his balance.

Rolls

Rolls can be supplied in a variety of materials, lengths and diameters or can be made to individual specifications by some firms. Some are made of rigid foam with brightly coloured washable plastic covers (Fig. 7.3) and may have a hanging cord for easy storage. The larger sizes have a rigid core to prevent 'bottoming out'.

Rolls are also supplied made of strong, clear, inflatable plastic. All rolls provide a soft stable base from which to exercise and are particularly useful for patients who find the less stable balls frightening. Patients can lie across them or sit astride them, both these positions being useful for controlling spasticity in the areas which are supported. The therapist or the patient can

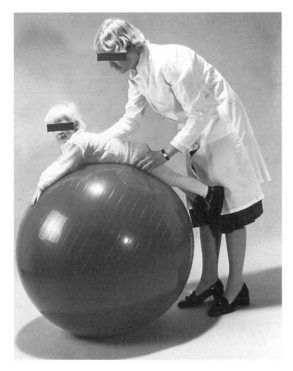

Fig. 7.2 A large soft inflatable being used for lying over.

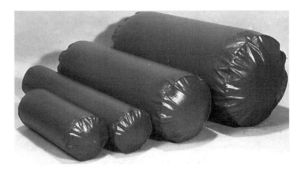

Fig. 7.3 A series of soft rolls.

initiate rocking movements, thus helping to re-educate balance, co-ordination and body awareness as the roll moves backwards and forwards. Patients can also use their legs and feet to propel themselves forward or backward along the roll as they sit astride it.

Wedges

Wedges are made in many sizes and with different elevations. They are made of rigid foam with a brightly coloured washable plastic cover and may be joined together with Velcro straps at the sides to make a continuous incline. Some manufacturers will make them to individual specifications.

Smaller wedges may be a true right angle triangle in cross section, but larger wedges need depth at both the front and back where the lesser depth accommodates the knees and allows some knee flexion (Fig. 7.4A). Some wedges have a vertical maximum height so that the patient can prop himself over the edge. Other wedges rise to a peak in the middle and have a large area of support so that the patient can recline across the peak with full support for the whole body (Fig. 7.4B), or when the wedge is small but tall at its peak the patient may sit astride it (Fig. 7.4C).

Wedges are useful in the re-education of walking. The plantar flexors and dorsi-flexors of the ankle may be strengthened by walking either up or down the incline, and the pliability of the foam promotes interplay between the invertors and evertors of the foot. These muscle groups can be strengthened by walking side-

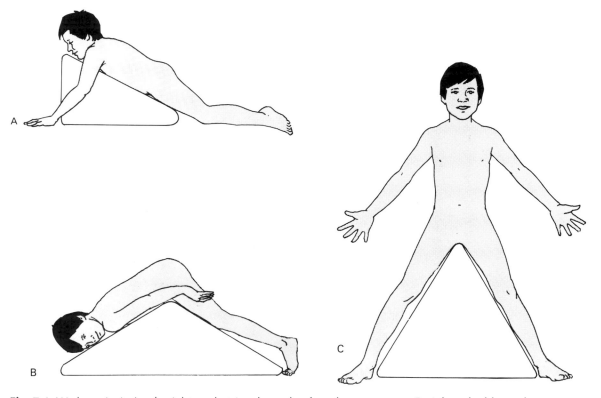

Fig. 7.4 Wedges. A, A simple right angle triangle wedge for a longer person; B, A low double wedge; C, A high double wedge.

ways along the wedges. Wedges also provide a soft surface for the stimulation of proprioception in the soles of the feet.

Wedges and rolls can be used in the same treatment area to provide a continuous uneven surface along which patients may crawl or walk, so providing a means of balance training in preparation for the uneven surfaces experienced in everyday life.

Soft therapy equipment for resistance

By using equipment which offers varying degrees of resistance, soft apparatus may be used to give an infinite variety of exercises gradually varying the resistance offered.

Figure 7.5 shows dumb-bells, handweights, a skipping rope, chest expander, tension bar, push up bars and power grips in various soft touch to semi-rigid materials.

All foam used in the manufacture of soft

therapy equipment is produced to the standard required by the fire safety regulations.

Silicone putty

Some modern materials such as silicone putty have the property of plasticity in that they can be deformed by pressure and will offer considerable resistance to the deforming force.

The major use for silicone putty is in hand exercises for regaining muscle strength, joint mobility and dexterity (Fig. 7.6).

The putty should be stored in a container between usages.

Large apparatus

Large apparatus can be space-consuming and good organization is necessary for its use. Patients who are moving it should constantly be

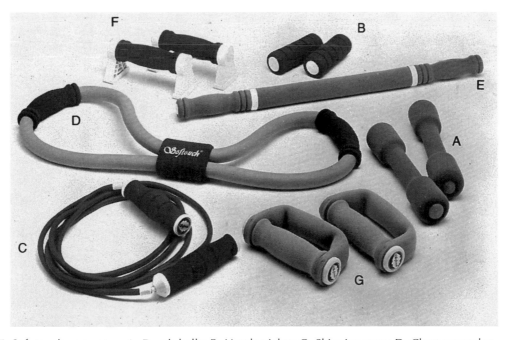

Fig. 7.5 Soft touch apparatus. A, Dumb-bells; B, Handweights; C, Skipping rope; D, Chest expander; E, Tension bar; F, Push-up bars; G, Power grips.

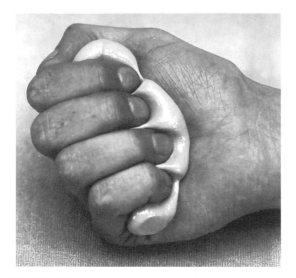

Fig. 7.6 Silicone putty being used for resistance to the hand muscles.

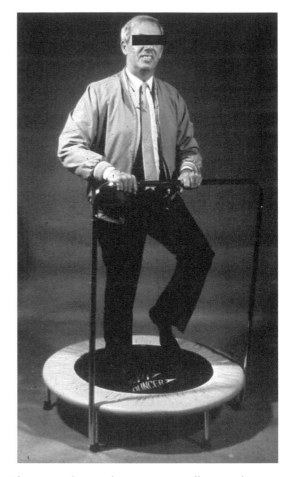

Fig. 7.7 A therapy bouncer or small trampoline. The handle is removeable.

aware of its potential danger to others in the room, e.g. when lowering a beam, although the patient's body will face the controlling rope, the face should be turned to look at the centre of the room ready to react to prevent other patients being hit on the head.

Wallbars

Wallbars may be fixed permanently to the wall or on hinges which allow them to be turned at an angle to the wall. In this position both sides can be used and they provide a climbing frame for suitable groups. Other uses are:

(1)   As a support for a patient's back
(2)   As a hand support to aid balance or to gain height in upward jumps
(3)   As a target for progressive upward stepping and jumping or for tying and aiming objects and for touching
(4)   For progressing height in landing training
(5)   For heaving and grasping exercises

(6)   As a support for other apparatus
(7)   As an attachment for pulley systems and springs.

Forms

Forms can be used with either the broad or narrow side uppermost. Patients should avoid stepping on the upturned feet as this will cause the form to tip sideways and throw them off. Forms have many different uses.

(1)   For retraining balance especially in weight-bearing positions

(2)   As a target for jumping over

(3)   As a platform for stepping and jumping on to and off

(4)   To stimulate a step or an incline

(5)   As a low seat

(6)   As an object for lifting (always use two people)

(7)   As a low target for aiming at or over

(8)   As an area divider.

Bouncers

It is important to distinguish between trampolines and bouncers. Trampolines can propel people to dangerous heights and are intended for use by the skilled gymnast. Bouncers have a more limited rebound capacity, are simple to use, fun for all age groups and small enough to be stored easily in the smallest gymnasium or even in the home. Patients may safely walk (Fig. 7.7), jog, run or jump on them and the more athletic may skip, or bounce and throw balls as they are exercising. Patients should be trained in the use of bouncers by the therapist and should not be allowed to work unsupervised until she is satisfied that they can use them safely.

Bouncers are particularly useful for re-educating the muscles controlling the knee and ankle joints. These muscles can be strengthened safely without the fear of joint trauma from landing on a hard supporting surface. Bouncing also helps in retraining balance, rhythm, speed, agility, proprioception and neuromuscular co-ordination. By gradually increasing the time spent exercising on the bouncer, the cardiovascular and respiratory capacities can be kept at an increased level for longer periods of time, improving cardiorespiratory endurance.

In the early stages of rehabilitation the therapist can help in initiating the bounce by standing astride the bouncer and giving an assistive upward thrust to the patient's forearms using a grasp immediately below his elbows. For those who need extra help with balance and stability, e.g. the elderly or children, rails for grasping can be attached (Fig. 7.7).

Chapter 8
SUSPENSION

M. Hollis

Suspension is the means whereby parts of the body are supported in slings and elevated by the use of variable length ropes fixed to a point above the body. Suspension frees the body from the friction of the material upon which body components may be resting and it permits free movement without resistance when the fixation is suitably arranged relative to the supported part.

All that is needed for suspension to be effected is a fixed point (hook) above the relevant part of the body and a suspensory unit which consists of a sling and an adjustable rope (Fig. 8.1).

The fixed point

It is common practice to fit stainless steel or plastic covered 5 cm metal mesh around the area of a plinth, i.e. 1 m or 2 m wide × 2 m long above it, perhaps 2 m × 2 m on the wall at the side of the plinth, and at the head of the plinth 1 m or 2 m × 2 m long and 2 m high (Fig. 8.2).

It is usual to suspend the overhead mesh from the ceiling joists at a height which will allow about 1.5 m clearance between mesh and plinth top. If it is impossible to fix mesh on to the ceiling because of the nature of the ceiling structure then a free-standing frame may be used (Fig. 8.3). This is a frame big enough to take a single bed, i.e. 2 m long × 1 m wide at the base and a somewhat narrower top frame which is serrated on the upper surface of both the frame and linking bars. Hooks on the side of the frame allow lateral fixed points and can be used to keep the small apparatus near at hand.

Storage
Storage of slings and ropes can otherwise be on a wall frame of suitable hooks or on a mobile trolley as in Fig. 8.4. Hooks that have a large and small curve are used (Fig. 8.5).

The supporting ropes

Ropes should be of 3-ply hemp so that they will not slip, and they can be of three arrangements: a single rope, a pulley rope or a double rope.

Single rope
A single rope has a ring fixed at one end, by which it is hung up. The other end of the rope passes through one end of a wooden cleat, through the ring of a dog clip and through the other end of the cleat (Fig. 8.1) and is then knotted with a half-hitch. The cleat is for altering the length of the rope and should be held horizontally for movement and pulled oblique when supporting (Fig. 8.6). The rope then 'holds' on the cleat by frictional resistance. The dog clip should be on a pivot to allow

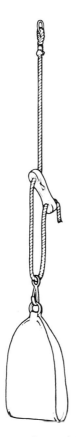

Fig. 8.1 A suspensory unit consisting of a rope and a sling.

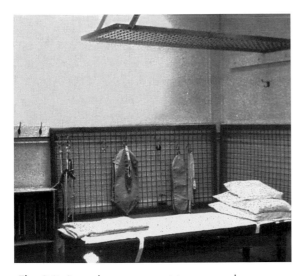

Fig. 8.2 A mesh arrangement to cover a large area and allow many variations in 'fixed points'.

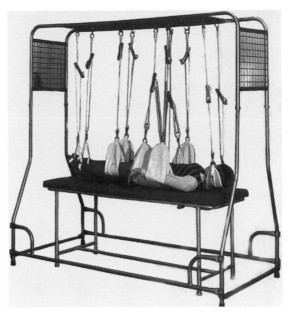

Fig. 8.3 A free-standing frame designed by the late Mrs Guthrie Smith MBE. The suspension is vertical for all body parts.

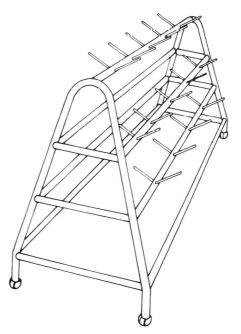

Fig. 8.4 One aspect only of an original design of a trolley to accommodate all the suspension equipment, pulleys, springs and handles needed for a large hospital. The trolley is shown minus equipment for clarity. Both sides have hooks for equipment and the hooks are arranged to allow the equipment to hang inside the castors and base frame.

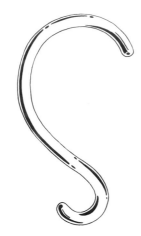

Fig. 8.5 An 'S' hook which may be used either end according to the size of the fixed points.

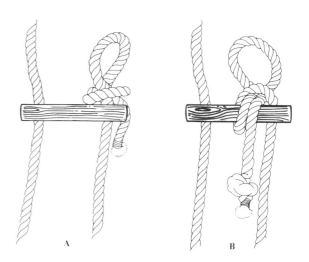

Fig. 8.7 Two alternative methods (A and B) of shortening a rope with the free end held in such a manner that a tug on it enables quick release.

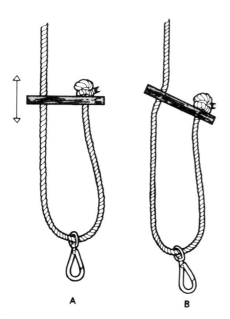

Fig. 8.6 A, The cleat in the horizontal position for changing the length of the rope; B, The cleat in the oblique position in which frictional resistance causes it to 'hold' its own position.

adjustments in position with minimum discomfort when the slings are attached. The total length of rope required is 1.5 m.

Further shortening of the rope may be brought about by knotting it about the cleat, as in Fig. 8.7, so that the supporting end is firm but the free end can be pulled out with no permanent knots made.

Pulley rope

A pulley rope has a dog clip attached to one end of the rope which then passes over the wheel of a pulley. The rope then passes through the cleat and a second dog clip as described above (Fig. 8.8). Like the single rope this rope is 1.5 m long. This arrangement is used for reciprocal pulley circuits; with one sling supporting a limb, and the ends of the sling attached to the two dog clips, it is used for three-dimensional movements of a limb, i.e. abduction or adduction with flexion or extension and medial or lateral rotation (combined, oblique, rotatory movements).

Double rope

A double rope consists of a ring and clip from which the rope is hung to create a compensating device permitting a certain amount of swivel on the rope. The rope then passes through one

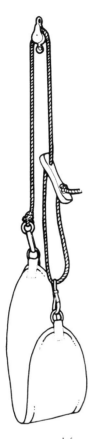

Fig. 8.8 A pulley rope – used for auto-pulley circuits or to allow rotation with angular movements.

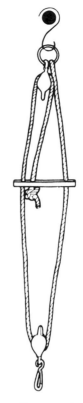

Fig. 8.9 A double pulley rope having a mechanical advantage of two.

side of a cleat, round a pulley wheel at the lower end, to the case of which is attached a dog clip, through the other end of the cleat and over the wheel of an upper pulley which is attached to the compensating device. The rope then passes down again through a centre hole in the cleat where it is knotted (Fig. 8.9). This device gives a mechanical advantage of two as two pulleys are used. The rope is shortened by pushing the cleat down, allowing the lifter to move with gravity at the same time as it offers a mechanical advantage of two. Such a rope is used to suspend the heavy parts of the body – the pelvis, thorax or heavy thighs when these are to be supported together.

Slings

Single slings

Single slings are made of canvas bound with soft webbing and with a D ring at each end (Fig. 8.10A). They are used open to support the limbs, or folded in two and as a figure of eight to support the hand or foot (Figs 8.11A,B and 8.12A). They measure 68 cm long by 17 cm wide.

Double slings

Double slings are broad slings measuring 68 cm long by 29 cm wide with D rings at each end (Fig. 8.10B) and are used to support the pelvis or thorax or the thighs together, especially when the knees are to be kept straight.

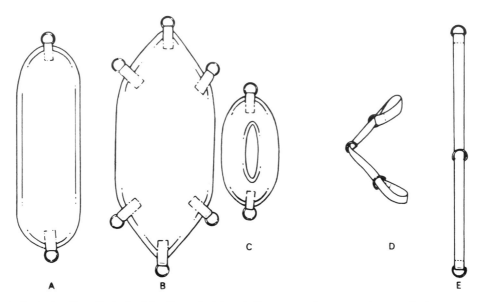

Fig. 8.10 A, A single sling; B, A double sling; C, A head sling; D, A three-ring sling ready for use; E, A three-ring sling ready for storage.

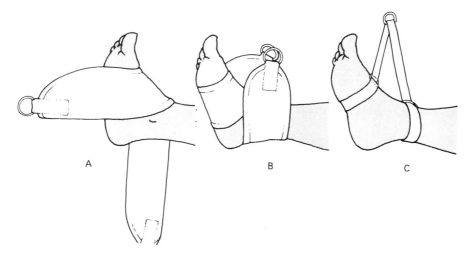

Fig. 8.11 A and B, A single sling folded and being made into a figure of eight for use on the foot and ankle; C, A three-ring sling on the foot and ankle.

Three-ring slings

Three ring slings are webbing slings 71 cm long by 3–4 cm wide with three D rings, one fastened at each end and one free in the middle. The centre ring is for attachment to the dog clip and the webbing is slipped through the end D rings to make two loops (Fig. 8.10D,E). These slings are used to support the wrist and hand or ankle and foot (Figs 8.11C and 8.12B).

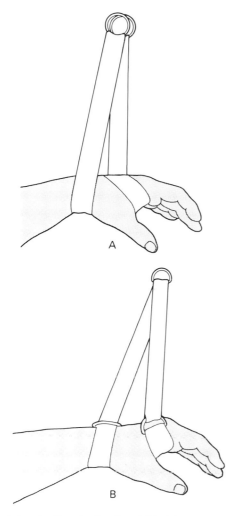

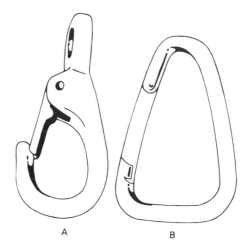

Fig. 8.13 A, A dog clip; B, A karabiner clip.

Fig. 8.12 A, The single sling folded for use as a figure of eight on the hand; B, The three-ring sling on the hand.

Head sling

A head sling is a short, split sling with its two halves stitched together at an angle to create a central slit (Fig. 8.10C). This allows the head to rest supported at the back under the lower and upper parts of the skull, or in the side lying position leaves the ear free. Skilful tilting of the sling when it is applied in side lying will arrange it so that the front ring lies at the level of the forehead and not over the eyes and nose, with the other half lying below the occiput.

Clips

Karabiner hooks (Fig. 8.13B) of 70 mm or 100 mm provide a convenient alternative means of clipping two pieces of equipment together.

Types of suspension

Vertical fixation

In using vertical fixation the rope is fixed so that it hangs vertically above the centre of gravity of the part to be suspended. The centre of gravity of each part of the body is, on the whole, at the junction of the upper and middle third. Vertical suspension is used for support as it tends to limit the movement of the part to a small-range pendular movement on each side of the central resting point (Fig. 8.14). It is advisable to carry out an experiment suspending the lower limb, for example, from two points, the

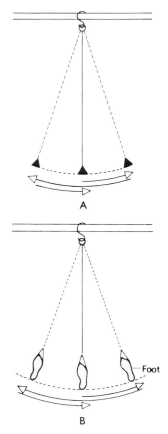

Fig. 8.14 A, A pendulum; B, The foot, supported at the centre of gravity of the leg, acts like a pendulum.

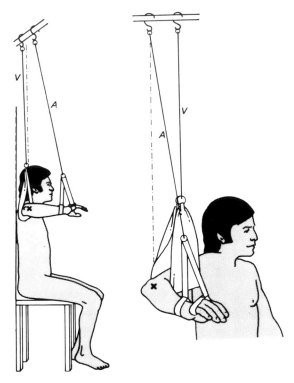

Fig. 8.15 Vertical fixation by rope *V* for the arm. Axial fixation by rope *A* for the forearm. ·—·—·— is the axis from the suspension point of rope *A* immediately above the elbow joint (×).

leg from above the tibia and the thigh from above the femur, and then attempting movement. It will be noted that the leg rises on each side in the lower sling and as it does so the thigh leaves the support of the upper sling. In other words, the support is partly lost and the movement is limited by the length of the ropes.

Vertical fixation is used primarily to support, e.g. the abducted upper limb when the elbow is to be moved is supported from above the centre of gravity of the arm and axial fixation is used over the elbow for forearm movement (Fig. 8.15).

Axial fixation

This occurs when all the ropes supporting a part are attached to one 'S' hook which is fixed to a point immediately above the centre of the joint which is to be moved, e.g. if the lower limb is to be moved at the hip joint, two ropes, one to the foot and one to the area of the knee, will be used and fixed at a point immediately over the axis of the hip joint (Fig. 8.16B). When such fixation is set up the movement of the limb will be on a flat plane level with the floor. In this way pure angular movements are obtained (Fig. 8.16A).

If some resistance to the muscle work is required, then the whole fixed point is moved away from the muscles which require resistance.

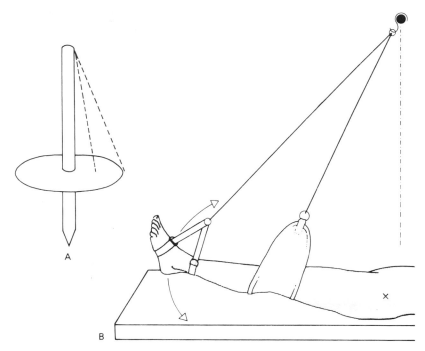

Fig. 8.16 A, The pencil pushed through a circle of paper demonstrates that when the pencil is pivoted the paper moves in a plane parallel with the floor, thus demonstrating the principle of axial fixation; B, Axial fixation for adduction and abduction of the hip (·—·—· axial line, X hip joint).

If abduction is to be resisted the fixed point is moved towards the adductors and the limb then falls towards that side, i.e. into adduction. On effort the limb will now rise into abduction brought about by isotonic shortening of the abductors, resistance being offered by gravity. Slow lowering into the resting position is controlled by isotonic lengthening of the abductors, with the movement assisted by the pull of gravity, and if at any time the abductors relax, the leg will drop into adduction. Figure 8.17 shows the method of finding the centre of gravity (A) and the axis (B).

Suspension for the lower extremity

The hip

Abduction and adduction
The starting position is lying with the opposite leg abducted to its limit, even if the knee has to

be bent over the side of the plinth and the foot supported on a footstool. The fixation point is immediately above the hip joint. One sling is put under the lower thigh and one three-ring sling on the foot and ankle; each is attached to a rope hung from the fixation point. The limb is lifted just clear of the plinth. Using this method of support the movements of abduction and adduction may be mobilized or the abductor or adductor muscles may be especially worked with or without manual resistance (Fig. 8.18).

Flexion and extension
The starting position is side lying with the underneath leg flexed as far as possible. The fixation point and sling arrangements are as above, with the limb lifted until it is horizontal. If the movement of flexion is to be

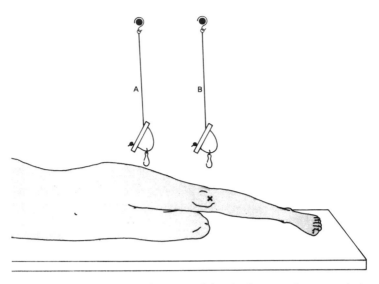

Fig. 8.17 Rope A, suspended over the centre of gravity of the thigh. Rope B, suspended over the axis of the knee joint and ready to support the leg and foot.

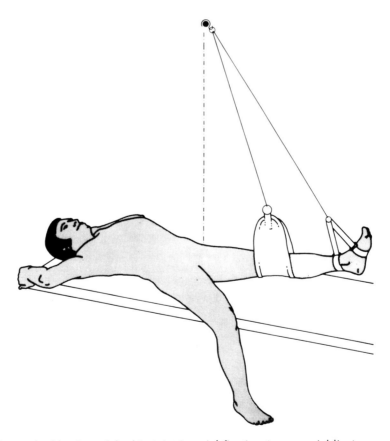

Fig. 8.18 Abduction and adduction of the hip joint in axial fixation (–·–·– axial line).

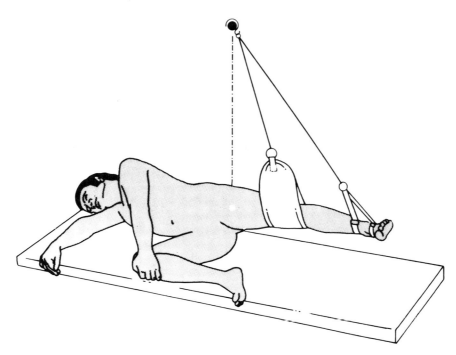

Fig. 8.19 Flexion and extension of the hip joint in axial fixation (—·—·— axial line).

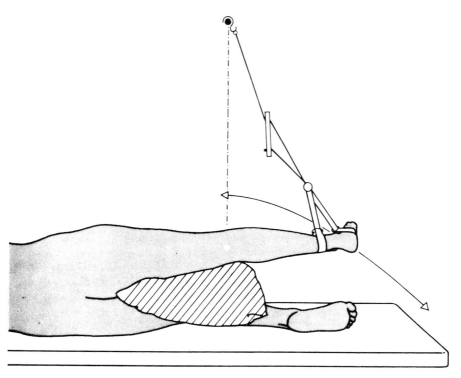

Fig. 8.20 A pillow is placed between the thighs for flexion and extension of the knee in axial fixation (—·—·—· axial line).

mobilized the knee and hip must be flexed together to overcome the passive insufficiency of the hamstrings. Equally, when mobilizing extension the knee should be extended to overcome active insufficiency of the hamstrings (Fig. 8.19).

The knee
Flexion and extension
The starting position is side lying with one or two pillows between the slightly flexed thighs. One three-ring sling is applied to the foot and ankle and one rope attached to a fixation point above the knee joint. By keeping the hip slightly flexed on the trunk the foot can be seen each time the knee is extended and part of the arc of movement is thus observed by the patient. This position may be used to mobilize the knee joint or to work the flexors or extensors of the knee (Fig. 8.20).

The ankle
It is rarely necessary to use suspension as in this case it is easier to perform supported movements by using a polished board.

Suspension for the upper extremity

The shoulder joint
Abduction and adduction
The starting position is lying, quarter turned towards the arm which is to be moved (Fig. 8.21A). This allows the normal anatomical movement to be performed in the plane of the scapula. Alternatively, the starting position is prone lying, quarter turned towards side lying with a pillow under the trunk on the side of the arm which is to be moved (Fig. 8.21B). The advantage of prone lying is that the therapist can see the movements of the scapula as well as those of the arm.

Two single ropes are required, one attached to a single sling under the elbow and one to a three-ring sling applied to the wrist and hand. The fixation point is over the shoulder joint.

If the movement is to be only of the glenohumeral joint, the therapist must stand on the opposite side with one hand on the point of the shoulder depressing the scapula. In this form of support either abduction and adduction of the glenohumeral joint, or movements of the shoulder girdle, may be mobilized. Glenohumeral rhythm may be re-educated and all the muscles performing shoulder girdle movements may be worked.

Flexion and extension
The starting position is side lying on pillows and quarter turned to the back. Female patients need two pillows under the head and one under the shoulder to allow the forearm to clear their wider pelvis. The slings and ropes are arranged as described above and again the movement may be limited to the glenohumeral joint and the muscles working over it, or movements of the shoulder girdle may be included.

If in addition to the angular movements it is desired to perform rotation of the glenohumeral joint, then only one sling should be used at the level of the elbow and a single pulley rope should be attached to the fixed point above the shoulder. The ends of the sling are attached to each end of the pulley circuit and it will then be possible to perform medial or lateral rotation with two angular movements (Figs 8.22 and 8.23).

It will be necessary to turn the patient further towards the side or more prone. It is then possible to perform flexion, adduction and lateral rotation alternately with extension, abduction and medial rotation, or flexion, abduction and lateral rotation alternately with extension, adduction and medial rotation.

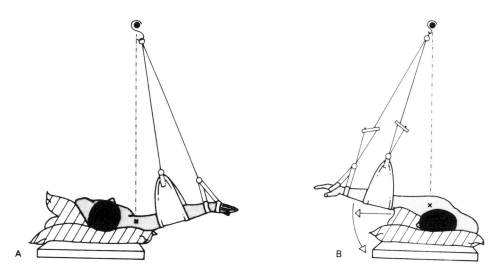

Fig. 8.21 Shoulder abduction and adduction in axial fixation. A, Quarter 15° turned from lying; B, Quarter 15° turned from prone lying. This position may also be used for protraction and retraction of the scapula (·—·—·— axial line).

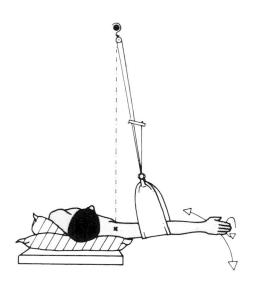

Fig. 8.22 Using axial fixation over the right glenohumeral joint and a single pulley rope the movements of extension/adduction/medial rotation and flexion/abduction/lateral rotation can be performed with the patient quarter 15° turned to the right (·—·—·— axial line).

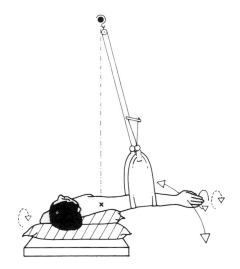

Fig. 8.23 Using axial fixation over the right glenohumeral joint and a single pulley rope the movements of extension/abduction/medial rotation and flexion/adduction/lateral rotation can be performed with the patient quarter 15° turned to the left (·—·—·— axial line).

Elbow joint

Flexion and extension
Because of the carrying angle of the forearm it is easier to perform these movements when the arm is suspended in abduction. The starting position is sitting on a low-backed chair. A single sling and rope supports the arm in vertical fixation, and a three-ring sling and single rope are fixed to a point above the elbow joint (Fig. 8.15). The therapist should stand behind as she may need to give additional support by holding the arm with a grasp inside the sling, which will allow palpation of the flexors and extensors which are covered by the supporting sling. Alternatively, a folded single sling under the palm, attached to a single pulley rope, will allow pronation and supination to occur with extension and flexion of the elbow joint.

Wrist
Flexion and extension
This is more usually and conveniently performed on a polished board or table.

Flexion and extension of the whole arm
As a functional movement this may be performed with the patient in the sitting position, e.g. practising taking the hand to the mouth may be done by using two single slings attached to two single pulley rope circuits. One sling is placed round the arm and one round the forearm. If the ropes are sufficiently tightened the patient can grasp, supinate and flex the elbow and shoulder while adducting and laterally rotating.

This sort of support is used for patients who have difficulty in performing personal facial toilet, feeding, turning the pages of a book fixed at eye level, or working in front of themselves.

Chapter 9
SPRINGS, THERA-BANDS, PULLEYS, WEIGHTS AND WATER

M. Hollis

Springs

Springs are elastic and therefore may have any of the properties of elastic materials. Three of the types of elasticity are used therapeutically, i.e. extensibility, compressibility and torsion.

When springs are extensible they offer resistance to muscle work as they are stretched and as they recoil they offer assistance to movement. During recoil they may be controlled by working muscles in isotonic lengthening.

Compressible springs are used in the form of three springs placed between two halves of a hand grip and are used for exercising the gripping muscles of the hand (Fig. 9.1A). A similar device is a Z-shaped piece of flat spring steel with the flat outer parts of the Z being covered in wood or plastic to form a gripping surface (Fig. 9.1B). These two types offer resistance by compression.

These devices are used for increasing the power of the coarse grip. Any type of spring device can be replaced by any compressible material (see section on small apparatus in Chapter 7).

Short tension springs of heavy weight resistance have less elasticity and are only suitable for use to give buoyant suspension when a heavy part of the body is to be supported in suspension for a long time. Long tension springs made in a softer metal are the most common type.

Thera-Bands

Another means of elastic resistance is a Thera-Band. These are supplied as 15 cm (6 in) wide rolls of latex in eight strengths and in eight colours. The required length can be cut and one end attached to a fixed object. The patient can be attached to the Thera-Band by means of the handle, by a sling or he can just hold it (Fig. 9.2). The Thera-Band may be used as a single band or a loop and Fig. 9.3 shows the resistances offered by the different strengths.

The weight of a spring

The mean coil of the wire and the wire diameter can be varied so that springs can be made to offer different quantities of resistance expressed in pounds or kilos. This is usually

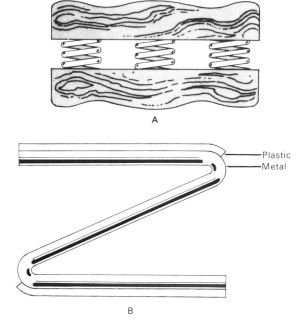

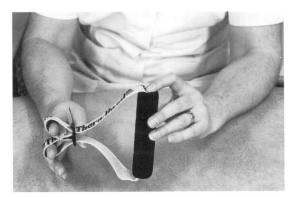

Fig. 9.2A The Thera-Band handle, showing the two loops into which the band can be threaded.

Plastic
Metal

Fig. 9.1 Two types (A and B) of compressible springs.

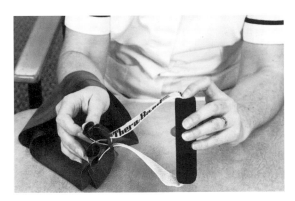

Fig. 9.2B The band being threaded into the loops.

noted on the tab at the end of the spring. The 'weight' or resistance offered ranges from 5 kg (approximately 10 lb) to 25 kg (approximately 50 lb) by 5 kg (10 lb) gradations. When the cord inside the spring is taut, the marked weight resistance is reached. A pull beyond this length will overstretch the metal and cause deformity by separation of the coils. Such deformity is also caused by bending springs round plinth ends and by allowing two springs stretched side by side to interlock and remain so.

Springs in parallel
If two springs are arranged side by side attached to the same point, i.e. in parallel, the weight of the resistance will be the sum of the two (Fig. 9.4A).

Springs in series
When two springs are joined end to end, i.e. in series, the resistance offered is the same as if

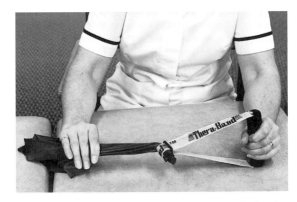

Fig. 9.2C When the retaining device is pulled tight the band is anchored, yet may be detached with ease.

These tables show the pounds of pull required to stretch a single length or a loop of Thera-Band resistive exerciser to various lengths. Pulls were measured using a pull-spring scale.

Single length (starting length of 6 in wide × 12 in long band)

US	Pull in pounds for various weights or thicknesses							
Extended length (in)	Tan Extra thin	Yellow Thin	Red Medium	Green Heavy	Blue Extra heavy	Black Special heavy	Silver Super heavy	Gold Max.
14	.500	.75	1.00	1.25	1.50	2.00	5.00	7.20
16	1.00	1.50	2.00	2.50	3.00	4.00	9.00	11.20
20	1.50	2.25	3.50	4.25	6.25	7.50	12.00	16.20
24	2.00	2.50	4.50	5.00	7.50	9.00	15.00	20.70
28	2.50	3.00	5.50	6.00	9.00	10.00	17.50	24.30
32	2.70	3.50	6.50	7.00	10.25	11.25	20.00	27.70
36	3.00	4.00	7.50	8.00	12.00	13.00	23.00	30.60

Metric	Pull in newtons for various weights or thicknesses							
Extended length (cm)	Tan Extra thin	Yellow Thin	Red Medium	Green Heavy	Blue Extra heavy	Black Special heavy	Silver Super heavy	Gold Max.
35	2.25	3.25	4.50	5.50	6.50	9.00	22.25	32.00
40	4.50	6.75	9.00	11.00	13.25	17.75	40.00	49.75
50	6.75	10.00	15.50	19.00	27.75	33.25	53.50	72.00
60	9.00	11.00	20.00	22.25	33.25	40.00	66.75	92.00
70	11.00	13.25	24.50	26.75	40.00	44.50	77.25	108.00
80	12.00	15.50	29.00	31.25	45.50	50.00	89.00	123.25
90	13.25	17.75	33.25	35.50	53.50	57.75	102.25	136.00

Loop (starting length of loop 12 in)

US	Pull in pounds for various weights or thicknesses							
Extended length (in)	Tan Extra thin	Yellow Thin	Red Medium	Green Heavy	Blue Extra heavy	Black Special heavy	Silver Super heavy	Gold Max.
14	1.00	1.50	2.00	2.50	3.00	4.00	10.00	14.40
16	1.50	3.00	4.00	5.00	6.00	8.00	18.00	22.40
20	3.00	4.50	7.00	8.50	12.50	15.00	24.00	32.40
24	4.10	5.00	9.00	10.00	15.00	18.00	30.00	41.40
28	4.50	6.00	11.00	12.00	18.00	20.00	35.00	48.60
32	5.50	7.00	13.00	14.00	20.50	22.50	40.00	55.40
36	6.00	8.00	15.00	16.00	24.00	26.00	46.00	61.20

Metric	Pull in newtons for various weights or thicknesses							
Extended length (cm)	Tan Extra thin	Yellow Thin	Red Medium	Green Heavy	Blue Extra heavy	Black Special heavy	Silver Super heavy	Gold Max.
35	4.50	6.75	9.00	11.00	13.25	17.75	44.50	64.00
40	6.75	13.25	17.75	22.25	26.75	35.50	80.00	99.50
50	13.25	20.00	31.25	37.75	55.50	66.75	106.75	144.00
60	18.25	22.50	40.00	44.50	66.75	80.00	133.50	184.00
70	20.00	26.75	49.00	53.50	80.00	89.00	155.75	216.00
80	24.50	31.25	57.75	62.25	91.25	100.00	178.00	246.50
90	26.75	35.50	66.75	71.25	106.75	115.75	204.50	272.25

Fig. 9.3 The table of weight resistances offered by Thera-Band.

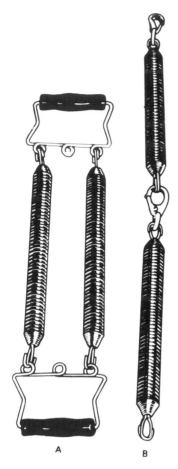

Fig. 9.4 A, Springs in parallel; B, Springs in series.

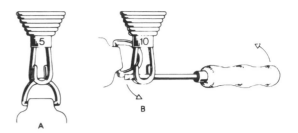

Fig. 9.5 The method of: A, attaching a spring to a split ring; B, detaching a spring from a split ring.

ring end on a spring is shown in Fig. 9.5A and the method of removal is shown in Fig. 9.5B.

A karabiner is also a very easy method of clipping springs to handles or slings. Some springs are now supplied with a dog clip already attached (Fig. 8.13A and B)

Methods of use

Rules for the application of forces

The most efficient angle at which a muscle can pull on a bone is one of 90° as then all energy is directed to producing the desired movement (see Figs 2.10 and 2.11). When the angle between the working muscle and the bone is less or greater than 90°, some of the energy will be expended in either approximating or separating the joint surfaces. When applying an external force to a moving bone, the same law relating to application of force will operate. Therefore, when force is applied it should be as nearly parallel with the line of movement as is possible and at right angles to the bone. However, as the bones of the body describe an arc of a circle during movement it is only possible to achieve this right angle at one point on the arc; the centre of the arc is usually chosen for the right angle application of the force or the middle range of the contraction of the muscle. In this position the force will be most nearly parallel to the line of motion for the

only one spring was used, e.g. if two 10 kg springs are attached end to end the resistance offered will be 10 kg, but the range through which movement must occur to stretch two springs fully would be twice as great (Fig. 9.4B). If the same range as would be required to stretch one spring fully is considered, then the force applied to the two in series would be half the weight resistance of one, i.e. 5 kg. Connecting springs in series, therefore, is indicated if either the range over which the springs must stretch is great, or a spring of sufficiently low weight resistance is not available.

The method of attaching rings to the split

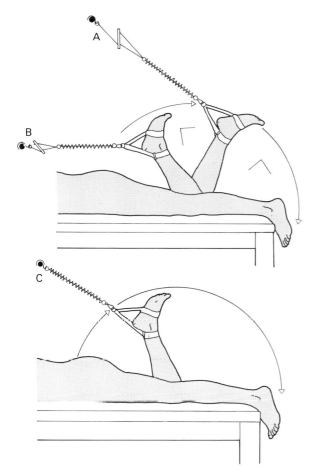

Fig. 9.6 A, The rigging to resist inner range of quadriceps contraction; B, The rigging to resist outer range quadriceps contraction; C, The rigging to resist the total movement produced by the quadriceps. Maximal only in middle range.

largest part of the arc of motion and the strongest part of the muscle pull.

Figure 9.6A (90°) and B (165°) show that when force is applied, whether it be a spring or weight and pulley circuit, it is possible to resist a range producing an arc of movement of more than 90° by using two springs each positioned to resist in an arc of movement of 90°. A less effective way of resisting in an arc of movement of 165° would be to position the spring as in

Fig. 9.6C when resistance is maximal in middle range for the quadriceps.

Sometimes it is desired to resist movement of more than one joint, as in extension thrusts of the upper or lower limb, in which case the resistance is applied so as to be parallel to the path of movement of the limb.

It should be noted that when an elastic material is applied to offer resistance it will *assist* the return movement unless this movement is controlled by the same muscles working in isotonic lengthening. When springs are rigged to offer resistance the following rules should be applied:

(1)   The patient's starting position should be considered and arranged with sufficient support so that the muscle work occurs where it is required.
(2)   The movement should be started with the elastic material slightly stretched and this may also call for modification of the starting position.
(3)   A suitable weight resistance should be selected relative to:
      (a)   The strength of the muscles.
      (b)   The part being supported and also resisted by the elastic material, e.g. in Fig. 9.7 the weight of the limb must be supported by the elastic material when the limb is flexed at the hip and yet it must be possible to achieve full range extension.
(4)   The correct angle of attachment should be worked out or experimented with to get the resistance in the required range, remembering also that the resistance will be greatest when the elastic material is most fully stretched.
(5)   To 'lengthen' the distance between the points of attachment a single rope may be used. It should usually be attached to the fixed point and the elastic material

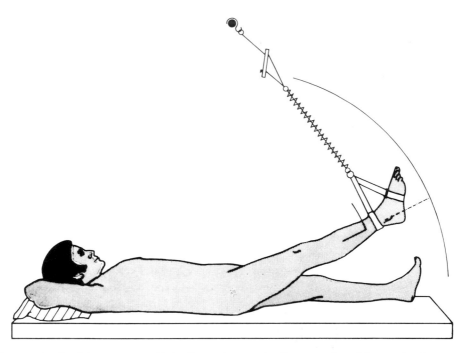

Fig. 9.7 Resistance for the hip extensors. Note: the spring must offer enough resistance also to support the limb.

attached either to the sling which is attached to the patient, or to the handle which he grips. In this way the patient is more likely to see and hear the spring and sensory stimulation is thereby increased. Exceptions are made when springs are attached for movements of the head and the noise so near the ears is irritating, or when the spring passes across the naked body and may catch hairs or pinch skin when it recoils. In these cases Thera-Bands are better.

Resistance for the lower limb

Hip abductors

These muscles may be worked in lying and in suspension with the spring attached to the medial side of the foot, or in yard grasp half standing (Fig. 9.8). A low weight resistance is used as the weight arm is long (try 5–10 kg). Alternatively use a Thera-Band (Fig. 9.8B).

Hip extensors

These muscles may be worked in lying as in Fig. 9.8 when allowance is made for the weight of the leg in selecting the spring (try 15–20 kg), or in reach grasp standing when a much lighter weight resistance is used (try 5–10 kg) (Fig. 9.9).

Hip adductors

This group of muscles may commonly need to be re-educated when an above knee amputation has been performed. The patient may be in lying or, later, in half sitting or standing. The difficulty lies in keeping a sling on the stump. The weight resistance should start low (5 kg) and increase as the patient becomes stronger.

Knee extensors

These muscles may be retrained in any of the three selected ranges – inner, middle or outer –

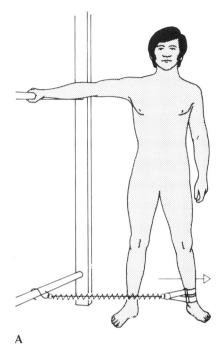

A

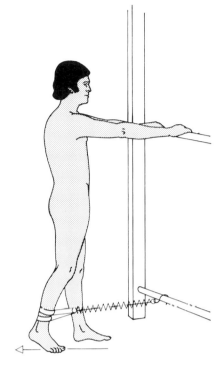

Fig. 9.9 Resistance for the hip extensors.

or simultaneously in all ranges by leaving springs A and B in Fig. 9.6 in position but reducing the weight resistance, as the total resistance offered by both springs will be greater than that by either of them separately.

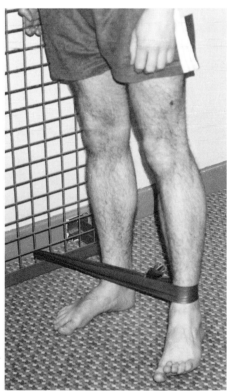

B

Fig. 9.8 Resistance for the hip abductors: A, by a spring; B, by Thera-Band.

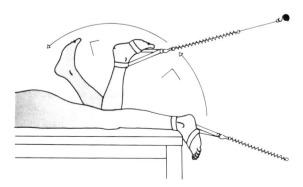

Fig. 9.10 Resistance for the knee flexors.

Knee flexors

The rigging is similar to that for knee extension except that the resistance will be in the opposite direction (Fig. 9.10).

Foot plantarflexors

The patient can hold the spring by means of a handle (Fig. 9.11) and so also perform an isometric arm activity. The turns of the three-ring sling must be round the forefoot (try a 10–15 kg spring). Remember here the distance the material will be pulled out will be small.

Foot dorsiflexors

The turns of the three-ring sling must again be round the forefoot. Try a 5–10 kg spring and prevent cheating by giving the patient a back support. Thus suitable positions are half lying or sitting on a chair with the legs straight and resting on a footstool (Fig. 9.12).

Foot invertors

These should be rigged as for dorsiflexion but the resistance should be attached to the lateral aspect of the foot. Alternatively a three-ring sling may be attached to each foot with a 5 kg spring fixed between them. The patient crosses his knees and he can practise inversion of both feet at once (Fig. 9.13).

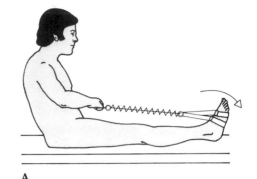

A

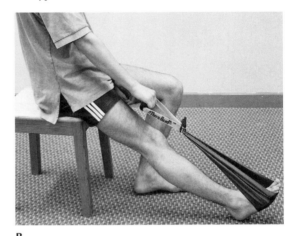

B

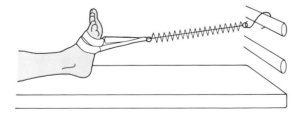

Fig. 9.12 Resistance for the dorsiflexors.

C

Fig. 9.11 Resistance for the plantarflexors: A, by a spring; B and C, by Thera-Band.

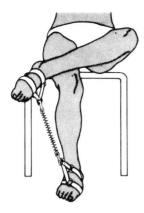

Fig. 9.13 Resistance for the foot invertors.

Thrusts

If a resistance is rigged as in Fig. 9.14 a combined hip and knee extension can be performed, and if rigged as shown in Fig. 9.24 hip and knee extension with leg thrusting downwards (lateral pelvic tilting) can be practised. The same rigging can be used for a hip flexion with knee extension followed by hip extension and slow hip and knee flexion; thus a bicycling movement is done

with isotonic shortening and lengthening being performed.

Resistance for the upper limb

Shoulder abductors, extensors and flexors

These muscles can be resisted by putting the patient into stride standing and anchoring a sling under his foot on the side of the arm to be exercised. A 5–10 kg spring may be attached to the sling and the patient holds the other end by means of a handle. Varying the angle at which the arm is raised will allow the same rigging to be used for arm abduction, arm extension, arm flexion and many intermediate movements (Fig. 9.15).

Shoulder rotators

The arm should be supported in a sling attached to a single pulley rope and the patient should hold a handle to which is attached a 5 kg spring or Thera-Band. If the other end is attached to the floor below the hand, inner range lateral rotation is resisted, and if it is attached to a point above the hand, inner range medial rotation is resisted (Fig. 9.16).

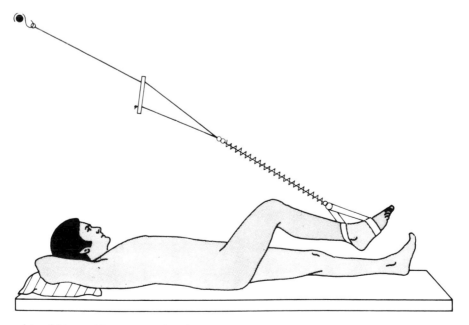

Fig. 9.14 A combined hip and knee extension thrust.

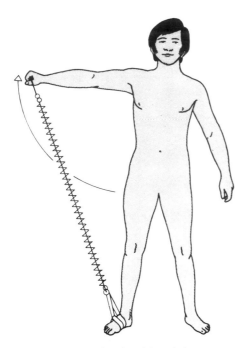

Fig. 9.15 Resistance for shoulder abductors.

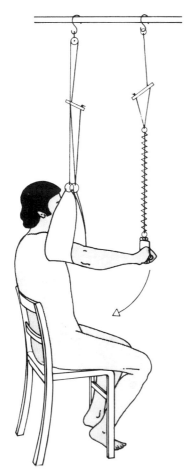

Fig. 9.16 Arm suspension, resistance for the medial rotators of the shoulder.

Thrusts for serratus anterior
The patient should be prone at the edge of the bed and hold a handle attached to a 10 kg resistance, the other end of which is attached to a fixed point above his shoulder. He should thrust to the floor protracting his scapula. The same exercise may be performed in sitting, with the arm supported in slings (Fig. 9.17) if necessary, or in lying with the spring fixed to the floor.

Elbow flexors
The patient is in toe support sitting at the wallbars and holds a spring with a handle. The other end of the spring should be attached in front and to his right for right arm work. He can supinate and flex simultaneously against possibly a 5–10 kg spring.

Elbow extensors
The patient can be standing or lying holding a handle with a 10–15 kg spring attached to a point above and behind the head (Fig. 9.18).

Pronators and supinators
Fix two 5 kg resistances to a handle, one to each of the outer of the three rings on the handle. Stretch both slightly and fix one above and one below the level of the hand when the elbow is bent. The patient can be standing or sitting facing the wallbars. The handle will be held vertical by the tension on the springs and the patient should fix his elbow by tucking it into his waist, grasp the handle and try to pronate in inner range and supinate in inner range.

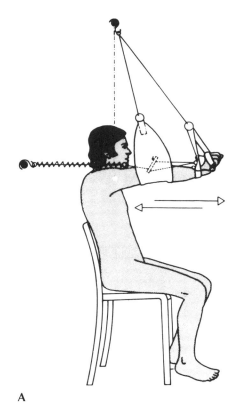

A

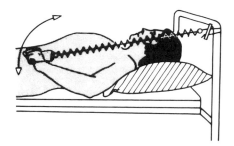

Fig. 9.18 Lying, resistance for the elbow extensors.

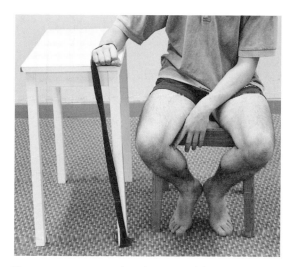

Fig. 9.19 Resistance by Thera-Band for the wrist extensors.

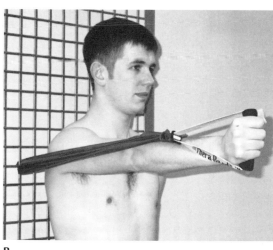

B

Fig. 9.17 Resistance for serratus anterior: A, by a spring; B, by Thera-Band.

Wrist flexors and extensors

Fix a three-ring sling on the palm and attach a 5–10 kg spring. The patient is in sitting at a table so that his hand is over the far edge of it. The spring may be fixed to the floor level by anchoring it with a sling under the patient's foot. The patient then either supinates the forearm to work the wrist flexors or pronates the forearm to work the wrist extensors. The three-ring sling should be slipped round on the hand when changing muscle work so that the pull is straight. Alternatively use a Thera-Band as in Fig. 9.19.

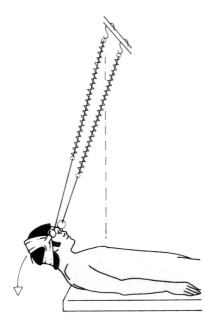

Fig. 9.20 Lying, resistance for the head and neck extensors.

Spring resistance for the head and trunk

Head and neck extensors

The most usual position for the patient is lying with a head sling under the head. A rope and a 10 kg spring are attached to each side of the sling. The fixed points are a head width apart and over the manubriosternal junction to allow for natural flexion. The patient pushes the head backwards when the stool, which initially supports the head, is removed (Fig. 9.20).

Trunk flexors

The abdominal muscles may be worked as in Fig. 9.21A by using 10–15 kg resistances, one to each hand. This has the effect of offering resistance to the abdominal muscles of up to 20–30 kg as the springs are being used in parallel; or with the patient sitting holding a pole to which are attached two springs (Fig. 9.21B).

Trunk rotators

The springs of similar weight resistance for flexion should be used alternately as in Fig. 9.21, or may be fixed above and behind the patient when he is sitting on a low-backed chair.

Combined spring resistance

A sequence of bed exercises may be performed in preparation for crutch walking by using the springs attached to the bed head and:

(1) Working the elbow extensors (Fig. 9.18)
(2) Continuing to thrust to work the shoulder depressors
(3) Arching the back and working latissimus dorsi and the back extensors (Fig. 9.22)
(4) Taking the hands over the thighs, thrusting and raising the head to work the abdominal muscles (Fig. 9.21A)
(5) Thrusting one arm at a time down by the side and working the trunk side flexors (Fig. 9.23)
(6) Thrusting one arm at a time across the trunk and working the trunk rotators (Fig. 9.24).

The above regime is suitable for any long-stay patient who must have lower limb rest or who may have to transfer all activity to the upper limbs and trunk. If eventually the patient will bear weight on one leg, the rigging as in Fig. 9.14 but attached to the bed head will allow:

(1) Leg extension from flexion
(2) Bicycling
(3) Resisted plantar flexion
(4) Thrusting and lateral pelvic tilting.

Three simultaneous limb thrusts as in Fig. 9.25 simulate the 'stance' phase of one leg weight bearing on crutches.

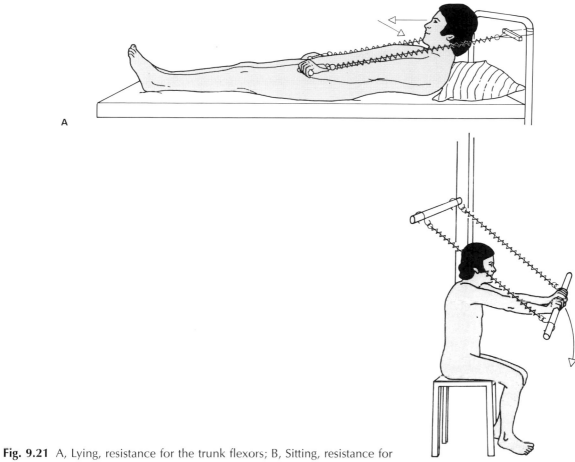

Fig. 9.21 A, Lying, resistance for the trunk flexors; B, Sitting, resistance for the trunk flexors.

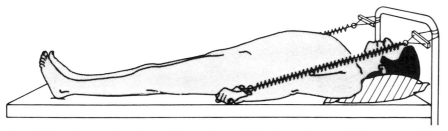

Fig. 9.22 Continued thrust into adduction and extension with back arching works latissimus dorsi and the back extensors.

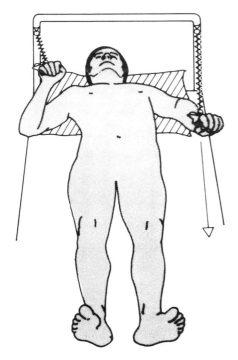

Fig. 9.23 Thrusting with one arm down to the side works the trunk side flexors.

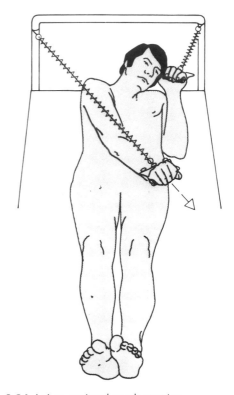

Fig. 9.24 Lying, resisted trunk rotation.

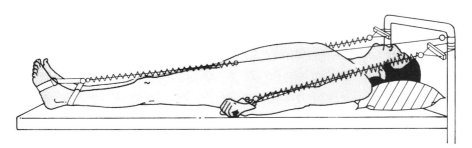

Fig. 9.25 Simultaneous thrust with one leg and both arms as in the 'stance' phase of crutch walking.

Resisted PNF patterns may be performed using springs, provided:

(1) The rigging is suitably arranged
(2) The patient is properly instructed and supervised.

Pulleys

Pulley circuits may be used to change the angle of pull either as auto circuits or as weight and pulley circuits, or to give mechanical advantage (see the section on pulleys in Chapter 2).

To change direction of pull

Auto circuit (reciprocal circuit)

The circuit consists of one pulley and a rope (Fig. 8.8) with a shortening device and may be used as an auto-pulley circuit for facilitating reciprocal movements of limbs (Figs 9.26, 9.27 and 9.28). In Figs 9.27 and 9.28 note the sloping support to allow the body weight to keep the rope taut and prevent cheating.

The method of use of an auto circuit is:

(1) Position the patient to prevent unwanted ('trick') movement
(2) The strongest limb or that with the greatest range is put into the position to be achieved by the disabled limb
(3) The slings/handles are attached and the rope just tightened
(4) The patient is then told to reverse the limb positions slowly initially until he familiarizes himself with the equipment and builds up confidence. Then there are several methods of use:
   (a) Increase the tempo so that the movement is carried past the point of pain by momentum
   (b) Tell the patient to make a 'reaching' or overstretch effort at the present limit of his range so that he hurts and helps himself
   (c) Teach the patient to use the sound limb to apply the stretch or overpressure, so that if he is caused discomfort it remains within his limit of tolerance
   (d) Instruct him to resist each reversal of movement so that he builds up muscle effort and then he can do an extra reach at each end of the cycle of events.

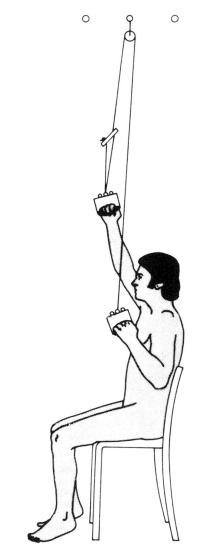

Fig. 9.26 An auto-pulley circuit for reciprocal arm movements.

Pulley and weight circuits

More than one pulley in the circuit will allow loading of a movement to occur. Such devices as the Nomeq Multitrainer allow exercises resisted by weights fixed to pulleys, yet the unit can be wall mounted and folded away. An optional free standing platform is available where wall mounting is not feasible, and allows repositioning of the unit (Fig. 9.29A and B).

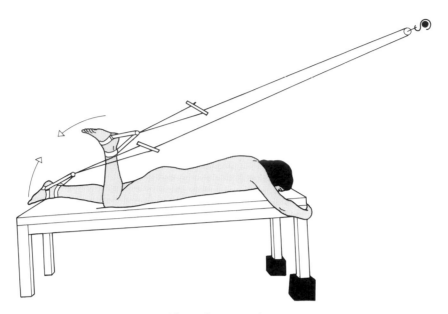

Fig. 9.27 An auto-pulley circuit for reciprocal knee flexion and extension.

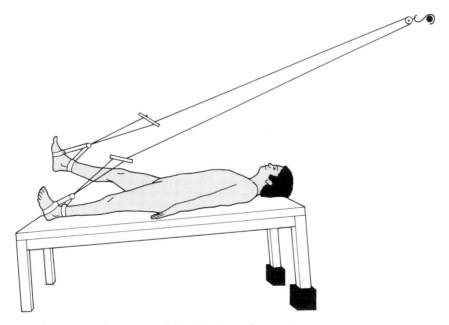

Fig. 9.28 An auto-pulley circuit for reciprocal hip flexion and extension.

The patient can lift a 'known and often visible weight' and thereby is stimulated to perform better in order to progress to greater loads on succeeding days or weeks.

In the absence of a proprietary device a pulley circuit can be rigged with fixed points as indicated in Fig. 9.30A and B.

In each of these cases care should be taken to allow the weight to travel up and down without either resting on the ground or hitting

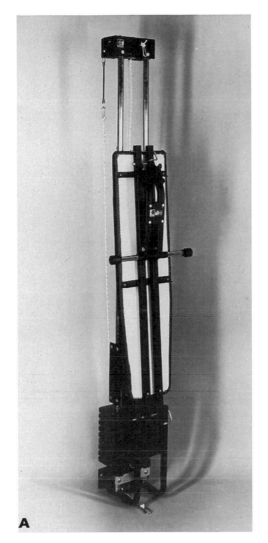 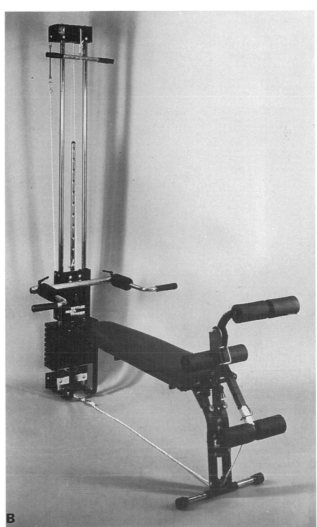

Fig. 9.29 A multitrainer which is wall mounted. A, Folded; B, Opened out to provide exercises resisted by weights using compact pulley circuits as well as by direct loading.

the first pulley in the circuit. A 'stop' is also usually introduced in the form of a cleat fitted to the circuit between the patient and the first pulley, so that on isotonic lengthening of the muscle, failure of control on the part of the patient does not allow his joint to move through an excessive range (Fig. 9.31). This is most important when the patient suffers

from both limited range and weak muscles acting over the same joint.

Weight loading

This is a type of loading which may be applied directly to a part by placing a weight in a

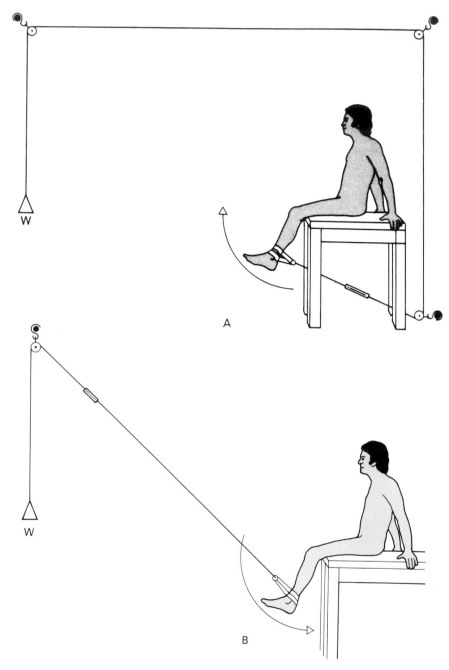

Fig. 9.30 A, A pulley and weight circuit to resist knee extension; B, A pulley and weight circuit to resist knee flexion.

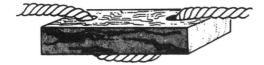

Fig. 9.31 The 'stop' inserted into pulley and weight circuits.

suitable position using either a special device such as the Variweight or de Lorme type boot (Fig. 9.32), or a bar, a barbell, a sandbag or a bag of shot. Alternatively a pulley and weight circuit may be used as in Figs 9.29 and 9.30. In rigging the apparatus as in Fig. 9.30A and B the weight can be placed so that it can be seen to move whenever the patient makes an effort.

The advantage of any of these types of loading is that the patient is moving a known weight with every endeavour. The disadvantages are that secure anchorage is sometimes difficult to achieve and the patient may not make a maximal effort at each attempt.

Any one of the three regimes outlined on pages 153–4 may be used in this type of loading.

Techniques

Using the de Lorme type or Variweight boot
This consists of a metal foot plate and straps weighing 500 g. A bar of varying weight may be supplied and it is essential to know the weight of the bar in calculating the load. The boot may be used for loading the quadriceps or hamstrings when the bar is placed in the rear slots on the foot plate and anchored by *both* of the securing screws. For loading dorsi- or plantarflexion of the foot, the bar is placed in the front slot on the foot plate and anchored by *one* screw.

The order of events in applying the boot is:

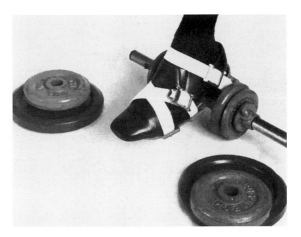

Fig. 9.32 The Variweight boot.

(1) Position the patient correctly supporting the distal part initially
(2) Apply the unloaded boot and secure it to the patient's shoe
(3) Position and fix the bar
(4) Load the weights equally on each side of the bar
(5) Secure them with the end stops which must be screwed into position so that the weights cannot move
(6) Remove the limb support if necessary and immediately require performance of the exercise.

The quadriceps are exercised with the patient in high sitting on a backward-sloping surface preferably padded under the knee (Fig. 9.33) so that the body acts as a counter-weight and the patient does not slip forward.

The anterior tibials are exercised in the same position but a back slope is not so necessary (Fig. 9.34). In both the above cases the limb should be supported on a stool until the boot and weights are fixed and the stool should be re-inserted under the boot at the end of the performance.

The hamstrings are exercised with the patient in prone lying but the range of

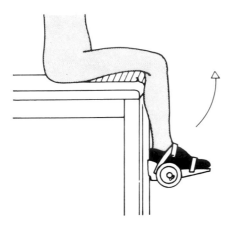

Fig. 9.33 High sitting, quadriceps exercise using the Variweight boot.

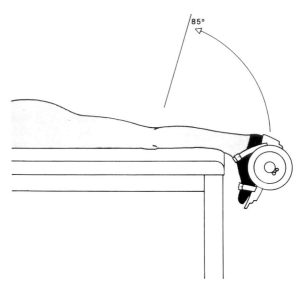

Fig. 9.35 Prone lying, hamstring exercise using the Variweight boot.

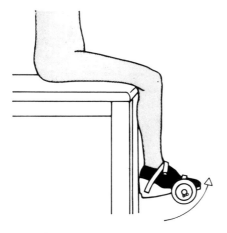

Fig. 9.34 High sitting, exercising the anterior tibial muscles. Note the bar is to the front of the boot.

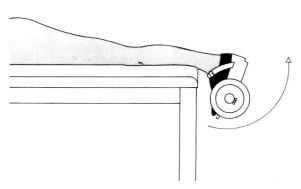

Fig. 9.36 Prone lying, exercising the calf muscles. Note the bar is to the front of the foot.

movement allowed at the knee should be just less than 90° (Fig. 9.35) and it may be necessary to change the length of the bar at each side of the boot to take into account variations in strength between the medial and lateral hamstrings.

The plantarflexors are also exercised in the prone lying position. In both the above cases the foot should rest over the end of the support (Fig. 9.36).

In using a de Lorme boot for treatmemnt of the thigh muscles, the foot is the area to be loaded and the anterior tibials and calf muscles must have adequate power to tolerate the load. This equally applies if a sandbag is placed on this region. Direct loading of the hamstrings or quadriceps only can be obtained by using a weight and pulley circuit and fixing the sling to the lower leg above the ankle joint (Fig. 9.30).

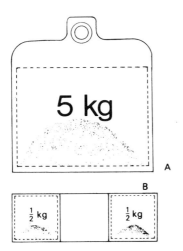

Fig. 9.37 A, A canvas bag weight; B, A canvas saddle weight.

Using weights of canvas and sand or shot
The canvas should be strong and of closely woven mesh and should be double stitched at the edges to keep the fine contents in place. The total weight of canvas and contents should be marked on each container – usually 500 g, 1 kg, 1.5 kg, 3 kg, 5 kg. Two styles are made:

(1) A bag (Fig. 9.37A) with a flat area at one end in which a metal eyelet hole is inserted allowing the weight to be suspended.

(2) A saddle in which a long strip of canvas has weights in pockets at each end. The centre (unloaded) area rests on the part to be loaded. Half the total contents should be inserted in each end of the saddle (Fig. 9.37B). The advantage of this type is that it can be laid across the area to be loaded, or the unloaded centre portion may be grasped.

Fixing weights such as sandbags to the lower limb can be done by using a band, which is placed round the back of the ankle. The weights are placed on the front of the ankle and held in position by crossing the band in front of

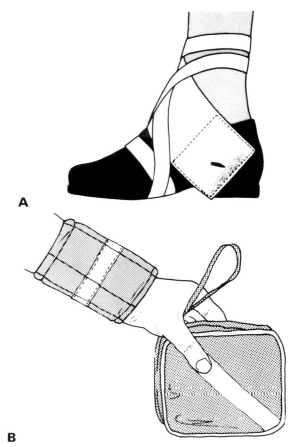

Fig. 9.38 A, A saddle weight held on the foot by the use of a band repeatedly crossed; B, A cuff weight attached to the wrist. The carrying case is also shown.

them. By crossing the band under the foot and continuing to cross the band around the foot the full length of the band is used up and the weights will be firmly secured (Fig. 9.38A).

Using weighted bands
Cuff weights are weighted bands made of artificial fibre fastened with Velcro. The bands have pockets in which lead shot is placed and are made in two sizes and weights, 794 g and 1134 g. They are supplied in pairs in a carrying case (Fig. 9.38B).

The bands are placed round the limb to be exercised and held securely with the Velcro fastening. More than one band may be applied to any part to obtain greater loading. It is also possible to join the bands to give a greater length for application to the waist when loading is required for neurologically disabled patients.

Bars and dumbbells

The bars from the de Lorme boot can be grasped and used to exercise the muscles of one hand or arm, or special dumbbells of weights varying from 1 kg to 5 kg may be used.

Barbells

These are long bars and heavy weights as used in weight-lifting training. They should be used by reasonably fit patients to strengthen the arms, trunk or legs. It is essential that a clear area of adequate size is in front of the patient before a lift is attempted, that the hands are coated with resin and that the patient knows exactly what to do. The bar may be lifted by the arms with the patient in lying. It may be lifted using arms and legs (the snatch) with the patient in walk crouch, but should not be raised above the head unless the patient is capable of *both* extending the elbows and flexing the shoulders fully as well as thrusting the pelvis forward so that the hips are fully extended to allow the high centre of gravity to fall within the base. The base changes in the course of the lift from walk to stride standing.

Isokinetic or accommodative resistance

Any form of resistance applied to a part of the human body varies in value as the part moves through its arc of movement. The angle of application of the resistance is only fully effective at a right angle to the part (see Chapter 2, 'Resolution of forces') so for those parts of the arc of movement at which the angle of application of the resistance is less or greater than a right angle, the output of the muscle will be less effective (see Fig. 9.6).

The problem is overcome by the Cybex machine which is capable of giving dynamic resistance by controlling the speed of the movement and accommodating the resistance to the force produced at every point in the range of action. An isokinetic contraction is dynamic, but the speed of the contraction is held constant so that the resistance is in direct ratio to the varying force applied throughout the full movement.

The speed of movement is pre-set. The lever arm of the machine, which is attached to the part to be moved, first moves a few degrees without resistance. When the moving part of the body achieves the pre-set speed, the moving arm of the machine continues to move at this speed. The arm of the machine may be stopped or reversed at any point in the arc of motion with the action sequence being reversed by the antagonistic muscle group(s).

Maximum muscular force applied to the lever arm of the machine moving at this pre-set speed is called an isokinetic contraction. The machine offers resistance to match the muscular output of the person exercising. The phrase 'accommodative resistance exercise' may be used for this type of exercise.

The machine will accommodate to limitations in joint range as well as to muscle weakness. Single joint movements or complex movement patterns may be performed, as well as training action patterns for specific athletic functions.

The machine can be used as a dyamometer as part of its basic facility.

Water

Exercises in water may range from the use of a bowl, bucket or domestic bath of warm water to exercise the hands or feet to the use of a fully equipped therapeutic pool. Obviously in either case the water should be at a temperature tolerable by and comfortable to the patient. Therapeutic pools are usually maintained at a temperature of 34°–37°C (94°–98°F), whereas in the domestic situation the water will cool and may need to be topped up. In either case the warmth will enhance the value of the treatment by causing relief of pain, relaxation of muscles and thus improving joint range.

Cleaning
Therapeutic pools require complex machinery and procedures to:

(1) Maintain the temperature
(2) Cleanse the water by filtration
(3) Sterilize the water by chlorination
(4) Turn the water over every four hours.

Therapists using such pools should ensure the above procedures are followed.

Surfaces and facilities
All surfaces in and around the pool should be of cleansable but non-slip material with adequate drainage to the surrounds to prevent pooling of water. All pools should have:

(1) Adequate surrounding heat and dehumidification facilities
(2) Undressing cubicles for ambulant and non-ambulant patients and for the staff
(3) Shower and footbath facilities for everyone who enters and leaves the pool
(4) Hot, dry-towel/sheet and pack facilities for patients and washing, sterilizing and drying facilities for clothing

(5) A hoist for both a chair and a stretcher
(6) Walk in steps at one side
(7) Variable and adequate depths for walking patients of different heights. The usual adult maximum depth is 1.37 m (54 in)
(8) Fixed rails at the pool walls and moveable rails to create walking bars
(9) Draining trolleys and mesh, wall mounted containers for the equipment such as floats, paddles and bats.

Flotation equipment

Assistance to buoyancy can be provided by the use of either:

(1) Air inflated containers such as are commonly seen in the form of rings, limb cuffs and horseshoes (Fig. 9.39A–D). Their advantage is that they can be deflated gradually to reduce the additional buoyancy offered and thus reduce the support if necessary.
(2) Polystyrene floats which are used in many shapes and may be attached to the patient by straps inserted into the swimsuit or, when threaded through by rods, used both for buoyancy and to keep a floppy head from falling to the side (Figs 9.39 and 40).

It should be understood that buoyancy equipment is not only used to sustain the patient floating on or near the surface of the water, but can be used to give extra resistance/assistance to movements in the water.

All equipment to be immersed and remain in the water in contact with the bottom of the pool must be weighted. Thus teak stools and wooden crutches both need weights on the under surface or near the leg tips. Metal equipment such as plinths or half plinths is likely to be heavy enough to maintain position or may

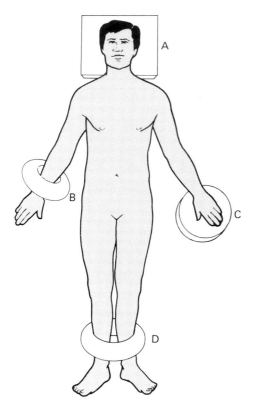

Fig. 9.39 Floats in use: A, Polystyrene floats with rod help to stabilize the head; B, Cuff limb float; C, Polystyrene float under palm; D, Swimming ring used as a float.

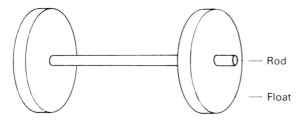

Fig. 9.40 Polystyrene floats with connecting rod.

be affixed to the side rails as a support. Most such supports should incline so that the patient lies with the face out of the water, but the feet will be totally immersed (Fig. 3.9A and B).

Contra-indication for pool exercises

(1) Skin infections especially Tinea pedis (athlete's foot).
(2) Those prone to sudden attacks of unconsciousness, e.g. poorly controlled epileptics or the older person prone to 'drop' episodes.
(3) Patients with ischaemia affecting the heart or brain although some hypertensive patients are suitable. Individual medical decisions should be made.
(4) Patients with poor respiratory function should be carefully selected.
(5) Those with perforated eardrums who are to have vigorous exercise which may make splashing inevitable.
(6) Patients, especially adults, who are afraid of water. Children can sometimes be coaxed out of their fear by careful progression from a 'ball pool' (see Fig. 7.1) to a very small pool and so into a larger therapeutic pool.

Balance

Balance in water is maintained by both buoyancy and hydrostatic pressure. The latter is equal in all directions and slight movement makes the body subject to the turning force which may be attempting to return the body back to the original position, or allow it to fall over. If a patient remains still in water then balance, either of the whole body, e.g. in standing, or of any other part is maintained. Deviation from the stationary situation causes loss of balance of forces on the body or body part and is especially noticeable in the standing position in water.

Any factors which increase the pressure on any one aspect of the body will cause loss of balance and create a need for recovery. We especially notice this when standing in natural water which has waves. In the pool, turbulence caused by the therapist or patient using hand movements will cause loss of balance and a need to react by using appropriate muscle work, e.g. turbulence on the patient's right will cause him to fall to that side and the muscles of his left will work to prevent him doing so.

The starting positions which may be used in the pool are discussed in Chapter 3, re-education of muscle in Chapter 11 and mobilization of joints in Chapter 12.

Special techniques in water

Bad Raqaz techniques

Proprioceptive neuromuscular facilitation (PNF) techniques described in Chapter 23 have been developed at Bad Raqaz in Switzerland so that functional movement patterns can be used in water. The techniques involve using buoyancy for flotation with the therapist as the fixed point, and moving the patient to achieve the selected oblique pattern of movement.

Method

The therapist must be in the pool with the patient and have a stable position from which to work. The water level should be no higher than the waist level or lower thoracic spine of the therapist. The patient is supported by his neck and trunk or by pelvic floats and limb floats as necessary. The size and density of the floats are varied according to the resistance required.

The therapist grasps the patient in such a manner that she offers resistance to the appropriate pattern of movement, remembering that the nearer the grasp to the point of buoyancy the less the resistance. By moving her grasp more distally the therapist can progress both strength of muscle action and range of movement. The therapist remains still and fixes the part in the required position. She asks the patient to move, controlling the type of muscle action by using the techniques described above and in Chapter 23. Thus a slow reversal is performed when the patient moves away from and then towards the therapist. Stabilizations are performed if the range of movement is minimal, and the amount of resistance can be varied through the combined actions in accordance with the muscle strength, to gain irradiation from strong to weak muscles using repeated contractions.

Stabilizations (see Chapter 23) are isometric contractions performed alternately on opposite aspects of a joint by opposing muscle groups. As on land, the joint is moved to a pain free position or to the position of muscle weakness. The patient is moved away from the therapist's holding hand first, then towards the holding hand to gain contraction in first one muscle group and then their opponents. The range of the movement will decrease as the muscles co-contract to stabilize the joint. On land the primary use is for co-ordination and balance and the exercise is of similar value in water.

Chapter 10
RE-EDUCATION OF WALKING

M. Hollis

Walking, together with its variants – running, going up and down stairs – is a skilled co-ordinated action which we acquire in infancy and improve with practice. It is an action which involves many joints and muscles, but which is performed by each of us without conscious effort until one of the muscle or joint components involved is disordered. As we walk we move our body components in an orderly manner, adapting to the surface trodden upon and to the space and hazards around us. The whole sensory input is involved and when any part of the sensory system is disordered, gait may also be affected.

Analysis of the disorder and examination of the whole patient may reveal one small cause which, when treated, will resolve the disorder of gait. It is no part of this book to analyse all the gait disorders, but in order to teach the use of walking aids and the return of a patient to the use of normal gait it is necessary to consider all of the muscles and joints which may be involved unless use of a wheelchair is to be a longer term, interim or permanent measure.

The propulsion muscles are the flexors of the toes, the plantarflexors of the ankles and the extensors of the knee and hip. The 'swing-through' muscles are the extensors of the toes, the dorsiflexors of the ankle, the flexors and extensors of the knee and the flexors of the hip.

The abductors and medial and lateral rotators of the hip and side flexors and rotators of the trunk also work in weight transference and pelvic movement. Without adequate pelvic movement in both rotation and hip hitching, correct walking is impossible. The upper trunk and head rotators also work, so that the face and upper trunk maintain a forward facing direction. The range of work of each of these groups will depend upon the length and height of the step.

With so many muscles involved in the act of walking it is necessary to maintain their strength, especially those of the weight-bearing limb. In the trunk the additional muscles must also be retrained and/or strengthened and the normal swing of the arms when walking must not be forgotten.

The following regime of exercises should be given to a patient who is in bed and will eventually use crutches or a partial weight-bearing walking aid. All exercises should be resisted by the use of springs or weights when possible and some of those in the sequence may be practised during the course of a ward class or even set to music.

For the arms
- gripping
- wrist extension

- elbow extension
- shoulder extension
- shoulder medial rotation
- shoulder depression

For the trunk
Upper trunk – rotation
                     extension
                     flexion

Lower trunk – rotation
                     extension
                     flexion
pelvic side flexion or hip hitching.

For the legs
- toe and foot flexion and extension
- knee flexion and extension
- hip flexion and extension
- hip abduction and adduction
- hip medial and lateral rotation

Some of these exercises may be performed isotonically, others isometrically and some may be performed together. For example, with the patient in slight crook lying the therapist may stand at the foot of the bed and, resisting on the soles of the feet, command the patient to perform first a bilateral extension thrust using hip and knee extensors and ankle plantarflexors, followed by the reverse movement, with the resistance on the dorsum of the foot. If the resistance is strong enough the patient will slightly extend the lower trunk on the thrust and flex on the pull up.

Alternate leg thrusting with a straight hip and knee will cause the patient to perform hip hitching and thus side flex the trunk on the opposite side and use the hip abductor on the thrust side. If the therapist maintains pressure on the soles of the feet or uses a foot board on the bed, or the temperature chart board, then the plantar reflex will be stimulated and

the muscles which normally work on the 'stance' phase of walking will all tend to work simultaneously.

Some of the exercises shown in Figs 9.21–9.25 are very suitable for the patient to practise alone. The patients should be encouraged to reach down to the side and across the bed to use their locker and so work the arms and trunk and maintain some balance reactions.

Progression
A patient who has spent a long time in the low half lying position (three pillows) will take a little time to accommodate to the upright position and should be taught to pull in the abdominal wall or to take several deep breaths to ensure good venous return and an adequate supply of blood to the brain before being sat more upright. Patients who are suspected of poor balance reactions may be given 'rhythmic stabilizations' or 'tapping' (Chapter 23) in half lying, crook sitting, high sitting on the side of the bed, feet resting on a stool, or preferably in sitting in a wheelchair in which the patient will feel more secure, to ensure they are ready to start standing practice.

Retraining plinths are of great value for those patients who need to be re-introduced to weight bearing following injury to the lower limbs. The plinth can be tilted gradually from the horizontal to the upright so that there can be a gradual increase in the weight borne on the affected part (Fig. 10.1).

Preparation for walking

The patient should, if possible, be taken to a retraining area fitted with parallel bars and steps. The wheelchair is placed between the parallel bars, the brakes applied, and the patient moved to the front of the chair, the footrests

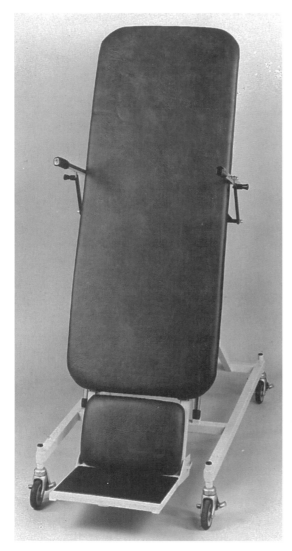

Fig. 10.1 A re-training plinth for gradual introduction of weight-bearing.

more distant from her with the palm (thumb out) of the other hand, or by exerting assisting pressure with the axillary grip using the palm only of each hand in the axillae (with the thumb out – one hand across the front to the far axilla, one hand at the back of the near axilla), while blocking the foot and knee from the side. Alternatively the therapist may stand in front of the patient and block the foot with one foot and pull on either the waistband or under the buttocks, thus bringing the patient into standing. The method chosen will depend on the relative heights of patient and therapist, on the stoutness of the patient and the length of the therapist's arms and on the balance ability of the patient.

The patient should now practise balance, and 'rhythmic stabilizations' may be practised with pressures on either the shoulders or the pelvis or both. The patient must be encouraged to perform small range flexion and extension of the standing leg and to move the arms in turn forwards and backwards on the bars. If he can bear weight on both legs he should practise transferring his weight first from side to side in stride standing and then forwards and backwards in walk standing. Pressure from the therapist on the pelvis of the side towards which he is swaying will encourage him to push the pelvis in that direction over the base and so transfer weight to the leg and support of that side. He should be allowed to have several rests as required.

After explanation and perhaps a demonstration he may attempt to progress along the parallel bars using initially a swing-to gait (Fig. 10.7A) and eventually may be given one or both of his walking aids to use in the parallel bars. He should, if the parallel bars are wide enough, walk first inside them, so that he has something to grasp if he feels unstable. He may use one bar and one walking aid, then both aids, then proceed outside the bars, but perhaps walk

raised and, by pulling with his arms on the parallel bars he is encouraged to stand up bearing weight wherever he is permitted to do so. The therapist should stand at the side and block the standing shoe toe with her instep and the knee of that leg with her knee. She should assist the patient to rise either by pressure on the sacrum with one hand and under the axilla of the side alongside them provided there are no floor obstructions.

Eventually he will walk free of the bars but a distance target should be given to him. 'Walk to the door' with the therapist perhaps holding his clothing at the back or putting a steadying hand on his sacrum and one shoulder, until he is more confident and capable of walking with just an escort. The target of distance walked should be constantly revised and the therapist should not hesitate to suggest frequent rests for patients who are afraid or frail or weak. Equally, as the patient performs better and more strongly, not only should the daily distance walked be increased but the rests should be less frequent.

Turning must be taught early unless the bars are of inordinate length and the wheelchair can be taken inside them. In taking the patient any distance inside or outside the bars it must be remembered that he must traverse a similar distance to return to his wheelchair.

Turning

In the parallel bars
The foot is hopped through 45° or less and the now rear arm is moved to the bar the patient is turning to face. A series of hops complete the turn beyond 90° and the arm on the side of the turning direction is moved to behind the patient. Further hops complete the turn.

With walking aids
The direction of turn is decided and agreed. The aid on that side is moved backwards and that on the opposite side is moved forwards with a small hop of the appropriate foot as described below. The sequence of moves for a patient weight-bearing on only one leg and turning to the right should be: right aid back, hop leg to right, left aid forwards, hop leg to right, and repeat until the turn is complete. For a patient

weight-bearing on both legs and able to move them separately the sequence for a turn to the right would be: right aid back, left leg forwards and turned to the right, left aid forwards, right leg back and turned to the right, and repeated to complete the turn.

Some strong patients will complete the process in possibly one or two moves.

Walking up stairs
The patient walks close up to the bottom step, takes his injured limb backwards and, leaning on his walking aids, hops up one step. His walking aids are now brought up on to the same step and the process repeated. Alternatively he may take both walking aids in one hand and use the banister rail. The procedure is as above, i.e. sound leg first, walking aid last.

Some patients may have to go upstairs backwards on their bottom, in which case the hands are put flat on the step above and the trunk raised on to the same step.

Walking down stairs
The patient walks close to the top of the stairs and puts his injured limb in front of himself. He places his walking aids on the step below, lowering by flexing his standing limb. He now hops this limb down to join the walking aids, or he may put both walking aids in one hand and, using the banister rail follow the above sequence of moving his walking aid first and his leg last, or he may sit on the floor and lower his bottom on to the step below his hands.

The disadvantage of climbing up or downstairs on the bottom is that either two sets of walking aids are needed, one at each end of the flight of stairs, or the aids have to be moved up and downstairs by an assistant or the patient hooking them on to one forearm.

Walking aids

Walking aids are appliances which may be a means of transferring weight from the upper limb to the ground or which may be used to assist balance. They fall into the following categories: single point or multipoint, tripod or quadruped (Figs 10.2–10.4).

Each point or tip should be rubber or plastic shod with a ferrule of material having a high co-efficient of friction and which fits well. Some ferrules are multiringed and depressed to form a vacuum when in contact with the ground; others have multiple small protuberances (Fig. 10.2A).

All should have a metal washer inside to prevent the tip of the aid from piercing the ferrule.

Sticks

The upper ends of sticks are of several designs as in Fig. 10.2B, C, D and E. The 'crook' top is usually a wooden stick (Fig. 10.2D) and the flat top and swan-neck top are usually of light metal. Wooden sticks cannot easily have multipoint tips whereas the metal sticks can and they can also be of adjustable length (Figs 10.2B, C and E and 10.3A and B), as can frames (Fig. 10.6A, B, C).

The correct length of stick allows 15° of flexion at the elbow when the patient is upright, the arm is by the side and the stick is a short distance in front of and to the side of the foot on that side. Measurement is taken with the patient lying or standing with the arm by the side, from the proximal wrist crease to the shoe heel or the ground 15 cm lateral to the shoe heel. This degree of flexion allows the elbow to straighten when a 'thrust' is made upon the stick as it is used to propel the body forwards. Figures 10.4A and B show correct positions for a stick in use.

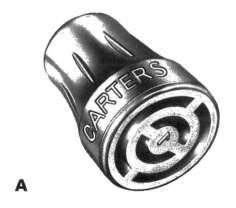

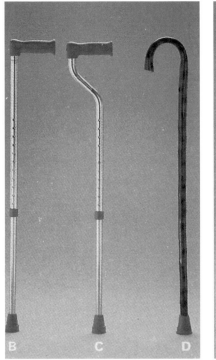

Fig. 10.2 Sticks and ferrules; A, A vacuum type ferrule; B, Adjustable metal stick; C, A Swan-neck stick in adjustable metal; D, A wooden walking stick; E, An adjustable metal walking stick with an ergonomic handle.

Crutches

Crutches may also be of wood or metal and should be adjustable both in hand grip to ground length and in axilla to hand grip length (Fig. 10.5A–E).

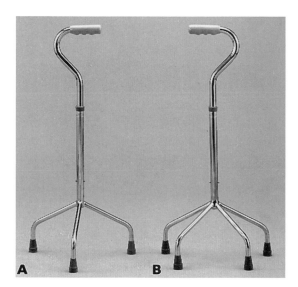

Fig. 10.3 A, A Swan-neck handled tripod; B, A quadripod.

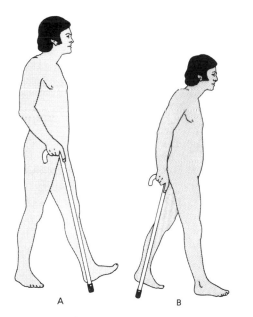

Fig. 10.4 A, B. The correct positions for a stick in use. The figure shows the correct walking pattern using one stick.

Axillary crutches

These should be used when weight must be relieved from one leg and can be used to train partial weight bearing before progressing to sticks.

The length is important as the axillary pad must not push up into the axilla, but must be high enough to allow it to be held between the upper arm and the chest wall when weight is put on the crutch. Measurement should be made with the patient's shoes on from the shoe heel to 5 cm below the posterior axillary fold. If the shoes cannot yet be put on, measurement is made from the tip of the medial malleolus to the posterior axillary fold. The position of the hand piece should be adjusted as for a pair of sticks, i.e. to allow 15° of flexion of the elbow when the crutch is held in to the side and is resting 15 cm out from and in front of the shoe toe.

Elbow crutches

These are essentially sticks of adjustable length with a horizontal hand grip and a metal forearm rest which may be in the form of a spring band which is sufficiently elastic to allow the arm to be put through the opening, but tight enough to stay in position on the forearm should the patient release his grip on the hand piece. These crutches are not as stable as axillary crutches, and are more frequently issued for long-term use as, with practice, it is possible to achieve balance and to let go of a crutch without losing it, in order to perform some manual task, e.g. opening a door, putting shopping in a bag (Fig. 10.5E).

Forearm bearing (gutter) crutches

These are metal adjustable crutch legs with a gutter splint mounted on the top with, usually, a handle at the front which can be set at an adjustable angle. The forearm is held in the

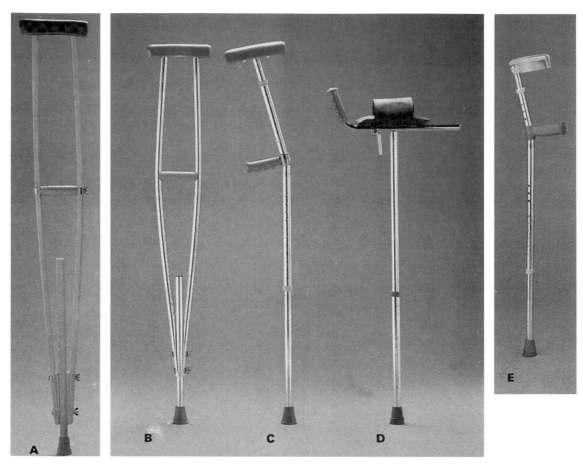

Fig. 10.5 A, A wooden axillary crutch – length and handle adjustable; B, A metal axillary crutch – length and handle adjustable; C, French type axillary crutch; D, A gutter crutch, length adjustable; E, An elbow crutch adjustable above and below the hand grip.

gutter splint by straps of Velcro or leather and the hand grips the adjusted handle. These crutches are used when weight cannot be taken through the forearms and hands, e.g. in fractures of these parts or in rheumatoid arthritis of the wrist and hand (Fig. 10.5D).

Pick-up aids or frames

These are essentially large-based frames having four points and two or three sides. They are used by picking them up, moving them forwards, putting them down, leaning upon them and walking into the frame. They should be adjustable in height (Fig. 10.6A, B and C). Variations may have:

(1) A reciprocal mechanism which allows right hand movement with left leg movement, but this type is often disliked by unsteady patients
(2) Two front legs and two rear casters
(3) Two front legs and two rear wheels with brakes which operate on downward pressure on the wheels

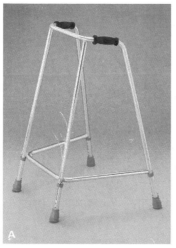
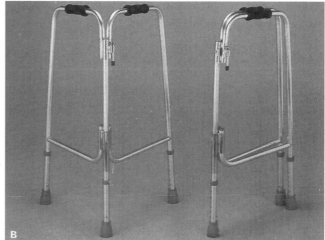
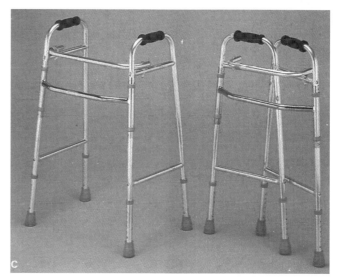

Fig. 10.6 Pick-up aids or frames: A, with three fixed sides; B, with two fixed sides and folding; C, with three fixed sides and folding.

(4) Wheels on all four legs, with or without brakes

(5) 'Square' wheels

(6) A mechanism which allows them to be folded. This facilitates travelling with an aid and also allows the aid to be carried up and down stairs (Fig. 10.6B and C).

The disadvantage of all except the reciprocal frame is the normal pattern of heterolateral limb movement cannot be used, and they cannot be used up and down staircases.

Crutches may be used to allow mobility when one leg must be non-weight bearing, when both legs may bear weight but cannot propel in normal walking action, or they may be used for partial weight bearing. The strength and needs of the patient will determine the method of use.

Sticks may be used to relieve a small amount of weight or to help with balance, and multipoint pick-up aids are used primarily to help with balance.

Patterns of use

Crutches

Three-point walking

Swing-to

The crutches start in front of the supporting leg. They are lifted and placed further in front, weight is taken on them and the sound leg is bent and swung to just behind the crutches. The disabled leg should be held clear of the ground and in front of the body (Fig. 10.7A).

Swing-through

The above procedure is followed but the sound leg is swung through the crutches and the foot is put down in front of them. This technique is for stronger patients (Fig. 10.7B).

Both these techniques may be used with any type of crutch.

Four-point walking

Both legs swing-to or swing-through

Both legs are swung forwards together and placed either just behind or just in front of the crutches. This technique is more likely to be used by the paraplegic patient and it will depend on his ability and strength whether he will move one crutch at a time, but the legs may be moved together or separately (Fig. 10.8A and B).

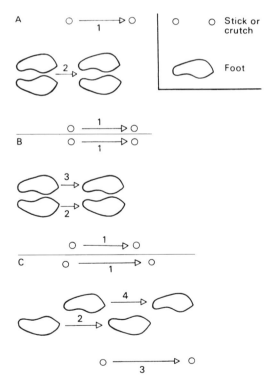

Fig. 10.8 Four-point gaits. Numbers indicate order of swing-through. A, Crutches moved together. A 'swing-to' pattern; B, Crutches moved together, then each leg in turn. A 'swing-to' pattern; C, Correct walking sequence. One crutch or stick, opposite leg, other crutch or stick, opposite leg.

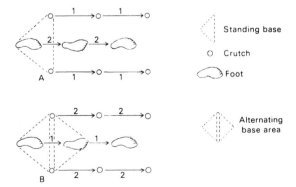

Fig. 10.7 Three-point gait. One leg non-weight-bearing. A, The swing-to gait: 1, crutches moved; 2, foot moved. B, The swing-through. The numbers denote the sequence of 'swing-through'.

Three and one pattern

The crutches and partial weight-bearing leg go forward together and the able leg alone, while weight is distributed on the other three points which are resting on the ground. This technique is used following non-weight bearing for a limb and when full weight may not yet be taken on an injured limb.

Sticks

Two sticks

(1) Both sticks may be taken forward with the injured leg, then the sound leg is brought through. This is a progression on the above type of crutch walking (four-point walking – three and one pattern).

(2) The sticks may be used reciprocally in a normal walking pattern. Right stick, left leg, left stick, right leg. Patients sometimes take a little time to achieve this, but its advantage is that the normal walking pattern is used ready for discarding the aids, or is maintained if the aids have to be used for some considerable time (Fig. 10.8C).

One stick

(1) With the stick held on the opposite side from the disablement, the walking pattern can be preserved when the only disablement is of one leg. The sequence is: disabled leg and stick, then sound leg and free arm swing forward together and in turn (Fig. 10.9A).

(2) With the stick held on the opposite side from the disabled arm and leg, the best pattern is: stick and disabled leg, then sound leg. The disabled arm may not be able to swing. Sometimes this sequence proves impossible and a more 'crab-like' gait has to be permitted, advancing first the stick, then the sound leg, and the dis-

abled leg last. The disabled arm will trail even more. In these cases a multi-point stick would almost invariably be used (Fig. 10.9B and C).

(3) Occasionally a patient may use one stick in the hand on the same side as the disabled leg. This is commonly done when severely disabling pain is suffered, when the stick and leg are moved forward together.

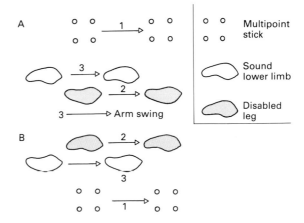

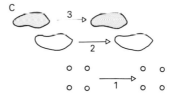

Fig. 10.9 A, A multipoint stick held in the hand opposite to the disabled leg. They move together, then the sound leg and free arm move together; B, A multipoint stick held on the opposite side from the disabled leg and arm. The desirable gait is stick and disabled leg move together, then the sound leg. The disabled arm may not be able to swing; C, The stick is held as in B, but the stick and sound leg move together leaving the disabled leg to 'trail' behind. An undesirable gait as the disabled arm will 'trail' even more than in B. The numbers denote the probable sequence of the 'swing-through'.

Pick-up aid

The patient puts the aid forwards and walks into it. He should be encouraged to try to take two small even steps – one with each leg – in moving into the aid, otherwise a more disordered gait may develop.

Wheelchair

Some patients may require exercise while in a wheelchair for temporary disablement, e.g. amputation until weight-bearing with confidence and endurance, or permanent disablement such as paraplegia. Thus a therapist may be confronted with deciding on the possibility of giving suitable activity to patients of very varying needs who are using a self-propelled wheelchair. After the patient has been introduced to the wheelchair and has learned basic management so that it acts as a substitute for his legs, he may perform other activities from it. The freest exercise and greatest choice of exercise activity can be taken if the chair arms can be removed and the chair back is sufficiently low to allow arm and upper trunk movement; greater limitations will be imposed if this is not so.

Wheelchair safety

The brakes must be efficient, the seat surface must not be too slippery and there should be no adjacent obstructions: the surrounding floor may need to be covered with mats to soften a fall if vigorous exercise is planned. Mechanical factors to be considered not only involve friction (brakes and seat) but the size of the base of the chair related to the patient's height and bulk. A tall, top heavy patient with no leg control and poor balance should not, for example, be encouraged to throw a heavy ball overhead and a long way. This courts loss of equilibrium.

To assess capacity to exercise in a wheelchair ask the following:

• Can the patient grasp and let go?
• Can the patient reach forwards, sideways, upwards and behind (one- or two-handed as appropriate)?
• Can the patient displace and recover the trunk in movements of trunk rotation, side flexion, flexion and extension?
• Does the patient understand and is he able to perform braking, use of footrests, removal of chair arms, use or removal of special fittings?

From a wheelchair the following may be possible:

• Balance exercises for head, upper trunk, lower trunk
• Loaded (by weights) exercises for the hands, elbows, shoulders, upper trunk (all movements) leading to ability to lift own body weight in chair
• Loaded (by pulleys) exercises for the arms and perhaps the knees
• Loaded (by springs) exercises for the elbow, shoulders, upper trunk, ankles
• Speed exercises using small apparatus which does not roll away.

When team exercises are used, a mixed ability group (some chairbound and some agile) will allow a greater choice of equipment as the agile can act as retrievers initially. Eventually the wheelchairbound will be able to participate in many sporting activities which will increase their co-ordination and physical capacity. Involvement in competitive sport will fulfil their emotional needs and allow, if they wish, participation up to international level.

Chapter 11
EXAMINATION, ASSESSMENT AND RECORDING OF MUSCLE STRENGTH

M. Hollis

Muscle malfunction may be easy to identify if disablement is very apparent; on the other hand only complete examination will reveal the exact strength of muscle and its endurance.

Muscle strength is recorded using the Oxford Scale in which:

0 = No contraction is present.
1 = There is a flicker of contraction.
2 = The muscle is capable of performing the full available range of movement with gravity counterbalanced.
3 = The muscle is capable of performing movement against the resistance of gravity into the fullest available range.
NOTE: It may not be possible to arrange the patient so that gravity offers resistance throughout the full range. Those muscles which perform over joints having a range much greater than 90°, such as the quadriceps or hamstrings, will have to be tested through the available gravity-resisted range.
4 = The muscle is capable of performing movement against the resistance of gravity and

an added resistance, which should be measured.
5 = The muscle functions normally.

In order to carry out an examination the part should be adequately undressed and compared, if possible, with the other side of the body if that is normal.

Observation will reveal loss of muscle bulk, although this may be irrelevant to loss of power. Passive movement should then be performed to test the passive length of the muscle.

Grades 0, 1 and 2 can be identified by placing the part so that movement can be performed in a gravity neutral situation. The therapist should be able both to see and feel the muscle belly and/or tendon and should not apply manual control to the part moved by the muscle under test, although consideration should be given to placing the muscle in a situation of mechanical and physiological advantage, e.g. use the middle range, ask the muscle to perform its own normal method of working – isotonic shortening or lengthening as the case may be – stretch the muscle slightly first, then release the grasp at once. If there is any contraction but little or no movement, then the grade is 1, and if movement through the full available range occurs then the grade is 2.

The position is then changed so that gravity offers resistance to the greatest possible range of movement and again a stretch may be applied before the patient attempts the movement. If the patient can perform a movement through the maximum available range the grade is 3, but care must be taken when testing for this grade that the muscle is isolated and the patient cannot cheat or perform 'trick' movements.

Grade 4 is tested by using the antigravity position as above and adding a known load in the form of weights (see later section on loading). A Grade 4 test may involve testing a 1 repetition maximum (1 RM). In such a test a muscle is required to lift a maximum load *once* only through most of its range. The 1 RM is only used for recording and testing purposes and once performed may exhaust a muscle for a time. A patient should not be required to perform a 1 RM more than once a week.

Normal muscle Grade 5 can perform any of the four roles outlined in group muscle action, i.e. act as agonist, antagonist, synergist and fixator. It can act slowly or quickly and stop as well as start movements. It can work equally well isometrically and isotonically, whether shortening or lengthening, and it has endurance for normal daily activities.

Endurance

This implies the capacity of a muscle to perform normally throughout a day's activities and at the end of the day be no more fatigued than any other muscle in the body. Endurance is tested by subjecting the patients to a full day's activity and observing their state at the end of the day, although in fact endurance may be a subjective assessment made by the therapeutic team

consisting of the patient and all those who work with him towards his recovery. It may involve sending him to a rehabilitation and/or training centre where he is subject not only to therapeutic procedures but also to workshop practice both with regard to his working day and the demands of a productive job.

Recording

A sample record of voluntary muscle power is shown in Table 11.1.

Re-education of muscle

When a muscle which has apparently lost all power is to be re-educated it is necessary to give it both physiological and mechanical advantage so that if it is possible for the muscle to contract it will be able to do so.

Mechanical advantage may be offered by positioning the patient so that either gravity offers assistance to the movement which the muscle normally performs, or preferably so that the part is in a position in which gravity is neutral and offers neither resistance nor assistance to the movement to be performed.

The patient should have a demonstration of the movement which is to be performed and should watch intently while this is being done. Clearly audible commands and instructions should be given before and during the training regime.

The movement should be done in middle range if this is the point at which the muscle will act at right angles to its bony attachment. A choice will have to be made between either an isotonic shortening or an isotonic lengthening as the first attempt at muscle action and it is more usual to choose the normal activity of the muscle; if normal activity is an isometric contraction then this is used with the therapist's hand offering resistance in the normal position

Table 11.1(a) Record of voluntary muscle power: upper extremity.

NAME					DATE OF BIRTH	
DIAGNOSIS						

RIGHT	Date	UPPER EXTREMITY			Date	LEFT
		Nerve	*Roots*	*Muscle*		
		Accessory	$A_cC_2C_3$	sternomastoid		
			$A_cC_3C_4$	trapezius ⎰ upper		
			$A_cC_2C_3C_4$	trapezius ⎨ middle		
			$A_cC_2C_3C_4$	⎱ lower		
		Brachial plexus	$C_3C_4C_5$	levator scapulae		
			C_4C_5	rhomboids		
			$C_5C_6C_7$	serratus anterior		
			$C_5C_6C_7C_8T_1$	pectoralis major		
			$C_4C_5C_6$	supraspinatus		
			C_5C_6	infraspinatus		
			$C_6C_7C_8$	lattissimus dorsi		
			C_6C_7	teres major		
		Axillary	C_5C_6	teres minor		
			C_5C_6	deltoid ⎰ anterior		
			C_5C_6	deltoid ⎨ middle		
			C_5C_6	⎱ posterior		
		Musculus cutaneus	C_5C_6	biceps brachii		
			C_5C_6	brachialis		
		Radial	$C_6C_7C_8$	triceps ⎰ long hd.		
			$C_6C_7C_8$	triceps ⎨ lateral hd.		
			$C_6C_7C_8$	⎱ medial hd.		
			$C_5C_6C_7$	brachioradialis		
			C_6C_7	ext. carpi rad. long.		
			C_7C_8	ext. carpi rad. brev.		
			C_5C_6	supinator		
			C_7C_8	extensor digitorum		
			C_7C_8	ext. digiti minimi		
			C_7C_8	ext. carpi ulnaris		
			C_7C_8	abd. pollicis longus		
			C_7C_8	ext. pollicis longus		
			C_7C_8	ext. pollicis brevis		
			C_7C_8	ext. indicis		

Table 11.1(a) *cont.*

RIGHT	Date	UPPER EXTREMITY			Date	LEFT
		Nerve	*Roots*	*Muscle*		
		Median	C_6C_7	pronator teres		
			C_6C_7	flex. carpi radialis		
			C_7C_8	palmaris longus		
			$C_7C_8T_1$	flex. dig. superficialis		
			C_8T_1	flex. dig. prof. 1 & 2		
			C_8T_1	flex. pollicis longus		
			C_8T_1	abd. pollicis brevis		
			C_8T_1	opponens pollicis		
			C_8T_1	flex. pollicis brevis		
			C_8T_1	lumbrical 1		
			C_8T_1	2		
		Ulnar	C_7C_8	flex. carpi ulnaris		
			C_8T_1	flex. dig. prof. 3 & 4		
			C_8T_1	abd. dig. minimi		
			C_8T_1	opp. dig. minimi		
			C_8T_1	flex. dig. min. brev.		
			C_8T_1	lumbrical 3		
			C_8T_1	4		
			C_8T_1	interossei palmar 1		
			C_8T_1	2		
			C_8T_1	3		
			C_8T_1	4		
			C_8T_1	dorsal 1		
			C_8T_1	2		
			C_8T_1	3		
			C_8T_1	4		
			C_8T_1	add. pollicis		

Notes:

Table 11.1(b) Record of voluntary muscle power: lower extremity.

NAME   DATE OF BIRTH
DIAGNOSIS

RIGHT	*Date*	LOWER EXTREMITY			*Date*	LEFT
		Nerve	*Roots*	*Muscle*		
		Femoral	$L_1L_2L_3$	ilio-psoas		
			L_2L_3	sartorius		
			$L_2L_3L_4$	quadriceps ⎰ rect. fem.		
			$L_2L_3L_4$	vast. lat.		
			$L_2L_3L_4$	vast. med.		
			$L_2L_3L_4$	vast. inter.		
		Obturatori	$L_2L_3L_4$	add. longus		
			$L_2L_3L_4$	add. magnus		
			L_2L_3	gracilis		
		Inf. glut.	$L_5S_1S_2$	gluteus maximus		
		Sup. gluteal	$L_4L_5S_1$	gluteus medius		
			$L_4L_5S_1$	gluteus minimus		
			L_4L_5	tensor fasciae latae		
				lateral rotator group		
		Sciatic	$L_5S_1S_2$	semimembranosus		
			$L_5S_1S_2$	semitendinosus		
			$L_5S_1S_2$	biceps femoris		
		Tibial	S_1S_2	gastrocnemius		
			S_1S_2	soleus		
			L_4L_5	tibialis posterior		
			S_2S_3	flex. dig. longus		
			S_2S_3	flex. hall. longus		
		Deep peroneal	L_4L_5	tibialis anterior		
			L_5S_1	ext. dig. longus		
			L_5S_1	ext. hallucis		
			L_5S_1	ext. dig. brevis		
		Sup. peroneal	$L_5S_1S_2$	peroneus longus		
			$L_5S_1S_2$	peroneus brevis		
		Plantar	S_2S_3	abductor hallucis		
			S_2S_3	lumbricals		
			S_2S_3	interossei		

Table 11.1(c) Record of voluntary muscle power: trunk.

RIGHT	Date	TRUNK			Date	LEFT
		Nerve	*Roots*	*Muscle*		
		Intercostal	T_{1-6}	intercostals upper		
		Intercostal	T_{7-12}	intercostals lower		
		V.R.	T_{6-12}	rectus abdominis		
		V.R.	T_{6-12}	ext. abd. oblique		
		V.R.	$T_{7-12}L_1$	int. abd. oblique		
		D.R.	$C_{3-8}T_{1-12}L_{1-5}$	erector spinae		
		Lumbar plexus	$T_{12}L_1L_2L_3$	quadratus lumborum		
		D.R.	$C_{4-8}T_{1-12}L_{1-5}$	intrinsic back muscles		

Notes:

in the range in which the muscle normally contracts isometrically.

The therapist's hands should be placed so that one can control the proximal part, i.e. the origin of the muscle and the joints proximal to this part, and so that the same hand can palpate the muscle belly.

The more distal hand will have to carry out several functions. In the first place it must offer resistance, especially so if a gravity-assisted movement is being used. The distance along the limb at which this hand is placed will control the length of the weight arm. Secondly, it may possibly have to initiate the movement, as it may be feasible for a muscle to continue a movement once inertia has been overcome; and thirdly, this hand will have to introduce some of the all-important physiological factors which facilitate the muscle's contraction. In other words, pressure on the 'leading' surface and stretch to the muscle to be worked will be applied by the distal hand.

With the patient concentrating mentally and having a mental picture of the movement to be performed, looking to see what is happening, listening to the therapist's clear commands, and the muscle being stretched rapidly immediately

prior to the command to work, there will be physiological summation of stimuli at the anterior horn cells supplying that particular muscle, more especially so if the muscle can contract and resistance can continue to be offered throughout the active movement.

Timing is very important at this point in the proceedings as the therapist must apply the stretch and immediately move the part so that the muscle can operate at a maximally satisfactory angle of pull and she must also immediately, if necessary, change the pressure on the part so that she resists, not assists, the movement. Practice will make the therapist more skilled in this particular technique.

Progression

Progress can be made in one of several ways based on the above points:

(1) The range through which the muscle works may be increased gradually.
(2) The amount of resistance offered by the therapist may be increased gradually.
(3) The length of the weight arm may be increased gradually.

(4)   The muscle may be required to initiate the movement as well as to continue to perform it.

(5)   The muscle may be required to work both in isotonic shortening and in isotonic lengthening in succession. This may be termed two-way innervation or continuous demand. The muscle is thus increasing its endurance as it is now working for twice the length of time of a single one-way contraction.

(6)   The muscle may be required to work isometrically at different points in the range. When the muscle can perform an isometric contraction as a true 'hold' it can be required to act as part of a team; that is, it can undertake each of the activities of group muscle action. By this time it would be anticipated that a muscle would be capable of carrying out a contraction at about Grade 2 on the Oxford Scale.

There is no reason whatsoever why, during the stage of recovery prior to this point being reached, the muscle should not be stimulated by being included in group activity or mass movement patterns as described in Chapters 20 to 22. When this is done the mass movement pattern is more usually done by the stronger proximal muscles which are then required to 'hold' (isometric muscle work) at the strongest point in the mass movement, while the therapist 'plays' on the paralysed or weak muscle – stretching it, concentrating the patient's attention on it and attempting to make it participate in the mass activity. If the therapist succeeds in persuading the muscle to work then the remainder of the mass movement pattern is continued, with the muscle included in the activity, but the quantity of resistance offered to the weak muscle will be less than that offered to the stronger muscles in the pattern of mass movement.

Table 11.2 Modified scale of assessment for use in water.

1	= Contraction with buoyancy assisting
2	= Contraction with buoyancy counter-balanced
2+	= Contraction against buoyancy
3	= Contraction against buoyancy at speed
4	= Contraction against buoyancy plus a light float
5	= Contraction against buoyancy plus a heavy float

(From *Duffield's Exercise in Water*, with permission).

When a muscle is learning to work as both an agonist and an antagonist, the technique known as 'slow reversals' is used. The muscle first works as an agonist and then, without pause, the movement is reversed so that the opposite muscles work and the former working muscle now relaxes reciprocally.

The muscle may do this in single joint movement, such as flexion and extension of the elbow or in a mass or group movement pattern such as taking the arm from the extension/abduction/medial rotation position to the flexion/adduction/lateral rotation position with the associated movements of the elbow, radio-ulnar, wrist, finger and thumb joints (associated flexion of elbow, supination and flexion of wrist and fingers). In this example, biceps brachii can thus be re-educated in its flexion of elbow/supinator role and also as a flexor of the shoulder via its short head; or the extension/adduction/medial rotation pattern with its associated movements may be used for opponens pollicis to be re-educated in its 'grasp' function.

Progressions of exercises for regaining muscle strength using the pool

There is no reason whatsoever, provided the patient is able to be immersed, that the pool should not be used for part of the muscle re-education.

First prepare the patient by following the routine set out in Chapter 9, 'Water'. The therapist must have completed a land assessment of muscle power and be aware of the patient's condition but may need to make the assessment shown in Table 11.2.

The scale in Table 11.2 is not the equivalent of the Oxford Scale, as normal, i.e. Grade 5, cannot be tested in water as this is not our normal environment for 24 hours a day and both increased speed and increased load make bigger demands on muscles in water.

The factors concerned in progress of exercises in water are:

(1)   Buoyancy
(2)   Length of weight arm of the part
(3)   Length of weight arm by added use of a float
(4)   Streamlining and speed of movement
(5)   Manual resistance or assistance by the therapist.

Buoyancy

If the part to be exercised is immersed in the water and allowed to move upwards to the surface assisted by buoyancy then

either there will be little or no muscle work
or the working muscles will be those reducing the speed of the movement by performing an isotonic lengthening.

To work the muscles on the superior surface of the part the therapist must offer minimal finger tip resistance, initially near the joint then further away, thus lengthening the weight arm. Positioning the patient so that buoyancy is neutral will be a small progression but will still require

either manual resistance from the therapist to ensure the required muscle work is performed
or the use of a bat to lengthen the weight arm and the use of slow speed of movement first
or an increase in the required speed of the movement to increase turbulence, first without a bat then with a bat.

Further adjustment of the patient's position can make greater use of buoyancy as a resistance. Turbulence (see above) can be used as a further progression. When the streamlining of the part is maximal, resistance is less; if the streamlining is less, resistance is greater. As the speed of movement is increased, resistance is also greater, e.g. the straight hand with the ulnar or radial borders leading in the direction of movement is streamlined maximally for arm movements. Turning the hand so that the dorsal or palmar surface lead, will decrease streamlining and thus increase resistance. If a bat is held, it too can lead with its narrow border, being turned to present maximum surface in the direction of movement to increase resistance. Turbulence will offer greater resistance if the speed of movement is increased in any of the dispositions of the hand and/or bat for streamline variation.

Initially the individual muscle or muscle group should be exercised and, when the patient is aware of what is required and strength is increasing, then special techniques may be used so that the weaker muscles are worked as part of a mass movement pattern. To use these techniques the therapist should first be familiar with the movement patterns described in Chapters 20, 21 and 22 and with the techniques described in Chapter 23. The following may be used.

Repeated contractions (see Chapter 23) when used in water, as on land, will act to increase strength in the weak part of the muscle range initially, thus building up full range strength and going on to greater endurance. Turbulence can be used so that the movement and the 'hold' are affected by it, and buoyancy and turbulence can be used together to obtain greater resistance. Turbulence is increased by either increased speed of movement or by use of a bat.

Stabilizations (see Chapter 23), can be used in water as on land to produce co-contractions. The part is first moved to the position of muscle weakness and the patient is moved first away from the therapist's holding hand and then towards the holding hand. Small movements are performed to gain a co-contraction.

A muscle needs to be re-educated at frequent intervals during the day so that short bursts of treatment are given rather than one long treatment in which the muscles and the patient become over fatigued. A well planned programme of re-education would start with the strongest group of muscles to be retrained, continue with the weaker groups and move from one part of the body to another so that each affected part is treated in turn, rests while another part works and then there is a return to work the strongest part again.

In addition to re-education of single actions, muscles must be re-educated to work in patterns, so that perhaps the first treatment may be of single actions, the second treatment of group or mass patterns (see Chapters 20 to 22), the third treatment may be in a change of medium, e.g. in the hydrotherapy pool with single and oblique patterns combined, whilst the fourth treatment could be a functional activity in which the weak muscle has to undertake perhaps objective work repetitively in order to increase endurance.

A programme such as this will not be possible for a very weak muscle below Grade 2 on the Oxford Scale, but once a muscle has

achieved Grade 2 then effort and endurance can rapidly be progressed through a programme as outlined above. In addition to the manual loading which the therapist will apply and constantly adjust, a regime of mechanical loading can be started.

First gravity is the resistance, then the weight arm is lengthened, then, as weights are added to the part, the weight arm may be first shortened and again lengthened.

Once a weight can be applied to a part it is important to use a weight which is known and recordable and a training regime for which the patient is partly responsible. The 10 repetition maximum (10 RM) is found for each muscle or muscle group. It can be estimated in several ways:

(1) Use is made of a spring balance which is attached so that it is at right angles to the middle of the arc of movement produced by the muscle. An effort is made by the patient to stretch the spring balance and a reading is taken. Three efforts are usually made and the average result taken as the 10 RM.

(2) The 10 RM may be known, as the training regime may have started with, for example, a $\frac{1}{2}$ kg weight and been increased daily.

(3) The therapist may place her hand on the part and ask the patient to make an effort against her resistance. If she then immediately takes sandbags in her hand until she feels the same 'load', then this weight can be used as the 10 RM.

If the patient can make ten efforts with that weight and the muscle just quivers with fatigue on the tenth attempt, then the therapist has made a correct estimate. If the muscle quivers after less than ten attempts the load is too heavy and if it does not quiver on the tenth attempt then the load is too light. After a rest the load should be adjusted and a further attempt should be made.

Once the 10 RM is known there are three training regimes which may be used.

De Lorme and Watkins

10 lifts of half 10 RM

10 lifts of three-quarters 10 RM

10 lifts of 10 RM

30 lifts four times weekly. Retest the 10 RM once weekly.

Macqueen

10 lifts of 10 RM repeated four times – total of 40 lifts three times weekly. The 10 RM is progressed every 1–2 weeks.

Zinovieff or Oxford

10 lifts of 10 RM

10 lifts of 10 RM – $^1/_2$ kg

10 lifts of 10 RM – 1 kg

10 lifts of 10 RM – $1^1/_2$ kg

10 lifts of 10 RM – 2 kg

10 lifts of 10 RM – $2^1/_2$ kg

10 lifts of 10 RM – 3 kg

10 lifts of 10 RM – $3^1/_2$ kg

10 lifts of 10 RM – 4 kg

10 lifts of 10 RM – $4^1/_2$ kg

100 lifts fives times weekly. The 10 RM may be progressed daily, but the 1 RM is usually tested and recorded less frequently. It is purely a measure of progress. If the 10 RM is less than 5 kg then reductions are made by making use of $^1/_4$ kg and $^1/_2$ kg units. Endurance is built up by the use of lesser resistances than the 10 RM and a higher repetition regime.

Although these regimes are most commonly used for building up large groups such as the extensors of the knee using a weight directly applied, there is no reason why the repetition maxima type of programme should not be used using a pulley and weight circuit or using a spring as the resistance.

In addition muscle re-education in circuit training must be included as part of the daily regime. Circuit training will have the advantage that a specially devised system of exercises for the particular patient with those especially weak muscles, will make those muscles work in a functional way. It will load the muscle in different ways and will give the patient a regime he can practise alone and in which he can aim at a weekly improvement in performance.

Circuit training

This is a means whereby a patient is given a series of exercises to be performed regularly, e.g. weekly or several times a week in a gymnasium, or up to three times a day unsupervised.

The object of using a circuit is to improve cardiovascular performance and muscular endurance. Regular testing and recording is essential. This involves both patient and therapist in some paperwork, especially in setting up the initial circuit.

A circuit usually consists of between six and eight exercises and may vary from simple, free exercises to those involving the use of as many pieces of apparatus as there are exercises in the circuit. Each patient must learn to perform each exercise adequately before he is allowed to use it in his circuit, and to this end uncomplicated exercises should be given. Circuits are not measures of skill and it is better to have good performance of an easier exercise than poor and reducing performance of a more complex exercise.

Circuits may be arranged either for activity of the whole body, to build up general fitness and endurance, or may be aimed at a more specific objective, e.g. strengthening one group of muscles by making those muscles work in several different ways: slowly and with control, fast, heavily loaded, associated with more distal muscles, associated with more proximal muscles and in a whole-body activity. It is usual to keep the number of repetitions of each exercise at a figure between five and thirty.

When devising circuits with a high apparatus content the timing must be carefully organized to prevent bunching and queuing. Apparatus circuits or very difficult circuits may be graded, usually into three divisions when the number of repetitions of each exercise controls the degree of difficulty.

If a fixed equipment circuit is to be set up it is possible to devise large cards to be placed in clear view beside the apparatus. These carry the following information:

- The *name* of the exercise
- The *number* of the exercise in the circuit
- An *outline drawing* of the exercise
- The *number of repetitions* to be done by each *grade* of participant (usually in three different colours, one for each grade)
- The *name* and *place* of the *next* exercise.

Each participant needs a card indicating his grade (by colour), the exercise numbers and a date of each attendance. He inserts the number of performances of each exercise on that day and when he reaches an agreed level he is retested and/or regraded to a higher grade.

Circuits can be of three main types: fixed time, fixed repetition and beginners circuits with progressions.

Fixed time

Fixed time circuits in which a certain number of exercises, usually six, are performed, each one for a limited time, usually one minute, with a one minute rest between each. The number of times the patient performs each exercise is counted and recorded when the circuit is first given and then recounted weekly. The daily performance should consist of the circuit of exercises performed without conscious rest and repeated three times in succession. The number of repetitions of each exercise need not be the test rate but should be an agreed lesser rate initially, and the patient should attempt to gain a higher repetition rate in the third run through the circuit and try gradually to increase the number of repetitions in each run through the circuit. If improvement has occurred, the number of times each exercise is performed per minute will have increased. This type of circuit increases endurance. Table 11.3 shows sample tables of exercise for fixed time and fixed apparatus circuits.

Fixed repetition

Fixed repetition circuits, in which, usually, six exercises are each performed for one minute on the test day with a one minute rest between. The number of times each exercise is done is recorded and the patient then repeats the regime doing each exercise the test number of times without conscious rest, and the circuit three times. On retesting after seven days it may be found that the total performance time for the circuit has dropped to less than six minutes. This type of circuit tends to increase strength slightly more than endurance.

Progression of a fixed time circuit is made by allowing the patient to achieve the maximum number of repetitions, which will be indicated by the same result on two successive weeks, and then changing that exercise for a more difficult one. A fixed repetition circuit is progressed by increasing the number of repetitions on the test day until a minute has elapsed, and this is the new daily target for each exercise. Again, when the patient cannot increase the number of repetitions of any exercise in a minute the limit has been reached, and that exercise should be made more difficult.

Beginners circuits with progressions

This type of circuit is more useful for groups of very mixed ability patients when each person in the group must do the same exercises. The therapist teaches the exercises to everyone, in circuit order, and fixes the circuit time using knowledge gained from the teaching; this time should be approximately that in which a good performer may complete

three laps of the circuit at half the maximum repetitions as determined in a fixed repetition circuit. Lower repetitions are then given to the less able performers. The repetition numbers are put on cards for each exercise in the circuit and the cards can be put up in the gymnasium or handed to each patient. Each patient performs his own number of repetitions of the exercises in the circuit, does

Table 11.3a Sample table of exercises for fixed time circuit, e.g. for knee injuries. Test time of 11 minutes; 6 exercises of 1 minute each and 5 rests of 1 minute each.

Exs. No.	Exercise name	Test No. of repetition 20th Oct.	Rep. 1	Rep. 2	Rep. 3	Test No. of repetition 27th Oct.
1	Sit down and stand up	30	20	25	30	
2	Run on the spot w. High Kn. raise	40	20	30	40	
3	Step St. to $^1/_2$ High St. w. $^1/_4$ turn round stool	24	15	18	24	
4	Skipping	24	16	20	24	
5	High Jump to touch target	8	6	7	8	
6	Run as far as possible in 1 minute	200 yds	200 yds	200 yds	200 yds	
		Recorded by a counter	Recorded by patient on day of exercise			Recorded by a counter

Table 11.3b Sample table of exercises for fixed apparatus circuit. (This is also a fixed repetition circuit.)

Exs. No.	Exercise name	Repetition No. for Beginner	Middle	Fit
1	Std. St. A. Bd. and Str. u. w. wt.	10	20	30
2	$^1/_2$ St. Hop in and out of hoop	6	15	25
3	Rch. Gsp. Ly. (under beam). Pull ups	6	12	20
4	Wk. St. Bd. to pick up quoit and post in wall bar	8	16	30
5	Toe. Supp Ly. Sitt. ups.	6	15	25
6	Run up and down inclined form to touch targets u. an d.	8	16	25

Table 11.3c Fixed time circuit: patient's record.

Exs. No.	Day 1 X X X	Day 3 X X X	Day 5 X X X	Day 1 X X X	Day 3 X X X	Day 5 X X X
1						
2						
3						
4						
5						
6						

each circuit three times, and checks and records his performance time. As each patient reduces his performance time to less than that estimated for his grade (e.g. beginner, middle and fit) he should move up a grade. The fit patient increases his repetitions to three-quarters and then to the maximum number of repetitions, aiming at performing them in the original estimate of circuit time.

Patients should be told exactly when to do the circuits, and to eliminate doubt should be given a card with the regime written down. It is advisable to check that the patient has sight of a suitable clock for the fixed time and beginners' regimes, and it sometimes helps if patients are paired and act as counters or timekeepers for each other. They should be advised that it is important that they complete each circuit without resting and that they record accurately for themselves.

The value of circuits lies not only in the increase of the patient's endurance and strength but in their flexibility in use and the transfer of the responsibility for his performance entirely to the patient. A young fit man with a knee injury can do a circuit alongside a chronic bronchitic as each of them is performing to his own limit but within the same rules.

Muscle loading

A muscle will work maximally if it is maximally loaded, i.e.

work = load.

Thus when work is demanded of a muscle it should be given maximum resistance in order to produce fatigue. Fatigue is indicated by:

(1) A slower response to command
(2) A slower or lesser range of performance
(3) Quivering of the muscle belly
(4) No action – this is extreme fatigue and rarely occurs in the incapacitated except when a paralysed muscle recovers and 'flickers' for the first time since onset of paralysis.

A muscle may be loaded in many ways, and the therapist will have to decide at which point to build up strength by maximal loading associated with low repetitions or endurance by a lesser loading associated with frequent repetitions.

There are three regimes which may be used for self practice (see pp. 153–4). However, these require first an estimation of the 10 RM and then its weekly re-establishment. The advantage of these regimes is that the performance of each is patient triggered and controlled, once the patient has been taught what to do, and he can use one of these regimes as part of a programme of treatment. One disadvantage is that maximal effort can be avoided by poor endeavour. Another is that patients often progress much faster than the orthodoxy of the regimes allows for. When this happens the therapist should use the principles of establishing the load and should train the patient to use a regime compatible with his needs and the aims of his treatment.

Manual loading

The greatest advantage of manual loading of any muscle work, whether a single muscle, a group or a whole pattern of action, is that the therapist can use her own hands both to stimulate effort and to palpate and can be continually aware of the patient's response; thus a variable resistance can be offered in accordance with the varying strength of the muscle(s) as it works in its various ranges and with differing capacities according to its quality of strength and degree of fatigue.

Self loading

This is also called auto loading and is brought about when a patient offers self-resistance to his own muscle actions. These may be in three ways:

(1) By offering resistance to the movement of one part of the body by resisting directly with another part, e.g. the right arm resisting the upward movement of the left arm, or the right leg crossed at the ankle over the left offering resistance to knee extension. In both these examples the movement is also occurring against the resistance of gravity. Similarly auto-resisted pulley circuits may be used (see Chapter 9).

(2) Movement of the body weight itself may be called auto loading as in standing, slowly bending and straightening the hips and knees.

(3) By performing a movement in such a manner that it is weighted by the intensity of the muscle action. Slow dramatic movements will self load a muscle action.

Variable loading

By using a spring as a resistance the work performed by the muscle can be varied as the spring will offer maximal resistance only when it is maximally stretched. The muscle may not put the same effort into each contraction. Moreover, the recoil of the spring may either return the part to a resting position with no effort from the muscle or may be controlled by the muscle thus performing an isotonic lengthening. In other words the more control the patient exerts on the spring the greater the muscle effort and the longer it will be performed as the muscle must first shorten isotonically and then lengthen isotonically.

Direct weight loading

Weights may be applied to the part to be exercised, either by placing a weight on the limb adjacent to the part to be exercised or by using a special appliance such as a de Lorme type boot (see Chapter 9). A pulley and weight circuit may also be used (Chapter 9). An exercise regime such as those described on pp. 153–4 may then be selected.

To be able to return for the next treatment session and perform at the same and a progressed level is the object of any exercise. An overloaded muscle will not do this and the demands on it should be lessened to allow slower strengthening.

Chapter 12
MOBILIZATION OF JOINTS

M. Hollis

To examine and test a joint prior to mobilization

The medical history should give enough information to allow the therapist to start by observing the patient arriving, undressing both sides of the body and taking up a well-supported position.

Relevant questioning will elicit more information, following which the therapist can observe the joint in detail for irregularities and palpate for change of temperature, state of swelling and painful areas.

Testing active range of movement, passive range and resisted range, should be followed by accurate recording. Tests of muscle power must also be made and recorded.

When the limitation of movement is not due to pathological causes within the joint but to neurological hypertonus, recording of range is irrelevant, but it will be necessary to record the abnormality of the muscle(s) working over the joint.

A joint may be immobile due to three main causes. It may be held still due to protective muscle spasm when severe pain is present. It may be held still and possibly in abnormal posture due to neurological hypertonus (spasticity). It may have little or no range due to pathological causes when changes have taken place to cause shortening of the peri-articular soft tissues or bony block as in osteoarthrosis.

Each of these requires a slightly different approach. In the first two cases it is necessary to relieve the spasm by reducing the tone to regain the range. In the case of soft tissue shortening these structures must be stretched, preferably by the patient. This third group includes those patients who lack the last few degrees of movement due to injury to or surgery upon joints or stiffness due to joints being held still for long periods by fixation. All three are amenable to exercise in water.

To relieve painful spasm

The patient is placed in a fully supported position using as large a base as possible. As the patient can often move at another joint and appear to be moving at the painful joint it is frequently necessary to fix joints in which undesirable movement could occur, so that 'trick' movements and 'cheating' are prevented. For example, in abduction of one hip unwanted movement in the contralateral hip is prevented by taking the leg to the side of the bed and flexing the knee over the side with the foot supported. Similarly, for extension of the hip unwanted movement is prevented by the patient fully flexing the contralateral leg and, if possible, holding the thigh against the abdomen.

For movement of the glenohumeral joint the patient should be in crook lying or sitting on a seat with a back support to prevent unwanted movement of the lumbar spine. The shoulder girdle is held still by the therapist, so that it is possible to isolate the anatomical movements of abduction and adduction, flexion and extension and medial and lateral rotation.

The best method of stabilizing the patient is by appropriate positioning. The therapist may give further support by using her hands. These methods are better than the use of straps or mechanical devices which should rarely be resorted to. The limb is allowed to rest in its position of minimal pain. If advisable it may be carefully supported in that position by the use of suspension or water (see later in this chapter for use of pool therapy).

The technique of 'hold relax' is applied (see Chapter 23) to the muscles which are in protective spasm without allowing any movement to occur at the painful joint, and the technique is repeated until some spasm is relieved and a pain free range of movement becomes possible. It is very important that the movement which is achieved is maintained by the therapist and that repetitive swinging movements of the part are not allowed to take place. In other words, following each relaxation, a little more range is gained and held, and at the end of the treatment the patient will have performed only one movement in that particular direction, but it will have been as full as possible, and the pain–spasm cycle pattern of events will have been broken.

If the 'hold relax' is applied in suspension it may be necessary and indeed is usually advisable to use the following procedure.

(1) Obtain a maximum 'hold' (isotonic contraction of the muscles in spasm).
(2) Grasp the part with the more distal of the two resisting hands.
(3) Apply traction and immediately give the command to 'relax' while continuing to increase the traction. The application of traction will prevent the limb from 'leaping' as the muscles relax and is especially essential when suspension is used as the supporting medium and when the muscle action is strong.

Once a range of movement has been achieved, the patient may be asked to perform the required movement actively to come out of the protective spasm position. He is asked to perform a normal movement against the resistance of the therapist, thus working the muscles which are antagonistic to those in spasm. In this way these muscles now become the agonists and the muscles which are in spasm become the antagonists and relax reciprocally as reciprocal inhibition is brought about.

At this point in the proceedings the patient may be asked to make frequent active resisted attempts at performing the desired movement at the limit of the available range, while bearing in mind that if a joint has been protected by pain–spasm, there may still be some condition existing at that joint for which too frequently repeated movements are undesirable.

Rhythmic stabilization (co-contraction of muscles) is a particularly useful technique in such conditions as periarthritis of the shoulder when there may be no movement of the glenohumeral joint, but isometric contractions may be given alternately to the various patterns of movement of the scapula (see Chapter 23). They should be followed by 'hold relax' to the muscles of the glenohumeral joint which may gain a little range.

Accessory movements

Sometimes joints are so stiff that anatomical functional movements are not possible. It may be feasible to mobilize the accessory movements before attempting an anatomical movement. By grasping the two components of the joint as near as possible to the joint surfaces and applying firm but gentle pressure in alternate directions, a gliding of the joint surfaces on one another may be possible. The range may be very small and the movements given should be repeated rhythmically and with some speed. Only the accessory movements should be attempted in this way.

Stretching soft tissues which are too tight

This is usually best brought about by the patient attempting to stretch the tissues himself. There are several techniques which may be used. The patient may make repeated efforts at achieving the difficult movement by working the muscles which would bring about the desired movement, e.g. if abduction is limited by tight medial structures the patient works the abductors, or if the last few degrees of elevation of the arm are lost then the patient should make repeated resisted attempts to gain the last few degrees of elevation. The resistance could be given by the therapist, or the patient could push a weight (sandbag) up the wall.

A second technique which may be used is pendular swinging in which the alternations of the pendulum will carry the limb past the limitation of movement and apply repeated minute stretch to the tight structures. The addition of a weight to the end of the limb will both distract the joint surfaces and increase the tendency of the pendulum to swing past the point of limitation. This technique is most commonly used for the shoulder and hip joints, but is equally valuable as a method for the smaller joints such as the wrist and ankle. At these joints rapidly alternating movements are performed and, although the limb of the pendulum is short, the effect of rapid alternations of direction will be to increase momentum in each direction and bring about stretch on tight structures and increase in range. The use of this technique for stiffness of the vertebral region is usually confined to movements of the lumbar spine by swinging the pelvis and legs in suspension, thus avoiding dizziness due to alternations in head movement. This is dealt with in Chapter 8.

However, free mobilizing activities for the trunk given in suitable starting positions with the use of the arms to add length to the pendulum may result in a gain in range by the judicious use of self-applied overpressure. Stride standing trunk side flexion with overpressure and stretch stride standing alternate toe touching with the opposite hand are examples of such exercises and are suitable for selected patients.

A third technique which may be used is that of an auto-pulley circuit (Figs 9.26 to 9.28), in which the patient may perform rapid alternations of the two limbs and so carry the stiff joint a little past its limitation each time. Or the patient may apply deliberate slight stretch to the tight structures by an added pull with the contralateral limb.

The fourth technique which is occasionally used is one of self-mobilizing by stretching tight structures using body weight. For example, to stretch a tight tendocalcaneous which is limiting full dorsi-flexion of the ankle joint, the patient may be put into step standing and lean forwards over the bent knee. If both heels are kept on their support the tendocalcaneous is stretched on both legs. This procedure should *never* be used unless the muscles acting over the joint being mobilized are already sufficiently strong to maintain the stability of the joint.

Following the relief of spasm or the regaining of range, any objective exercises may be used which will increase joint range, while interesting the patient and allowing him to forget his limitations. Some methods of working out such exercises are suggested in Chapter 7 on the use of small apparatus.

Mobilization of joints in water

Exercise in a pool may be of great value in increasing range of joint movement. The warmth of the water promotes relaxation and will also relieve pain so that protective muscle spasm may be reduced.

The routine procedure (Chapter 9, p. 131), for use of a pool should be followed and the therapist should be aware of the land assessment of the joint state and of the patient's general condition. The following rules should be observed:

(1) Good fixation of the rest of the body should be obtained by the use of supports or by the patient holding on the fixed apparatus or both.

(2) Starting positions should be selected to allow maximum range of joint movement without major alterations in the starting position, e.g. heave grasp prone $^{1}/_{2}$ support lying for hip extension. This allows maximum range of hip extension using buoyancy as an assistance. To progress, the $^{1}/_{2}$ plinth can be slipped along the rail into deeper water, thus allowing the movement to start from a more flexed position of the hips, yet still using buoyancy to assist in achieving hip

extension which is usually the most limited movement.

(3) Buoyancy should be used to assist or be neutral (counterbalanced), e.g. shoulder abduction can be started with the patient in low grasp sitting in shallower water. The range for the arm movement in water will be small and buoyancy will assist. The seat can then be moved into deeper water, or the patient may grasp at the opposite side and lean outwards towards the working arm. From full adduction the movement will then be first and briefly resisted by buoyancy, then assisted by it. To achieve buoyancy neutral movement the patient should be in float lying, but this position is more difficult to stabilize and fix than low grasp sitting.

(4) Slow movements should be used to minimize turbulence and thus resistance to the movement.

(5) Using a long weight arm (full length of the part perhaps plus a bat) will allow sweeping movements through the water. This may take the movement past the point of previous limitation.

The following may be used. Hold relax, repeated contractions and stabilizations can all be performed in water. Their use for strengthening muscles round painful joints is enhanced in water due to the effect of the water in reducing pain. Hold relax (see Chapter 23) is used in water, as on land, to increase range of movement. As buoyancy can be used to assist in obtaining the extra range on completion of the technique, the starting position should be chosen to permit this assistance.

Chapter 13
ASSESSMENT OF A PATIENT'S SUITABILITY FOR GROUP TREATMENT

M. Hollis & B. Sanford

All patients should be assessed before being given any treatment but patients are not always assessed as to their suitability for inclusion in a group of people to exercise together. This omission often arises because the patient is already being treated somewhere other than the gymnasium, e.g. as an in-patient or in an individual therapy room. Such transfers tend to be based on unsuitable standards: there is a space in the group or there is a waiting list for his individual therapist.

Transfers or admissions to group work should be for positive reasons and should take into consideration all of the following points:

(1) Is the patient mentally suitable? In other words can he concentrate, work with others and comprehend and obey commands.

(2) Is he physically fit enough to work at the pace of the group? Has he the endurance to carry out exercise for a period of not less than 20 minutes without rests? In other words, are his cardiovascular and respiratory systems normal or will they present complications, needing a special group?

(3) Can the patient perform all the exercises which form the therapeutic core of the group he is to attend? This means all staff must be familiar with the basic exercises which comprise the penultimate parts of a table, e.g. a patient for the straight leg group must be fully capable of good quadriceps contractions and a patient for a joint mobilizing group must already have an agreed quantity of joint motion and the necessary muscle stability.

(4) Is the patient capable of working on his own without close supervision? If there is any doubt two patients with similar disability should be treated together so that the one-to-one relationship is reduced to two-to-one, and each only receives half of the therapist's attention.

(5) Has the patient used all or some of the types of equipment which will be used in the group? This means that the therapists

must know what sort of exercises are given and what equipment is used in each of the different groups in the gymnasium.

(6)   Is the patient sufficiently independent to get himself ready for and dressed after group exercise? This implies not only can he undress and dress the essential areas, but can he balance safely while doing so and possibly also can he walk about without shoes and socks?

(7)   As group work involves the use of the floor, stools and the fixed apparatus of the gymnasium, the patient must be capable of reaching all of these. Can he, with minimal help, get down on or up from the floor, sit down and stand up and walk the necessary distance?

(8)   Are there any special social circumstances which would prevent the patient arriving in time for the group? For example a 9 AM start is not feasible for a parent who has to see children to school.

(9)   Will the patient benefit psychologically from being included in a group? The extrovert patient often stimulates the introvert patient and the more advanced patient can encourage those new to the group by example. Groups that consist of patients of varying ages can be beneficial

to all in the group. The enthusiasm of younger livelier patients can often encourage the shy, older and less able patient, and equally the young patient making slow and laborious progress can be encouraged by an older patient.

To effect the transfer

At the very beginning of the treatment regime the patient should be told that he will have this treatment now and that later, and as he gets better, he will go into a group. He is thus prepared for and accepts group work as an improvement in his own performance. Some patients may need to be reminded at intervals that group work is a goal of good performance and is a progression.

Next he should be introduced to his new therapist and, if possible, be shown at least the room and at best some part of the activities he will be joining. He should be advised about special clothing in plenty of time for him to obtain what is needed if it is not provided.

Finally, if necessary, his appointment for any continuing individual treatment should be rearranged and his notes handed on for his new therapist to read before he enters the new sphere of treatment.

Chapter 14
GROUP EXERCISE

B. Sanford

Groups of people for exercise may be formed whenever there is a number of patients whose treatment in part or in total has a sufficiently common core to enable them to be treated safely in the same area and at the same time. This applies equally whether the treatment in the group is aimed at prevention of illness, e.g. general exercises for long-stay elderly patients, or at rehabilitation following injury or disease. Group therapy, if used with thought and skill for exercise programmes whether used for in-patients or out-patients, can never be counter-productive. Exercising a group without careful and positive identification of the patients who are likely to benefit from working with others, will always be counter-productive. (See Chapter 13, Assessment of Patients' Suitability for Group Treatment.)

For many patients the introduction of group exercise at a planned appropriate time can be psychologically uplifting as it represents the achievement of a new goal. Working in a group often helps a patient to feel less of an invalid, particularly if there are others in the same group who are at an earlier stage of recovery. The more advanced patients in the group can give hope and encouragement to those whose previous individual treatment has led them to question their ability to recover fully. Earlier despondency and consequent diminished effort can quickly be dispelled and a new enthusiasm created.

Human beings, with few exceptions, are naturally gregarious and group exercise can provide a social and therapeutic function, particularly for the elderly and for those brought from the isolation of living alone. Working in groups induces conversation and laughter, which in turn lead to relaxation of mind and body which is so essential for effective rehabilitation. Children treated in groups are less inclined to become hospitalized through too much adult attention and this stimulation could well lead to an increased effort to get better.

In all groups the therapist's attention has to be shared, thus giving patients more responsibility for their own achievements when exercising and for their own management when dressing and undressing. It may even inspire them to give help to those less independent than themselves, so boosting their own self-confidence.

In today's society working as part of a team is of utmost importance in both service and manufacturing industries. Adult patients whose ultimate goal is to be cared for at home, need to be mindful of their own and their carer's strengths and weaknesses to make this feasible. They must thus acquire sufficient independence to reduce the load on their carers if any. When exercising in groups, patients learn mutual inter-dependence as they work with and against each other. New and more interesting exercises can be introduced which may give an extra stimulus to those who have previously had individual treatment.

Although group exercise is economical of the therapist's time and thus of cost, the ultimate consideration when selecting group treatment should always be the patient's welfare and progress. In this chapter are suggestions to help the therapist prepare the climate for learning to which every patient is entitled. No one has taught anything until the pupil has learnt something and the degree of success of this communication will determine the satisfaction or otherwise of both teacher and patient. Teaching in a gymnasium presents its own special problems and attention to safety will minimize potential dangers.

Safety in the gymnasium

All unfamiliar gymnasia should be inspected by the therapist before she prepares a series of activities. The following points should be investigated and possible dangers noted so that exercises can be carried out safely. In the event of the construction of a new gymnasium, attempts should be made throughout planning and construction stages to minimize these hazards.

Construction of the gymnasium

Roof
Ideally, this should have all the supporting structures enclosed above a flat ceiling. This prevents the unexpected deflection of equipment, e.g. balls, beanbags.

Walls
These should be smooth to prevent grazing injuries; and free from unnecessary protruding structures, e.g. clocks should be recessed and covered with wire mesh, and mirrors should fold and reverse to form a flush surface when

not in use. Unavoidable protrusions should be carefully situated. A semi-gloss paint will reduce glare from the sun on those walls likely to be affected.

Floor
This should be constructed of suitable wooden laths running across the room. This type of floor gives some spring and if the direction of the laths is opposite to that of the general movement, slipperiness will be reduced. The floor should be cleaned in accordance with the builder's instructions and at no time should polish be applied.

Windows
These should be sufficient to provide adequate lighting with opening elements enough to secure reasonable ventilation. They are best situated well above the level of activity to prevent draughts on patients when they are opened to avoid a sleepy or unsavoury atmosphere. Protection from breakage by moving balls, etc., is also effected by high positioning. The incorporation of mesh-integrated glass is a good safeguard against injury from falling glass.

Lighting
Artificial lights should be adequate in number and spacing. They should not cast shadows and should be protected from the danger of moving small equipment. They are best built flush with the ceiling and protected by mesh-integrated glass.

Heating
The heating system should be unobtrusive but adequate for the size of the room. Hot air entering the room through adjustable grids seems to be the most practical solution and unavoidable radiators should be protected. A stuffy and therefore dangerously sleepy atmosphere should be avoided by using a thermostat.

Apparatus in the gymnasium

Fixed apparatus should be installed by experts and regular checks should take place (in accordance with the safety regulations of the Department of Health). Obvious faults should be dealt with immediately and such apparatus put out of use. Moveable apparatus, large and small, should be stored neatly in an easily accessible adjoining area, which allows simultaneous free entry and exit of a reasonably large number of people. Agility apparatus should be moved with care and patients should not use it until it has been checked for safety in its new position by the therapist. Small equipment should be moved about in suitable containers and not left lying around on the gymnasium floor while exercises are in progress. Apparatus involved in an accident should be retained for inspection.

People in the gymnasium

These include patients and therapists.

Punctuality
The therapist should already be in the gymnasium when the first patient enters. A full period of treatment is important to all patients and they may well start their own exercises using equipment which could be dangerous. Patients, too, should arrive punctually so as not to miss the early exercises to prepare them and to produce a good circulatory effect for safe, stronger exercises later.

Dress
This should be such as to allow safe, free movement, e.g. shorts for a knee group, a sleeveless garment for a hand group. The therapist should be easily distinguished by a uniform outfit. If worn, the footwear of both patients and therapists should be lightweight with non-slip

soles, and under no circumstances should socks or tights only be allowed. If hair is long, it should be suitably tied back and well secured so as not to swing. Watches, jewellery, etc. should be removed to prevent scratching injuries. These last points apply to both patient and therapist.

Other factors

The number of patients in any one group should not exceed eight to twelve (according to type of disability) and the therapist should know every patient by name. There is a special danger in teaching anonymous patients; they cannot be protected from individual hazards. Similarly, the therapist should be sure the patients know her name. Of primary importance is the firm mastering of the word stop. It ensures a quick control of a foreseeable accident. It is essential too that not only is each patient's diagnosis known, but also any other relevant medical factors, e.g. heart condition, deafness, etc. Finally, the therapist should know and apply all the basic rules of teaching (see later).

If, despite all reasonable care and attention to inherent dangers, an accident occurs, deal with it calmly and competently, then report the details in writing immediately to the appropriate department.

General teaching technique

It is often claimed that good teachers are born, not made. This is not so; only some good teachers are born and many more are created by determination and deep understanding between staff and student. Apprehension is an essential ingredient of good teaching and the fact that initially it often displays itself as a deep fear should be accepted as normal. Time and actual teaching practice expertly guided can put this to good advantage. It should be remembered that to the injured, exercise is not a reflex physical process, and it is necessary to stimulate the desire to perform. Only by complete involvement on the part of the teacher will this be successful. The following basic rules should be observed.

Teach firmly and positively but not aggressively. Tell the patients what to do, rather than ask them. 'Please' and 'can you' should initially form no part of the command. It is not easy and often feels rude and abrupt not to use these phrases in the early stages of learning to take a group, but patients who are often frightened and in pain should be given no hint that they may fail to perform what they are asked to do. To help achieve this the best use of the teacher's voice should be regarded as of extreme importance.

Voice

The correct use of the voice is an important factor in ensuring the success of the group activity. It should be stimulating and portray enthusiasm and enjoyment, while working at least as hard and keenly as the patient's muscles. The most carefully planned exercises may be rendered ineffective by poor vocal delivery.

Patients best hear sounds which come from their front or sides, and the therapist should bear this in mind when it is necessary to change her own position, or that of the patients, e.g. when patients roll over from lying to prone lying the therapist should move to the opposite end of the group. The voice should always be firm and audible and have clear diction and a variety of intonation. Words should be carefully separated and not allowed to run into each other. Particular care is needed at the end of the first word when the same consonant ends one word and starts the next, e.g. 'let your *leg go* forward', or when any two hard consonants come together, e.g. '*sit down*'.

The volume should vary to suit the size, nature and participants in the group. A rehabilitation group of boisterous young people will require greater volume than a group of older ladies. When working in the open air a greater volume will be needed due to the lack of throwback from walls.

The voice will be most clearly heard if the muscles of the neck, shoulder and shoulder girdle are relaxed and an effort is made to feel that the words come from the abdomen. Daily practice of deep breathing will help, making a long 'ah' sound in expiration. In this way deeper, more audible tones will be produced and the therapist will be spared a perpetual sore throat. If the size of the group is large the therapist should feel that her voice is thrown high to the back of the room.

How a movement is to be performed should be indicated by the therapist's voice. She may wish it to be done quickly or slowly and the speed of her voice should vary accordingly. Movements requiring prolonged effort should be helped by corresponding effort on appropriate words in the therapist's voice. When encouraging a patient to lift a heavy weight, the word '*lift*' should be prolonged and have a rising inflexion. When helping a patient to relax a limb, the therapist may use the word '*drop*', which should be sudden and have a falling inflexion. Movements to be performed lightly need a lighter tone. Words should be produced in a staccato manner for light, tripping movements.

Variety in the choice of words used is stimulating, but care must be taken to avoid the use of technical terms, e.g. '*bend*' not '*flex*', '*turn*' not '*rotate*'. Some knowledge of local words and phrases could be an asset, but should not be overused. Monotony will be avoided if important words are emphasized, usually verbs, adverbs or adjectives, e.g. '*push*' your partner over'; 'throw the ball *high* into the air'; 'make your jump *long*'.

The successful use of the voice will only be achieved if the therapist is completely convinced of the effectiveness of the exercises she is presenting. Careful preparation of all exercises is essential (see next chapter).

Positioning

Within reason, use all available space. The positioning of both patients and therapist should be such that observation of expected difficulties is easy. Movement of the therapist, any part of a patient or of apparatus should not present danger to anyone in the room. If the sun is shining into the room, place the patients with their backs to it; the therapist's position can be adapted more easily to a safe position in the shade.

Patients likely to need extra help should be at the sides of the group, so that as it is given, the therapist can, at all times, have the whole group in view. If using a circular formation the therapist should teach from the outside so that no patient is ever behind her. Patients who have special problems, e.g. the deaf or blind, should be positioned where they can most benefit from the group. The deaf may be able to lip read and the blind will need to hear well, so they should be near the therapist.

Teaching an exercise

All exercises used in teaching should be within the experience of the therapist. This does not necessarily mean that she must be able to give a perfect demonstration, but that she is at least aware of potential difficulties. There are four clear stages in teaching an exercise.

Starting position

This should be carefully chosen for each exercise, bearing in mind what the therapist is trying to achieve. That it is correct is of utmost importance. If it is wrong then any movement from it will inevitably be performed inefficiently and uneconomically. A starting position used for successive exercises should be checked before proceeding, and all starting positions should be observed continuously.

The exercise to be performed

This can be taught by words and demonstration or by a combination of both. Words should be clear, brief, to the point and above all audible, bearing in mind that several group and individual treatments may be in progress in the same room. Tell the patients what to do and get the exercise going as quickly as possible, remembering that ears 'shut off' fairly quickly. Demonstration can be of assistance in teaching those exercises which otherwise would necessitate lengthy explanations, but bear in mind that a full day's teaching in a gymnasium can be very strenuous – choose the demonstrations wisely. If this method of teaching is used, the exercise should be performed without fault and from a position (or series of positions) from which every patient can see.

Help, advice and encouragement

Should be given as the exercise is in progress with a view to improving performance (see section on observation and correction).

The termination

The exercise should finally be brought to a close when the therapist feels that the time is appropriate, and not when the patient feels like it. This should normally be when a further continuance of the exercise would result in reduced performance.

Observation and correction

This calls for tact and initiative. Always teach to avoid the necessity to correct. The need for too much correction indicates lack of care in preparation. A dynamic standing position is normally most suitable from which to observe faults. Teaching in other positions should be reserved for special occasions, e.g. if helping a patient or teaching children (see Chapter 16). If it is necessary to use other positions for demonstrating an exercise, return to the standing position as soon as possible. A teacher should change her position in relation to the group according to the faults an exercise is likely to present, but any movement should be for a purpose and not just a continuous irritating pace backwards and forwards.

Observation should be done systematically from side to side or front to back and the therapist should spend time learning to make full use of all her peripheral vision. This is easily done by fixing her eyes on any stationary object and increasing her awareness of other movement in the room. In the first instance, correction should be of the whole group. The therapist should pick out the more widespread mistakes and correct positively by encouragement and help as the exercise is in progress. Care must be taken to deal with one fault at a time, not forgetting the starting position. Individual corrections must be dealt with very tactfully in a group, and all improvement, not necessarily perfection, should be suitably rewarded with praise – remember success breeds success. The patient should always feel that the therapist's standard is high, but individual effort should not go unrewarded. Should all effort to correct an exercise fail, stop the group and re-teach, if nec-

essary breaking the exercise down into fewer components.

General points

It is important that groups are used for the benefit of patients and not because of a staff shortage. All patients should have had at least one individual treatment for assessment or teaching purposes and should have been selected for group work by the therapist in the gymnasium in consultation with other appropriate staff (see Chapter 13). It is essential to know the patient's previous and future intended occupation so as to have an idea of earlier fitness and strength and to be able to gear the treatment to that needed for the future.

The co-operation of the patient is vital. All successful teaching is based on this mutual trust both in the group and in the daily practice of exercises to be done at home (see Chapter 15). All exercises should be carefully chosen and suited to the age and sex of the patient. They should show variety, sometimes stimulating, sometimes quietening, perhaps rhythmic or to command, formal or informal. Every physical activity, e.g. entering or leaving the gymnasium, collecting and clearing away apparatus, should be used for teaching purposes. These activities give a useful knowledge of a person's independence away from the hospital and can provide natural breaks between physically exhausting exercises.

Should the therapist herself feel bored with the group activity then undoubtedly the patients will feel likewise. Boredom arises because she is not completely involved in making the exercises enjoyable, and from total involvement alone comes the satisfaction of a job well done.

Mixed ability groups

Mixed ability groups can be useful when there are small numbers of patients at different stages of recovery from similar disabilities, for whom group treatment would be beneficial. A typical group in a younger age group could consist of patients at different stages of recovery from knee surgery or injury. In the older age group hemiplegics or amputees could each form satisfactory groups. To prevent too much movement of patients, the room should be arranged so that apparatus needed for similar disabilities is adjacent. For example, patients with hand injuries or handling problems will need both tables and adjacent small apparatus, while those with balance problems will need to be near both parallel bars and stools.

Exercises from which all patients benefit should be taken at the beginning of a group activity and also for all at the end if time permits. For these collective exercises the patients should be positioned so that those needing extra help are together where the therapist can give help while watching the rest of the group. Some may need only a little help and can often be interspersed with the more advanced patients who will benefit from giving a little aid to the less able.

The middle of the treatment session should consist of exercises designed for specific disabilities and the patients should be repositioned in the appropriate area and possibly with the designated apparatus. At this stage they each may be performing a different exercise and the therapist should be constantly alert and ready to move to prevent dangerous situations developing or to improve a patient's performance. These exercises should be of a more functional nature and the patient should easily be able to move to another task if the room is correctly planned. Mixed ability groups inevitably need more time and supervising staff who can help the less able, than do groups of patients with more equal ability. They should not be attempted unless at least an hour's treatment time is available.

Patient orientated medical record

Each patient in a group should have a patient orientated medical record card (POMR) which should be filed in a conveniently situated safe place to which therapist and patient have access. Individual problems are defined and objectives laid down so that they are easily understood by the patient. These should be monitored at regular intervals.

Chapter 15
PREPARATION OF GROUP ACTIVITIES

B. Sanford

Confidence is the keynote to successful teaching and for this reason the therapist should always prepare the exercises in advance. If unavoidable circumstances make prior warning impossible, it is best to let the patients practise familiar exercises (e.g. those taught for use at home) for a few minutes. The therapist can then quickly work out a suitable series of exercises. It is never satisfactory for a therapist to be teaching one exercise while thinking out the next one.

Two types of preparation are necessary for teaching a group of patients: a scheme of treatment and an exercise programme.

Scheme of treatment

The scheme of treatment should be a long term plan setting out the broad aims of a particular period of treatment. The joints to be mobilized and in which ranges, the muscles to be strengthened and the type of muscle work to be used should be identified. At all times a scheme of treatment must be aimed at enabling the patient to live the fullest possible life which his immediate problems will allow. Therefore treatment at any stage of recovery must be related to the function of the body as a whole as well as to the specific disablement. Each scheme should cover the period of time from the patient joining a particular group to the time of his progression to a more advanced group or to discharge. Should the scheme of treatment be concerned with recovery immediately prior to discharge, it should lead to the patient being able to follow his chosen occupation.

Exercise programme

Each exercise programme should consist of a series of suitable exercises to be taught on any one day and should be based on the scheme of treatment previously worked out. The therapist should include at least one exercise for each aim with a second or third exercise for the more important aims. All exercises should be prepared with function in mind and care should be taken not to fatigue individual muscles or groups of muscles by using the same ones in quick succession. Easily accessible cards listing quick reminders of the order of exercises will ensure the planned programme is followed.

For a 30 minute treatment period it is advisable to prepare an average of ten exercises bearing in mind the tempo may vary each day and not all exercises will be completed every time. Undressing and dressing may have to be done in the time allocated and these are a common cause of extra consumption of time. Individual patients should be made aware of any exercise which is unsuitable for them to perform and should separately be instructed in a safe substitution. In this way patients with many different specific problems, but with the same basic re-education needs, can be accommodated safely in the same group. (See last section of Chapter 14.)

Regardless of the time available, all exercise programmes should present a similar pattern:

(1) An introductory exercise which should have a 'warming up' effect on appropriate areas. This should allow great freedom of movement, and unless injuries make it impossible, it is best taken in a standing position. It should involve movement of a large joint or joints related to the actual area of concern, e.g. in a hand group an exercise involving shoulder movement would be suitable. If the group is concerned equally with the whole body, then an exercise involving large movements of the whole body is appropriate, e.g. an easy game previously taught.

(2) The warming up active exercise can be followed by stretching of the muscles acting over the same joints. For example running on the spot can be followed by self-stretching for the hamstrings or the quadriceps.

(3) This should be followed by three or four exercises which localize movement if this is appropriate, and starting positions should be carefully chosen. If restricted movement is no longer a problem, the exercises in this section should not demand precision or too much strength; the body must work up to these. In a group involving exercises for the whole body large movements of the trunk, legs and arms are suitable, and, when dealing with more specific areas, the larger muscle groups should be used.

(4) The patients should now be ready for exercises demanding range of movement and greater strength, and/or precision, taken in the more dynamic positions of everyday life. These should include exercises involving quick movement and quick thinking. As the patients progress, the number of less specific exercises (as in (2) above) should be reduced and be replaced by more in this group.

(5) The climax should consist of a game or activities involving all the skills which have been taught, and if possible involving the interaction of all the members of the group.

(6) To cool down allow the treatment to end on a quiet note while individual lifestyle problems are dealt with.

The original exercise programme should be recorded and progressed systematically each day. One or two well performed exercises may be changed at each treatment, so that a good part of them always remain familiar to the patients. In this way all the exercises will eventually by progressed and boredom prevented. The therapist should at all times make sure that the progressions are within the scope of the patients or she may well find they 'give up'. Finally, any prepared exercises which, through lack of time are omitted, should certainly be included in the next treatment.

Progression of exercise

Carefully planned progression will ensure that the injured part of the body returns to the highest possible degree of function in the shortest possible time. Such progression can be judged to be successful when the injured area, having been worked to the point of fatigue in any one treatment session, recovers so as to enable the patient to take part fully in the next.

Most progressions can, and should if necessary, be tailored to accommodate individual members of each group. Only the observation of the therapist in charge can decide which type of progression is relevant and when this should be implemented. Constant reference to the original scheme of exercises will serve as a guide.

Starting positions

Progression is effected by changing the starting position so as to alter the effect gravity has on a muscle action when performing a movement. If gravity is counter-balanced, muscle work is easier than if gravity is resisting a movement, e.g. if a patient is lying on the floor lifting his arms sideways, the abductors of the shoulder will work less hard than if he is performing the same exercise sitting on a stool.

Change in the size of the base provided by a starting position alters the degree of difficulty of an exercise. A broad base, e.g. stride standing or walk standing, gives greater stability to a movement than a small base, e.g. close standing or toe standing. An exercise performed on a stationary surface is easier than the same exercise performed on a moveable surface because of the extra balance involved in the latter, e.g. bouncing a ball with the feet on a balance board is harder than bouncing a ball with the feet on the floor.

Endurance

There should be a gradual increase in the length of time spent performing each exercise. This may be controlled by measured time or by counting the number of repetitions, whichever is appropriate. The ultimate goal should be within the limits of the patient's ability and concentration. Endless repetitions of simple exercises may cause regression through loss of interest. The total duration of each session should be increased gradually. For instance, a new patient may get maximum benefit from just 20 minutes' daily exercise. This can be increased to 30 minutes, then to 45 minutes and eventually to an hour or a full day's treatment. This will depend on the needs of the patient and the lifestyle he is to resume. As the treatment time increases the therapist should ensure that exercises putting excessive stress on the cardiovascular and respiratory systems do not follow in rapid succession. In this way complete rest periods will be kept to a minimum.

Muscle loading (See Chapter 11)

Sandbags provide a useful and cheap means of muscle loading in group work and are most frequently used in the re-education of limbs. They can be used to resist both isometric and isotonic muscle work. Using considered judgment, the therapist should introduce weights in appropriate exercises to offer resistance in addition to that of the weight of the limb. Without added resistance such exercises would need an unacceptable number of repetitions in order for the muscle to reach momentary exhaustion.

Loading can be progressed according to the needs of the individual. An example of a suitable exercise is backward prop support long sitting, straight leg lifting and lowering. Weight bearing exercises for suitable lower limb injuries should be progressed alongside muscle loading and should replace it completely in the later stages of recovery. Lower limb joints are normally subjected to compression and to encourage normal functioning, weight bearing exercises must be introduced as soon as possible. In addition muscles should be re-educated to work in a functional capacity.

Levers (See Chapter 2)

A short weight arm is more easily moved than a long one and exercises can be progressed using this principle. For example, when working the back extensor muscles in prone lying, head and shoulder lifting, at first the arms should remain at the sides of the body. The exercise can be made harder by stretching the arms out in front to make the lever longer. If the starting position is changed to across prone lying (form) the lever is lengthened because the fulcrum is moved from the chest to the pelvis.

Range (See Chapter 1)
Muscles work most easily in their middle range and this is in many cases the range in which they produce functional movements. Weak muscles should be re-educated first of all in this range, progressing to the more difficult inner and outer ranges. Strengthening of muscles which control range should precede increase in joint range or control may be inefficient, e.g. if the knee joint has mobility without muscle strength the leg will collapse on weight bearing.

Speed
Alteration in the speed of an exercise is a useful means of progression. The speed may need to be increased or decreased to effect the desired progression. Walking may become harder if done more slowly because of the harder balance involved. Throwing a ball against a wall and catching it again becomes more difficult when done more quickly, demanding better co-ordination and speedier muscle actions.

The therapist should allow a gradually shorter time for changing from one starting position to another and for collecting and putting away apparatus. The patient should be encouraged to dress and undress at greater speed. In industry today, piece work on production lines makes the time taken to do a job of paramount importance.

The condition of the patient should be checked at each session. Any signs of regression should be investigated. Should pain, swelling, reddening of the skin or reduced ability to exercise be present, progressions in exercises introduced at the previous session should be omitted.

Music, rhythm and exercise

Whilst all human beings have their own natural speed which they use in all daily activities, rhythmical actions may be learned as co-ordination increases with motor experience. Suitable exercises performed to a rhythm have many therapeutic uses. When a rhythmical beat is needed to maintain activity at a particular tempo for a period of time, music provides a useful accompaniment.

Constant noise induces inattention as is exemplified by the way we ignore constant background noise. It is important to ensure that periods of silence interrupt repetitive noise so that attention is not lost.

Production of a beat

By using a musical instrument
This may vary from a rather immobile piano to a more portable orchestral instrument. Whichever instrument is chosen, a competent, reliable and sympathetic player must be available and the sound produced should be at the correct volume for the size of the treatment area, bearing in mind that other patients may be receiving treatment nearby. The therapist should be in overall control and the accompanist should be ready to make changes in the tempo and duration of the music as requested by the therapist.

By using recording equipment
Recording equipment, fixed or portable, may be used in most environments for exercising provided that a safe electrical socket of the correct voltage is available near at hand. It is dangerous to have long lengths of flex trailing across the floor. Suitable music recorded on tapes or discs can be bought in many shops or the therapist may record on tape melodies of her own choosing and of the required tempo

and length of time for any particular group of exercises.

By beating a rhythm with the hands or feet

A beat can be produced by tapping on a tambourine or by clapping the hands together. If the therapist needs to use her hands to give help to a patient the beat may be maintained by stamping on the floor.

By using the human voice

By singing or reciting words in a chosen rhythm or even by counting in rhythm the therapist or patient can produce a beat.

Rules for using music

The exercises should always be taught first, then the therapist can give encouragement and correct the patient's performance throughout the exercises whilst at the same time helping to maintain the set rhythm. The two ways of doing this are by the therapist:

(1)   Speaking in time with the beat
(2)   Encouraging and correcting whilst demonstrating the exercise in progress to help maintain the rhythm for those who cannot easily pick it out.

As the music alone will not stimulate the patient to produce his best performance of the exercise, the therapist should use her voice frequently but intermittently to maintain levels of performance and interest.

Uses of music

(1)   For most patients, music provides a mental stimulation. Many unco-operative patients can be persuaded to participate in exercises which are accompanied by a familiar tune. Older people may respond best to known melodies of their era; young men or women may enjoy tunes of more recent times and rhyming songs usually appeal to children. Reluctant participants may be stimulated to take part in exercises for which they have helped to choose the musical accompaniment, but the choice must always be acceptable to the therapist and the therapeutic need.

(2)   Psychiatric and mentally handicapped patients enjoy repetitive exercises and, as with older people, will often work at their own pace in time with the set rhythm.

(3)   Music may be used when treating groups of patients who are in hospital for long periods, e.g. orthopaedic or geriatric patients for whom exercises are needed to maintain muscle strength and joint range in uninjured areas.

(4)   Patients with chest problems often benefit by humming or singing to the music whilst performing easy exercises. In this way long expirations can be induced if these are required in their treatment.

(5)   Patients exercising at home often enjoy working to music on the radio or on their own recording equipment and suitable programmes can often be suggested by the therapist. For the more musically gifted patient, performing on a suitable instrument can be a useful therapeutic exercise, e.g. fingers may be exercised by playing the piano, or the playing of a wind instrument may be suitable therapy for patients suffering from certain chest conditions.

Home exercises

Unless patients are attending daily, for treatment to be fully effective, exercises carefully selected from those taught should be practised daily at home. It is not always easy for patients who are working full time to set aside special periods for exercise during the day and for such people some of the exercises chosen should be able to be practised at work, e.g. an office worker with a knee injury could practise isotonic quadriceps exercises under his desk, or perhaps he could walk to and from work.

All home exercises should have been taught very thoroughly and the therapist must be satisfied that the patient can perform them unsupervised. As each exercise selected for home practice is introduced, suggestions for recognizing improvement should be given to the patient, e.g. improvement in shoulder movement could be measured against the good arm with the help of a mirror. Improvement in errors of gait can be recognized with the aid of a mirror and improvement in muscle endurance can be measured by noting the length of time for which an exercise can be performed. Alternatively the number of repetitions of the exercise may be counted. The therapist should bear in mind that in modern houses, rooms are small and ceilings are low so the exercises should not need height, large areas of uninterrupted floor space or involve quick movement of dangerous apparatus, e.g. exercises involving running or high throwing of balls should be avoided.

Patients who are at home should be encouraged to practise their exercises for short periods throughout the day. A 15–20 minute exercise period at the beginning of the day when the body has been resting is advisable with further 10 minute periods spread throughout the day, e.g. mid-morning, lunchtime, mid-afternoon and in the evening. In the early stages of treatment when muscles are very weak, exercise periods could be shorter and taken more often, and in the later stages effort should be made to increase the time spent at each practice session. It is advisable for patients to stick to their routine unless special circumstances make this impossible. Fatigue due to inadequate rest

periods can make the exercises less effective. Patients who are working all day should make time for 15–20 minutes concentrated practice in the morning and in the evening.

Exercises practised at home should be checked regularly by the therapist and progress recorded. The patient should be told in what order the exercises should be practised and how many times to repeat each one, the latter being progressed as the patient improves. Circuit routines are particularly suitable for more advanced patients (see Chapter 11). If small equipment is to be used it should be cheap to buy, e.g. a small ball, or should be such that may be represented by objects found in the home, e.g. a rolling pin or a rolled up newspaper can be used instead of a pole, and weights for resistance can be made up of packs of household goods, etc.

In addition to practising exercises taught in the group, many daily activities serve as 'home exercises'. A shoulder may be exercised by a housewife each time she cleans a window if she is instructed to clean as large an area as possible before moving her feet to a new position. If she stands in a position giving a large base (e.g. stride standing) a large range of shoulder movement will be achieved. Post-natal exercises particularly should be incorporated into the mother's very busy new routine at home, e.g. trunk rotation may be practised when ironing if she collects the clothes from one side and puts them away at the other, provided she keeps her feet still.

The therapist should realize that patients are full of human failings and exercising at home will be conveniently forgotten unless the therapist is conscientious in checking progress each time the patient attends for treatment. Only by continuous effort both at home and at the treatment session can the patient expect a satisfactory recovery.

Chapter 16
EXERCISES FOR INFANTS AND CHILDREN

M. Hollis & B. Sanford

Infants

The term infant is applied to those capable of understanding play and vocal encouragement. A wide selection of toys is now available for the therapist to use for play/exercise for this age group.

It should be remembered that one can engage the attention of small children for only very short periods, i.e. the concentration span is shortest in the young and therefore a great variety of simple or ingenious exercises must be thought up. All exercises should be applied with the aims of treatment in mind.

Only three or four repetitions may be possible with very young infants, but some children like endless repetitions. A large selection of toys should not be displayed at one time but most of them kept out of sight until they are needed. The treatment should be given in the smallest available space remembering that to an infant big spaces are infinite and probably frightening. It may be better initially to play with a well-loved toy which the child may be using as an emotional prop for the temporary deprivation of his mother and normal environment.

In giving exercises to small children it is important to remember that ill health or dis-tress reduces the mental age and he should not be expected to perform at his normal age level even though the child is known to be socially, emotionally and mentally normal. This is very evident in a ward of sick children when normally independent children become either attention seeking or withdrawn due to the change of environment as well as ill health. Parental involvement in the treatment and any therapeutic activities may help to overcome the problem.

Most activities can be performed as a game, to nursery rhymes or rhyming songs. Skilled musical performance is not demanded, but lively vocal stimulation will usually produce a satisfactory performance when it is performed with enjoyment on the part of the therapist and the child's attention is still commanded. The moment the child's attention wanders a different exercise and a different song or rhyme pattern should be substituted and even a change of exercise to another part of the body. So long as there is constant return to the part that needs most work there is no harm in diversion. The same person should give the exercises at every visit if possible so that the infant feels secure in this social contact. The child should be encouraged and praised for each success.

It is easy to forget that children will become exhausted by effort and concentration, but that they will express fatigue differently from an adult. A fall off in performance, an increase in irritability or a refusal to perform at all will signal that it is time to go away for the time being and return later in the day. Always give the child something to do or he will find it for himself and may do neither the therapist's exercises nor his own.

For this group and those in the next age group, the clothing of the therapist may be important. Again hugeness is suggested by a person wearing all the same colour.

Older children

As children get older they often like to exhibit their skills especially to the parent who, unless they interfere in the treatment, should be encouraged to stay in the room. Mothers and fathers should be discouraged from resigning their parental role in the interests of becoming full time therapists in order to 'push' the physical progress of their child to a daily limit. Nevertheless, an understanding parent who can encourage from the other side of the room, who will learn the simpler exercises and is prepared to be instructed in the best method of carrying out the most fundamental tasks the handicapped child should perform, is the best friend of the child and the therapist.

Parents should be excluded from the treatment session when they interfere all the time or if they refuse to participate in the regime. Fortunately most parents are very willing to learn and eager to help.

With the slightly older child in the four to eight years age group there can be vast differences in the mental capacity and approach. Children up to about the age of five will play on their own in a group environment and over

the age of five will increasingly be willing to play with a partner. This development will increase the variety of exercises which can be used.

Children of this group will have developed interests and normal play patterns and enquiries should be made of the parents or the child observed in an assessment environment to allow suitable exercises to be chosen. The exercises should be briefly explained, but it will be necessary for the therapist to join in the activity and teach by example and thus by demonstration. Some children enjoy a challenge and others need cajoling or encouragement and sometimes a great deal of shyness has to be overcome. Whatever the emotional approach, the child should have a routine of exercises which is progressed regularly (and recorded). If no progress is being made the exercises should be altered if not progressed so that they do not seem to be in a rut. All children tend to have plateaux of performance in the same way that they have intermittent spurts of growing. Plateauing may be the explanation of lack of progress and approaching the exercise in another way may provide the required stimulus.

It is important to avoid the hazard of 'talking down' to children. A normal voice and manner of address appeal more to children, who are charmed to be talked to in an adult voice and manner. A special vocabulary is not necessary, only remember that children have a limited vocabulary and known language. Failure to understand what is said will cause the child to say 'I don't know what you mean' or to fail to carry out the task. Then the explanation can be simplified.

An authoritative manner is also part of the therapist's role. Firm physical handling of a baby and firm commands to older children are necessary as the children must do their exercises. The same sort of command as to an adult, telling the child what to do, will give re-assurance to a child who may, out of bewilder-ment, start to 'play up'.

Children from the age of eight upwards are really small adults and apart from simplifica-tion of language to suit the age, can be dealt with as adults. It is important to remember that to many children imitative activities, e.g. role acting of being parents, nurses or at school, is often not regarded as play. Play is, to some chil-dren, only going on when their own creative thoughts are being acted out with no relation-ship to the world of reality.

Children's groups (5–12 years)

The best teachers are those who learn most from their pupils and there is no better ma-terial to learn from than children. They do not tolerate boredom and never hide their feelings. Young children are extremely vociferous, and whilst adults and older children may think the same, young children will actually tell you quite firmly, 'I don't like you'. What they are telling you is that your method of communication does not please them. A therapist facing this situation would be well advised to investigate different methods, or communication will eventually cease altogether. The following hints should be of help.

Most children coming to hospital for the first time are tense and frightened and a big effort must be made to provide a familiar atmosphere. Parents, who are emotionally tied up with their children, share this fear and the therapist should not take offence if this results in their abruptness and apparent lack of co-operation at the first treatment. As they see their child happily accepting the new situation they will become more co-operative.

It is a good idea if a special room can be set aside for the treatment of children. They tend to identify and associate deformed adults with grotesque characters in fairy tales and this only adds to their fears. The room should be rea-sonably small as children see things as being much bigger than they actually are and they tend to feel lost in a large open space. If a sepa-rate room is not possible, curtains could be used to divide a suitable area from a larger room. The room should be decorated with bright colours and one wall could be covered with pictures or posters, just like the class-rooms at school. These will attract the child's atten-tion and may well provide a topic of conversa-tion between therapist and child, or between the new child and the other members of the class.

Overcoming the usual initial silence barrier in the very young is important. Children will chatter only when they feel secure and are therefore relaxed. In this atmosphere, they will be happy and co-operative. All children must have complete confidence in the therapist and she should have a little prior knowledge of each new child so that she can talk of familiar things and the child does not feel he is meeting a complete stranger. The therapist should make 'getting to know each other' her primary concern at the first treatment, and it is a help if a new child arrives a little before the rest of the group.

The therapist should take care not to tower over a child. It is a good idea to get down to his level by sitting or crouching adjacent to him and to greet him with a smile. She should try to encourage him to talk by asking questions about his family or pets so that he feels she is involved in his life away from the hospital. The therapist must take care to remember all she is told and the child's trust in her will gradually grow, although a young child may need a few visits before he is completely at ease. Some young children respond to physical contact and a new child may like to perform his exercises while holding the therapist's hand. He will let go of his own accord when he becomes absorbed in the simple painfree exercises that should be taken at the beginning of the group.

At the first treatment the parent should be invited into the room and the therapist should tactfully ask her not to interrupt the group and assure her that there will be an opportunity for her to ask questions later. It should seldom be necessary for a parent to be excluded from a group. Sometimes the child requests this and, as the parent may later be criticizing the child's performance, the therapist should accede to the request until she can talk to the parent and assure herself that it will no longer happen.

It is best to discuss problems whilst the child is otherwise gainfully occupied – perhaps when he is getting dressed – as it is not a good thing to discuss the child when he is listening. If he thinks his physical difficulties are attracting his mother's attention at home it might slow down his progress, e.g. an asthmatic child may well bring on an attack in order to attract his mother's attention more to himself than to her other tasks. Each parent should be involved in the supervision of the exercises to be done at home, and this should make them feel useful. Parents should be advised how routine actions at home could help the child's progress, e.g. a child with flat feet should hang his coat on a peg high enough to make him lift on to his toes each time he takes it off and on.

In children's groups the age range should be small. The 5- to 8-year-old children will work well together, and children from 9 to 12 years old can be grouped together successfully. (Some 8-year-old children may be better in the older group.) Children in the younger age group have a vivid imagination and will enjoy performing their exercises by acting out their own ideas of people and objects in a story told by the therapist. The children should be encouraged to add their own ideas to the story and the therapist should learn quickly to turn them into useful exercises. Many effective exercises for a chest group can be found in the story of a farmer riding on a tractor (the turning of wheels for shoulder mobilizing) to chop down trees and saw them into logs (trunk rotation and side flexion). The logs then float down the river (relaxation) and are finally thrown on to a lorry (trunk flexion and extension). Imitation of wind blowing can produced deep breathing. It is essential that the story is told with great expression with the therapist involving herself in the movements.

Opportunity for working with a partner for some of the exercises is a good idea, but team work should be reserved for the older children. Young children will enjoy games where one child is the focal point, e.g. 'What time is it Mr Wolf' could be used to exercise feet. In the older age group the exercises should be taught in a more adult way and in both groups vocabulary and ideas used should be within their comprehension. The 9- to 12-year-old children particularly enjoy games involving teams.

There should be a variety of available apparatus, not all on show at once. It is a good idea if some of it is identifiable by the child as that used at home or at school. Apparatus makes the exercises more interesting and takes the child's attention from the part being exercised. Extra care should be taken in making sure the exercises are performed in safety. All children demand keen observation as they are impulsive and move quickly and suddenly without thought for their own or others' safety.

The majority of exercises should allow freedom in standing positions unless the child's disability prevents this, and then the starting positions used should be the most active possible. The concentration span of children is limited so that exercises should be of short duration and the therapist should prepare a greater variety and more exercises than she would for adult groups. Children are always enthusiastic and the therapist should make sure there are no long gaps between the exercises as, if this happens, the children will find their own, often undesirable occupation and control of the group will be quickly lost.

The therapist should give very brief explanations of exercises and be prepared to demonstrate and join in many of the activities. Children are always anxious to please, and praise will lead to a big increase in effort. The therapist should look carefully for effort in those who find the exercises difficult and remember that praise is especially important to such children. Children like to be noticed; 'look at me' is a favourite phrase in the younger age group and the therapist should use this to encourage good and better work. All children like to demonstrate good work, but the therapist should take care that each child in turn is capable of demonstrating something or it could lead to unhappiness and a decrease in effort for

a few. 'Follow my leader' type of exercises with different children playing the leader according to the difficulty of the exercise are good for encouraging all ranges of ability.

Clothing

The therapist's clothing should be colourful. It is unusual for mother or teacher to be dressed completely in white and the therapist is in a similar relationship with the children. Parents should be advised to bring young children in clothing that is suitable for exercise as they are often reluctant to undress, particularly on their early visits. It is best to suggest they remove clothing as the exercises make them hot, and they are therefore more readily persuaded to discard their clothes. The older age group will enjoy changing into a special outfit for exercises.

Lastly, although some children will appeal to the therapist more than others, evidence of favouritism will quickly lead to disaster.

Chapter 17
SPECIAL REGIMES

M. Hollis

A regime for sensory ataxia (Frenkel's exercises)

Patients who suffer total or partial sensory ataxia will lose both cutaneous and proprioceptive sensation and therefore tend to exaggerate movements in an attempt to complete them. Their disability is easily tested because patients with sensory loss perform a simple movement less smoothly and well with the eyes closed than with the eyes open. Their movements are also arrhythmical and lack smoothness and precision.

The loss of proprioceptive impulses is compensated for by the use of vision and hearing. The movements must be performed accurately and with great precision and constant repetition of each movement is necessary until this is achieved. The patient must concentrate hard and watch the movement throughout while counting at a slow even tempo. No progression should be made until the first movement can be performed accurately. Adequate rest periods may be necessary during a treatment session as the patient may tire and lose the concentration necessary to achieve precision.

The rules are:

(1) Every movement he performs must be watched by the patient and a high degree of concentration is required.

(2) He must count out loud at first, then to himself at a slow even tempo, and try to perform the same range of movement for each count with great precision.

(3) The counting tempo must be the patient's own and not one imposed by the therapist.

(4) Large single movements are retrained first, followed by alternate movements of contralateral limbs, then more complex movements.

(5) Every movement made in the treatment session is counted at the same tempo and watched closely.

(6) During performance the patient should be guarded against falls.

(7) The worst limb should be exercised most.

(8) Progression should not be made until smooth accurate performance of the first exercise is achieved and this rule is followed for all progressions.

(9) Give the patient adequate periods of rest.

The regime starts when the order in which movements are to be trained has been decided. The patient is suitably positioned for both maximum support to allow the part to be moved easily, and so that he can see the part moving through the selected range. The range of movement performed need not be the fullest possible range of the part, but should be that which can be easily managed and is function-ally useful, e.g. in hip and knee flexion and extension, full extension is useful, flexion to 90°C is all that is functionally necessary for sitting down in a chair.

A polished board or reasonably slippery surface is used. The two extremes of the selected range are decided on and their posi-tions on the supporting surface are marked with chalk. The distance between these two points is then marked out according to the agreed count. If the count is to include 'start, 1, 2, 3, 4' at which point the end of the range is reached then five marks are needed, but only four marks are required if the movement starts on the count of '1' (Fig. 17.1).

The movement is first performed with the part supported. It is performed without pause during the movement, first in one direction, then in reverse and without wobbling. Next the patient can either lift the limb and touch each mark in turn or carry the limb through the air just off the support, passing each mark in turn.

Examples of movements

For the lower limb
Side lying – knee flexion and extension.
Side lying – hip flexion and extension.
Half lying – hip abduction and adduction.

Half lying – knee and hip flexion and extension.

For the upper limb
Sitting at a high table, arms held in abduction on the support:
Shoulder flexion and extension.
Elbow flexion and extension.
Elbow flexion with supination.
Elbow extension with pronation.
Wrist flexion and extension.

All the above exercises can then be practised:

(1) With a voluntary halt
(2) With a halt on command
(3) With the part unsupported
(4) With the part unsupported and with a voluntary halt
(5) With the part unsupported and a halt on command
(6) Placing the heel or fingers on specific points
(7) As 6 with a voluntary halt, e.g. heel on opposite toes, ankle, shin and knee; fingers on opposite fingers, wrist, elbow and shoulder
(8) As 7 but halting on command
(9) As above but the therapist points to the part to be touched
(10) As above but the therapist moves her fingers as the patient reaches the part.

Next, a less supported position can be used and the above stages used for each position and exercise such as:

- Sitting – knee extension and flexion.
- Sitting – hip abduction and adduction.
- Sitting – moving the foot over a numbered board or pushing a beanbag on the board (Fig. 17.2).
- Sitting – lifting objects about on a table.
- Sitting – personal toilet training.

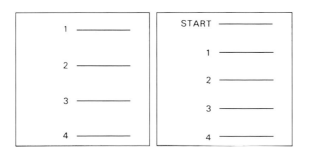

Fig. 17.1 The marks for counting; A, to a count of 4; B, to a 'start' command and count of 4.

Walking training follows

The patient stands using stride standing or oblique walk standing while holding on a firm hand support (wallbars or fixed parallel bars). Weight transference is practised first, remembering that counting must be maintained.

Sideways walking is practised first making the base narrower and wider in turn but never closing the base into close standing. A Frenkel mat can be used (Fig. 17.3) when the patient is first required to put the foot into a space and eventually on to the lines.

Forward progression is made to ordinary walking with a wide base using first a 'step to' gait, i.e. right foot forwards, left foot up to it. Then later the left foot can be carried through and forwards. The two outer sets of footprints on the Frenkel mat are used first followed by using one of the outer and the middle footprints.

Turning round may be performed by either step turning or pivot and step turning.

Step turning

The direction of the turn is decided, e.g. to the right. The right foot is lifted and turned through 90° and placed in the right-hand footprint. The left foot is lifted, turned and placed in the left-hand footprint (Fig. 17.4A). The above manoeuvres are continued

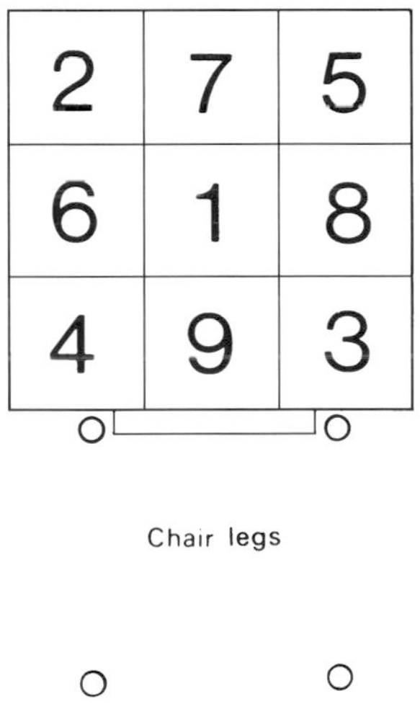

Chair legs

Fig. 17.2 The numbered board for co-ordinated lower limb movements in sitting.

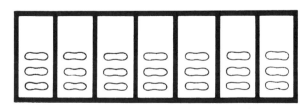

Fig. 17.3 A Frenkel mat.

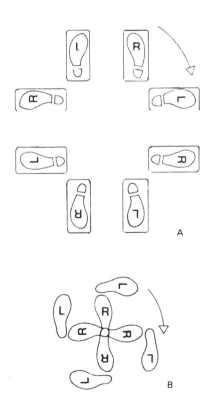

Fig. 17.4 A, Step turning; B, Pivot turning. A is easier than B. When using B the patient will not necessarily be in line with his stepping line on the Frenkel mat.

until the patient has turned through 180° or 360°.

Pivot turning

A decision is again made about direction but this method may be used when the turn must be made in the direction of the worst leg. The patient pivots to the right on the heel of the right leg. The left foot is then lifted, turned and placed a short distance away alongside the first foot. The manoeuvre is repeated (Fig. 17.4B). Pivot turning may also be used as a progression on step turning as the base may be narrower.

Vertigo

Vertigo occasionally requires a regime of exercises when it follows concussion as a post-concussion syndrome or when it is associated with space-occupying lesions or vascular accidents of the brain. This regime may also be used for conditions such as Ménière's disease which does not respond to drug therapy.

The regime of exercises is based on the principle of gradually inducing an attack of vertigo and then, when the patient recovers, carrying on with the regime. In this way the threshold of onset of an attack is pushed back and the patient learns both to accommodate to and to cope with an attack.

The regime starts with the patient performing eye movements while fully supported and continues through lessening support until the body movements can be made fast enough to evade moving obstacles.

The positions used are:

- Lying with minimal pillows for comfort
- Half lying
- Sitting in a corner of a room (i.e. using two walls for moral support)
- Sitting free in a space
- Kneel sitting
- Standing – stride or walk and eventually walking.

The objective is achieved by the therapist using a small coloured ball which she moves about in front of the fully supported patient asking him to follow the movements with his eyes. Next the range of the movement is increased so that head movements must be performed to keep the ball in sight.

In half lying a return is made to eye movements only and then to head movements again.

In sitting the same procedure is followed. The ball can be bounced by the therapist, then by the patient, starting with a single bounce and catch, continuing with repetitive bouncing with either hand and in different areas round the patient. Throwing between patient and therapist follows, with the therapist aiming the ball to make the patient move both or either arm to catch. In other words obtaining spontaneous displacement from the sitting and supported position and recovery to that position. Kneel sitting is a position of security in which total body displacement can take place as the patient is required to retrieve objects placed further and further away.

Similar procedures can be practised in free sitting plus getting up from the stool and walking round it, first without, then with ball bouncing or throwing it in the air and catching.

An obstacle course is then set up and the patient is required to thread his way in and out of the course, to walk in tight circles round some of the obstacles at first carefully escorted by the therapist and then to cover the course with other people simultaneously using it from other directions. Such a course may be set up first indoors and then outdoors, or alternatively the patient should be taken on a walk in the grounds of the hospital and through the adjacent streets.

This regime can be taught to a group of patients once they are all able to sit on a chair or stool.

Posture

Posture is an alternative name for position but in an exercise context is usually taken to be a dynamic position in which the body components relate to one another so that the centre of gravity is over the base and the muscle work to maintain the position is reduced to a minimum.

Good posture is also pleasing to the eye and is dynamically adapted to the size of the base and the circumstances in which the body is resting or working. Good posture should not throw undue stress on muscle or joints and should be automatically resumed after displacement has occurred.

Poor posture is frequently produced by bad habits, e.g. the slouching posture adopted by the adolescent following the fashion of walking and standing with their hands in the front pockets of jeans. The use of unsuitable equipment may induce poor posture, e.g. a too low working surface will cause a kyphotic posture of the back at its weakest point; and associated round shoulders and poking chin will follow.

Holding the head to one side in a 'listening' posture due to slight deafness may become a bad habit and lead to the adoption of resultant deviations of the relationships of pelvis to shoulder girdle or of the vertebrae to one another.

Standing with most of the weight on one leg will lead to lateral deviations of the vertebrae and pelvis–shoulder girdle relationship.

When the cause is shortness of the lower limb of more than 2.5 cm, correction will occur if raised footwear is worn, but if any of the above postural habits are allowed to persist they will become permanent disfigurements and adaptive shortening of the soft tissues will ensue.

Early detection of poor posture and retraining to good position can be most rewarding and may need the following procedures:

(1) The patient's interest must be gained and he must *want* to improve his posture.
(2) Local relaxation may need to be taught, preferably in lying.
(3) The patient is then 'straightened' by teaching the correct alignment of each body component to the other starting with the pelvis shoulder girdle relationship. At this point the patient may complain that 'It, or he, feels odd'. The new proprioceptive pathways are being stimulated and he will now have to learn that 'feeling odd' may be correct. During this part of the proceedings he should be encouraged to maintain maximum body length by feeling as though he was stretching like a piece of elastic between his feet and his head.
(4) It is now important to displace body components while maintaining the corrected position, e.g. perform an arm or leg exercise and *maintain* the new posture.
(5) Next he must be totally displaced into a vigorous activity or maybe a game and then he must lie down and *regain* his new posture.

This procedure can be repeated several times perhaps during the course of a class but at the first treatment the patient must also experience his corrected posture in sitting and standing and by constant reminder in all dynamic positions assumed during the course of that day's treatment session.

The treatment must include, for each patient, the adoption of their normal work or daily activity position so that the therapist can teach correction of what may be a poor posture adopted for the greater part of the day.

Chapter 18
NEUROPHYSIOLOY OF MOVEMENT

Phyl Fletcher-Cook

As functional beings, we make demands on our neuromuscular system which enable us to fulfil our daily activities. The motor activities which enable this can be considered in three categories: voluntary movements, reflex activity and rhythmical movements (Ghez 1991a).

Voluntary movements

Voluntary movements have purpose, are consciously initiated, are goal directed and are learned motor acts (Ghez 1991a). By virtue of this learning, voluntary movements may become more automatic, e.g. playing the piano requires less conscious thought as skill level improves.

Reflex activity

This occurs in response to sensory stimuli, e.g. flexor withdrawal of the leg when standing on a pin, or contraction of the quadriceps muscle when the patellar tendon is tapped. The movements involved in reflex responses are fairly stereotyped (Shumway-Cook & Woolacott 1995; Ghez 1991a). It is thought that reflexes are served by central pattern generators in the spinal cord and that, even in the absence of sensory stimuli from the periphery, central processes may generate reflex patterns when

required (Shumway-Cook & Woolacott 1995; Gordon 1991).

Rhythmical movements

Walking is an example of rhythmical movement and results from a combination of voluntary and reflex control (Ghez 1991a). We voluntarily begin and end the movement sequences but the sequence itself is under central pattern generator control in the spinal cord (Bear *et al.* 1996). For example, these central pattern generators control the crossed extensor reflex which appears to be the basis for locomotion (Bear *et al.* 1996).

Organization of the nervous system for motor control

All movement involves the integrated activity of several motor control systems (Cockell *et al.* 1995). Motor control systems are organized hierarchically and in parallel (Bear *et al.* 1996; Ghez 1991a; Shumway-Cook & Woolacott 1995).

In essence, the hierarchical model involves the integration and interpretation of sensory information in the association areas of the cortex to determine, for example, the current position of body parts relative to each other and to the environment. Information is shared between the cortex and basal ganglia in order to develop motor strategies for action. These aspects represent the highest levels in the hierarchy. The middle level is represented by the motor cortex and cerebellum which together determine the tactics for the action, i.e. the spatio-temporal sequences of muscle activity necessary to achieve the strategy (Bear *et al.* 1996). The lower levels, which comprise the brain stem and spinal cord, execute the movements via activation of motor neuronal pools for selective movements and postural adjustments (Bear *et al.* 1996; Shumway-Cook & Woolacott 1995; Ghez 1991a).

Parallel processing also occurs, whereby the same input is shared between several areas of the brain at the same time, for example, the cerebellum and basal ganglia process information from the cortex prior to signalling the motor cortex for resultant action (Shumway-Cook & Woolacott 1995).

Role of the spinal cord in movement control

The spinal cord is the lowest level in the hierarchy for movement control. It receives somatosensory information from muscles, tendons, joints and skin, which it processes and acts on. It also transmits such information to higher centres in the brain. Essentially, the spinal cord is concerned mainly with reflex activity which is moderated by descending influences from higher centres to produce movements appropriate to the task.

The spinal cord is organized into defined neuronal populations in the grey matter, surrounded by the white matter which is composed of ascending and descending tracts. In the intermediate area between the anterior and posterior horns of the grey matter lie populations of interneurons. These are essential in the processing of incoming sensory information from the periphery via the posterior horn, as well as descending signals from higher brain centres (Gordon 1991). It is here that divergent connections enable a signal to be relayed to several neurons at the same time and convergent connections enable stimuli from many sources, e.g. muscle spindles, descending signals from higher centres and collaterals from lower motor neurons, to target a specific neuron (Gordon 1991). These divergent and convergent connections enable spatial organization of reflex activity in the cord. Temporal organization also exists by virtue of central pattern generators which form reverberating circuits where the interneurons re-excite themselves and so prolong their activity over time (Gordon 1991). The latter form the basis for locomotion.

Inhibitory interneurons

The ability of the spinal cord to co-ordinate muscle actions is dependent on distinct populations of inhibitory interneurons. Group 1a inhibitory interneurons form the basis for reciprocal inhibition. Thus, when descending impulses from the cortex cause the agonists to contract, collateral branches from the corticospinal axons stimulate 1a inhibitory interneurons which then inhibit the alpha motor neurons to the antagonistic muscles (Gordon 1991).

The 1a inhibitory interneurons also receive both inhibitory and excitatory connections from all of the main descending tracts. By altering the relative balance of inhibition and excitation onto these interneurons, higher brain centres can integrate muscle activity. For example, if the task being performed requires co-contraction of agonists and antagonists, the summative influence on the 1a inhibitory interneurons to the antagonist will be inhibitory, thus disinhibiting the alpha motor neurons to the antagonist which then contracts along with the agonist (Gordon & Ghez 1991).

A second group of inhibitory interneurons are the Renshaw cells. These cells form a negative feedback system which smooths the firing rate of motor neurons (Gordon & Ghez 1991). When activated, motor neurons in the anterior horn send collaterals to adjacent Renshaw cells which then tend to inhibit the same motor neurons. This is known as recurrent inhibition. Thus, when the firing rate of a motor neuron increases, the Renshaw cells become more active to prevent large changes in the firing rate. When motor neuron firing rate decreases, so too does that of the Renshaw cells (Gordon & Ghez 1991). This helps regulate fluctuations in muscle contraction.

Renshaw cells also form inhibitory synapses with 1a inhibitory interneurons to antagonistic motor neurons. This tends to disinhibit the motor neurons to the antagonist muscles. A similar arrangement exists with motor neurons of synergistic muscles. Thus, integration and co-ordination of muscle activity can be achieved (Gordon & Ghez 1991).

A final population of inhibitory interneurons, 1b interneurons, also needs consideration. Golgi tendon organs lying at the junctions of muscle fibres and tendons transmit information to the spinal cord and connect with 1b interneurons to excite them. The 1b interneurons in turn tend to inhibit the motor neurons to the muscle in which the Golgi tendon organ lies. This forms a negative feedback loop for the regulation of muscle tension (Gordon & Ghez 1991; Bear *et al.* 1996).

It must also be remembered that these populations of interneurons are subject to modulating influences from higher centres via descending pathways which ultimately determine the summative outcome appropriate to the movement being performed.

Alpha motor neurons

The anterior horn of the spinal cord houses the alpha and gamma motor neurons via which movement and postural adaptations are executed. Each alpha motor neuron supplies several skeletal muscle fibres to form a motor unit. Each muscle comprises several motor units and movements are graded by recruitment of more or fewer motor units to suit the task (Bear *et al.* 1996).

Gamma motor neurons and the muscle spindle

In order to understand the effects of gamma motor neuron activity, it is first necessary to consider the muscle spindle. Muscle spindles lie within skeletal muscles, in parallel with their fibres. Each muscle spindle contains a dynamic nuclear bag fibre, a static nuclear bag fibre and several static nuclear chain fibres (Gordon & Ghez 1991). The ultimate purpose of the muscle spindle is to monitor the length of skeletal muscle and the rate of change in its length and to regulate muscle tone. To this end, all the fibres within the muscle spindle have primary nerve endings located around their central portions. The axons running from these receptors are rapidly transmitting 1a fibres (Gordon & Ghez 1991) which synapse directly onto the alpha motor neurons which supply the skeletal muscle. Once excited by stretch of the muscle, these primary receptors transmit impulses at a higher rate to the alpha motor neurons of the muscle and it then contracts to reduce the stretch. This is the phasic stretch reflex. This sensory information is also relayed to higher centres for the planning of motor activity.

The static nuclear bag and nuclear chain fibres are also served by another type of sensory ending which lies on either side of the primary endings. These are the secondary endings whose axons are group 11 afferents. They constantly transmit signals to the spinal cord and to higher centres about the static length of the skeletal muscle in which the spindle lies. The connections of the type 11 afferents are polysynaptic, exciting several interneurons (Gordon & Ghez 1991), which in turn excite the alpha motor neurons to the skeletal muscle. The tone of the skeletal muscle is therefore maintained by the excited alpha motor neurons. This is the static component of the stretch reflex.

The polar regions of each intrafusal fibre are composed of intrafusal muscle, which when contracted puts a stretch on the central regions of the intrafusal fibres. The neurons which drive this muscle are the static and dynamic gamma motor neurons of the anterior horn of the spinal cord. The static gamma efferents supply the static nuclear chain fibres and the static nuclear bag fibre. The dynamic nuclear bag fibre is supplied by the dynamic gamma efferents (Gordon & Ghez 1991).

The effect of gamma motor output is to increase the gain of the spindle by contracting the intrafusal muscle and therefore placing a small stretch on the central sensory regions of the intrafusal fibres. This increases the impulse traffic from the receptors and, via the stretch reflex, increases alpha motor neuron firing to the skeletal muscle, increasing its state of contraction, i.e. its tone.

Descending impulses from higher centres moderate the firing of the gamma efferents and can therefore moderate skeletal muscle tone to suit the activity being performed. Thus, movements and the associated background postural adjustments can be efficiently executed.

Role of the brainstem in movement control

One of the functions of the brainstem is to act as a conduit for ascending and descending pathways concerned with the control of movement. These include all somatic afferent pathways, e.g. the medial lemnisci and spino-thalamic tracts, and the descending motor tracts, e.g. the cortico-spinal tracts.

Reticulospinal tracts

In addition, some descending tracts originate in the reticular formation of the brainstem. These include the pontine reticulo-spinal tract which influences the alpha and gamma motor neurons of extensor muscles to increase extensor tone (Role & Kelly 1991; Bear *et al.* 1996). A second tract, the medullary reticulo-spinal tract, which originates in the gigantocellular reticular nucleus, influences neurons in the intermediate area of the cord grey matter and has an inhibitory effect on extensor muscle tone (Role & Kelly 1991; Bear *et al.* 1996).

Vestibulospinal tracts

Other motor tracts originate in the floor of the medulla where the vestibular nuclei are located. The lateral vestibulo-spinal tract originates in the lateral vestibular nucleus and drives the anterior horn cells to the anti-gravity muscles of the neck, trunk and limbs (Shumway-Cook & Woolacott 1995). The medial vestibulo-spinal tract arises from the medial vestibular nucleus and is involved in the control of neck muscles and in co-ordinating head and eye movements (Shumway-Cook & Woolacott 1995). The importance of these postural adjustment mechanisms is underlined by the fact that a feed-forward system exists so that the postural adjustments for a selective movement are made in advance of the movement beginning (Ghez 1991b). This system is augmented by rapid feedback compensatory adjustments as the movement progresses (Ghez 1991b).

Brainstem reflex activity

The brainstem is also the site of reflex activity. The reflexes consist of vestibular and neck reflexes which stabilize the head and neck and align the body relative to gravity (Ghez 1991b). Changing head position will elicit vestibular reflexes and bending or turning the head will elicit neck reflexes such as the asymmetrical tonic neck reflex and the symmetrical tonic neck reflex.

Vestibular reflexes

Vestibular reflexes are involved in postural adjustments to maintain balance, and as such they alter muscle tone in the neck and in the limbs. The otolith organs in the inner ear register changes in head position with respect to gravity and linear acceleration of the head, and the semi-circular canals detect angular acceleration of the head. This information results in tonal changes in groups of muscles, e.g. if a subject trips while walking, his head is tilted forward and the head extensors contract to return the head to the vertical. At the same time, the upper limbs extend and flexion of the lower limbs occurs in order to minimize the impact of the fall (Ghez 1991b).

Neck reflexes

The neck reflexes also induce tonal changes in neck and limb muscles. In the asymmetrical tonic neck reflex, when the head is rotated to one side, the extensor tone in the limbs on that side will increase, whereas flexor tone will increase in the opposite limbs. The neck muscles which are stretched will tend to contract to return the head to neutral. In the symmetrical tonic neck reflex, bending the head forwards will increase tone in the flexors of the upper limbs (Ghez 1991b). These reflexes are moderated by descending influences from higher centres such that they are not readily apparent, but they can be released to varying degrees when required. For example, when a tennis player reaches up to the side to hit a high ball, the asymmetrical tonic neck reflex is less inhibited to enable quick production of the movement to position the racquet for the ball.

Role of the cerebellum in movement control

Cerebellar structure

The cerebellum is an important centre for movement control. Structurally the cerebellum consists of an outer cortex where neuronal bodies lie, and an inner area of white matter formed by the axons of input and output neurons. Embedded in the white matter are three pairs of deep cerebellar nuclei: the fastigial nucleus, the interposed nucleus and the dentate nucleus (Shumway-Cook & Woolacott 1995). All inputs to the cerebellar cortex first send collateral branches to one of these deep nuclei before proceeding on to the cerebellar cortex. Once information is processed, the output from the cerebellum is relayed via the deep cerebellar nuclei to various motor systems in the brainstem and cerebral cortex (Shumway-Cook & Woolacott 1995).

Neuronal populations in the cerebellar cortex

There are distinct neuronal populations and circuits within the cerebellum. The cortex is basically composed of three layers.

The outermost layer (molecular layer) contains mainly axons of granule cells which are known as parallel fibres and which run horizontally in the molecular layer. Also, some stellate and basket cells lie here and act as interneurons. The final structures identifiable in this layer are the dendrites of Purkinje cells (Ghez 1991d).

The middle layer contains the cell bodies of the Purkinje cells which lie side by side in a single row. These cells' axons run downwards in the white matter, forming the only output from the cerebellar cortex. They are inhibitory neurons which influence the deep cerebellar nuclei (Ghez 1991d).

The innermost layer (granular layer) contains granule cells and some golgi cells.

Afferent fibres

In order to function, the cerebellum requires information from the spinal cord, brainstem and cerebral cortex. There are two forms of excitatory afferents to the cerebellum: the mossy fibres and the climbing fibres. Both send excitatory collaterals to the deep nuclei on their way up to the cerebellar cortex. The excitation of the deep nuclei is modulated by the cerebellar cortex via the inhibitory Purkinje cells.

The mossy fibres are more numerous, carrying information from the spinal cord via the spinocerebellar tracts and from brainstem nuclei. These fibres synapse onto the granule cells which in turn excite the Purkinje cells. The climbing fibres are afferents from the inferior olivary nuclei in the medulla. They make powerful connections onto the Purkinje cells, increasing their output (Ghez 1991d).

Functional divisions

Functionally, the cerebellum may be divided into three areas: the spino-cerebellum, the cerebro-cerebellum and the vestibulo-cerebellum. The two cerebellar hemispheres are joined by a central area called the vermis. The hemispheres themselves may each be functionally sub-divided into an intermediate zone and a lateral zone. The vermis and the intermediate zone together constitute the spino-cerebellum, while the lateral zone forms the cerebro-cerebellum. The vestibulo-cerebellum is formed by the flocculo-nodular lobe (Ghez 1991d).

The spino-cerebellum receives somatosensory information via the spino-cerebellar tracts, which signal the cerebellum about movements as they occur (dorsal spino-cerebellar tract) and about the activity of segmental interneurons in the spinal cord (ventral spino-cerebellar tract) so that the cerebellum is appraised of current neuronal circuits in operation (Ghez 1991d). These afferents make up the mossy fibre input. Another input is via the spino-olivo-cerebellar tract which constitutes the climbing fibre input (Shumway-Cook & Woolacott 1995).

The Purkinje cells in the two components of the spino-cerebellum project to different deep nuclei. Those in the vermis project to the fastigial nuclei which in turn project to the reticular formation and the lateral vestibular nuclei in the brainstem. From here, the reticulo-spinal and vestibulo-spinal tracts, i.e. the medial descending system, exert descending influences on the anterior horn cells of the spinal cord (Ghez 1991d).

The fastigial nuclei also project via the thalamus to the primary motor cortex to influence cortical output via the descending system (Ghez 1991d). Thus, the vermis regulates axial and proximal limb musculature. The intermediate parts of the cerebellar hemispheres project to the interposed nuclei which in turn influence the brainstem and cortical components of the lateral descending system (rubro-spinal and cortico-spinal tracts). Thus, the intermediate zone influences the action of distal limb muscles (Ghez 1991d).

Overall, the spino-cerebellum is involved in the execution of movements, by comparing intended movement with actual movement and by modulating muscle tone through its descending effects on gamma motor neurons to muscle spindles (Shumway-Cook & Woolacott 1995). In this way, it fine tunes movements.

The cerebro-cerebellum (the lateral zone of the cerebellar hemispheres) receives input via the pontine nuclei from the sensory and motor cortices and from the pre-motor and posterior parietal cortical areas of the cerebral hemispheres.

The Purkinje cells of the cerebro-cerebellum project to the dentate nuclei. These in turn project via the thalamus which relays information back to the motor and pre-motor cortices of the cerebral hemispheres, thus completing a feedback loop. The dentate nuclei also form a feedback link to the red nuclei which then project back to the cerebellum (Ghez 1991d).

The cerebro-cerebellum controls the precision of rapid limb movements and fine dexterity of movements. It is involved in the preparation for and the initiation of more complex, multi-joint movements as well as precision movements of individual fingers. It is this area which enables timed activity of agonists and antagonists to prevent overshooting of a target, a function which involves the cerebro-cerebellum in a motor planning role which it achieves by working with the motor and pre-motor cortices (Ghez 1991d).

The vestibulo-cerebellum (the flocculonodular lobe of the cerebellum) receives afferent input via the vestibular nuclei from the semicircular canals detailing changes in head position, and from the otolith organs which signal head position in relation to gravity. It also receives visual information. Output from the vestibulo-cerebellum is to the vestibular nuclei which activate the medial descending systems to the axial and proximal limb muscles which control balance (Ghez 1991d; Shumway-Cook & Woolacott 1995).

Motor learning

Finally, the cerebellum appears to serve as a memory site for motor skill learning (Raymond *et al.* 1996). It is thought that climbing fibre activity is increased during motor learning and this decreases the activity of the mossy fibres, thus correcting deviations in actual movement from the planned movement (Ghez 1991d). This is also thought to involve the cerebro-cerebellum (Shumway-Cook & Woolacott 1995).

Raymond *et al.* (1996) also hypothesize three elements to motor learning. Firstly, learning occurs in both the cerebellar cortex and the deep nuclei which both store memories. Secondly, the learning in the cerebellar cortex is essential for the timing of movements. Finally, the cerebellar cortex output initiates the learning in the deep nuclei which may be the site of long term memory.

Role of the basal ganglia in movement control

The basal ganglia comprise the putamen and caudate nuclei, the globus pallidus, the subthalamic nucleus and the substantia nigra. They are bilateral structures lying just below the cerebral cortex, except the substantia nigra which lies in the mid-brain. In addition to the basal ganglia role in motor control, they are also involved in cognitive function and behavioural aspects which are not related to movement. This section will concentrate on their input to motor control.

Almost all input to the basal ganglia is to the caudate and putamen (the striatum). The sources of this input include the entire cerebral cortex, in particular the motor, sensory and association areas. The motor cortex also projects to the striatum via the thalamus (Cote & Crutcher 1991; Connor & Abbs 1990; Shumway-Cook & Woolacott 1995).

The internal segment of the globus pallidus and the substantia nigra constitute the main output areas of the basal ganglia, projecting first to the thalamus from which excitatory relay fibres reach the pre-frontal and pre-motor areas of the cerebral cortex (Shumway-Cook & Woolacott 1995).

The motor loop

There are several circuits within the basal ganglia, one of them being the motor loop. This is the most direct pathway, with input to the putamen causing it to inhibit cells in the globus pallidus. The globus pallidus in turn makes inhibitory synapses onto cells in the ventro-lateral nucleus of the thalamus. The thalamus sends excitatory connections to the supplementary motor area of the cortex (Bear *et al.* 1996).

Thus, movement occurs when the thalamus is released from tonic inhibition allowing it to excite the supplementary motor and pre-motor cortex. This then signals the motor cortex to activate the descending systems to the spinal cord for movement execution (Cote & Crutcher 1991).

Motor programming

The supplementary motor area and the basal ganglia are thought to be involved in motor programming, i.e. the planning and execution of complex movement strategies (Cote & Crutcher 1991), and in the preparation for movement which may be why patients with Parkinsons disease have difficulty initiating movements (Connor & Abbs 1990; Contreras-Vidal & Stelmach 1995).

Role of the cerebral cortex in movement control

The cerebral cortex is a higher centre for movement control. It receives sensory data from the body, eyes and ears, which it uses to plan and initiate movements. It is also concerned with memory, emotions and intellectual ability (Young & Young 1997) which may also be linked to its motor functions.

Communication within the cortex

Different areas of the cerebral cortex fulfil different functions, e.g. Brodmann's areas 4 and 6 of the frontal lobe are labelled as motor cortex, but control of voluntary movement involves nearly all of the cerebral cortex (Bear *et al.* 1996). This is reflected in the fact that different cortical areas within the same hemisphere are linked by bundles of association fibres, e.g. the occipital and parietal lobes link with the frontal lobe via the superior longitudinal fasciculus, and adjacent gyri are linked by arcuate fibres. The two hemispheres are also linked by bundles of commissural fibres which pass between them, e.g. the corpus callosum and the anterior commissure (Young & Young 1997). Thus, a complex communication system operates at cortical level.

Functional areas of the cortex

In relation to movement, the cerebral cortex can be divided functionally into several areas, including the somatosensory cortex, the motor cortex and their association cortices.

The somatosensory cortex consists of a primary somatosensory cortex located in the post-central gyrus of the parietal lobe (areas 3,1 and 2 of Brodmann), a secondary somatosensory cortex which lies in the lower, lateral part of the post-central gyrus and forms the upper wall of the lateral fissure (Young & Young 1997) and a third area in the posterior part of the parietal lobe (areas 5 and 7 of Brodmann) (Martin & Jessell 1991).

The primary somatosensory cortex receives information on proprioception, touch, pain and temperature from the body which is relayed via the thalamus to the cortex (Martin & Jessell 1991). It is here that sensory information is represented in a somatotopic way, i.e. all the body parts are represented inversely and larger areas are devoted to the hands, lips, tongue and fingers. The various modalities of sensation are processed together, which allows integration of for example cutaneous and proprioceptive information to build a picture of the position of the body relative to the environment and the positions of body parts relative to each other (Shumway-Cook & Woolacott 1995). This integration is essential if co-ordinated movements are to occur. This area also registers the texture, size and shape of objects (Bear *et al.* 1996).

The secondary somatosensory cortex also has a rudimentary somatotopic representation and it is thought that this area also registers pain (Young & Young 1997). The posterior parietal lobe or parietal association area receives input from the primary somatosensory cortex, the motor and visual cortices and from association areas in the frontal, temporal, occipital and limbic lobes. The parietal association area processes visual and somatic information to enable recognition of objects (Bear *et al.* 1996). It is also thought to enable perception of the body in space and its relationships to objects around it. As such, this area may be important in the sequential performance of motor tasks, especially by the hands (Young & Young 1997).

The motor cortex lies in the frontal lobe. It comprises the primary motor cortex (area 4 of Brodmann), the pre-motor cortex (area 6 of Brodmann) and the supplementary motor area lying in the superior and medial parts of area 6 (Ghez 1991c). These motor areas communicate with the sensory processing areas in the parietal lobe as well as with the cerebellum and basal ganglia in order to plan and implement movement strategies (Shumway-Cook & Woolacott 1995).

The primary motor cortex is organized topographically, similar to the primary somatosensory cortex. The hands, fingers, mouth and tongue are also disproportionally represented, which reflects the need for precision movements of these parts (Young & Young 1997; Bear *et al.* 1996; Ghez 1991c). Activation of the primary motor cortex causes muscles to contract on the opposite side of the body. This is achieved by activation of the pyramidal cells in the primary motor cortex whose axons project to the spinal cord via the cortico-spinal tract.

The pre-motor cortex is also organized topographically and sends axons to the primary motor cortex as well as to sub-cortical structures and the spinal cord (Ghez 1991c). This area deals with motor activity to larger groups of muscles (Young & Young 1997) and is involved in the co-ordinated contraction of muscles acting over multiple joints on the opposite side of the body (Ghez 1991c; Shumway-Cook & Woolacott 1995).

The supplementary motor area projects to the same areas as the pre-motor cortex and essentially produces the same complexity of muscle activity over multiple joints, but this area stimulates movements on both sides of the body (Ghez 1991c) and is essential in the co-ordination of the hands during tasks which require both hands working together. Bear *et al.* (1996) support this but further claim that the pre-motor cortex connects mainly with reticulo-spinal neurons which supply proximal muscles, whereas the supplementary motor area innervates predominantly distal muscles.

Overall, the pre-motor and supplementary motor cortices appear to play a major role in the planning of complex movement sequences (Bear *et al.* 1996; Young & Young 1997).

Cognitive influences on movement

The pre-frontal areas of the frontal lobe, which lie anterior to the motor cortices, are concerned with decision-making, abstract thought and anticipation of the outcomes of actions (Bear *et al.* 1996). These areas connect extensively with the posterior parietal cortex and together they constitute the highest level of motor control in that they make decisions on what actions to take and what the consequences will be. Axons from these areas reach the pre-motor and supplementary motor cortices which both contribute to the cortico-spinal tract (Bear *et al.* 1996).

Plasticity of the nervous system

Plasticity of the nervous system is essential for an individual to function normally (Annunciato 1995). Plasticity is the ability of cells to undergo alterations in their form and function in response to significant changes in their environment (Kidd *et al.* 1992). Most importantly, plastic adaptation may occur at any stage in the cell's lifespan.

It is easy to imagine the developing brain of a child as having the capacity for neuroplastic adaptation, but it has also been established that the adult brain has a great capacity for '... structural and functional regeneration' (Goldman & Plum 1997). For example, Rauschecker (1997) reports that the Braille reading finger in blind subjects has an increased sensori-motor representation in the cortex. This is supported by Seil (1997) and Lee & Van Donkelaar (1995) who claim that both the motor and sensory cortex in adults (and children) can plastically adapt to altered neural firing patterns, thus showing that neuroplastic adaptation will depend on environmental influences.

One way of inducing neuroplastic adaptation is by manipulating the periphery to invoke a change in the target neurons' environment. For example, when a physiotherapy student first tries to palpate vertebral spinous processes the sensitivity of the palpating thumbs is not adequately developed for the student to be certain that her thumbs are indeed on the spinous process. The sensitivity of the thumbs is dependent on their somatosensory representation on the cortex. Through practice, it is hoped that plastic adaptation will occur in the sensory cortex topography as a result of the regular sensory input from the skin and pressure receptors of the thumbs.

Plastic adaptation of the cortex has also been shown to occur after central lesions. For example, in some cases of hemiplegia, other adjacent areas of the sensori-motor cortex were shown to assume the role of the damaged area to some extent (Seil 1997; Lee & Van Donkelaar 1995; Stephenson 1993).

Mechanisms of plastic adaptation

There are several physiological mechanisms by which neuroplastic adaptations can occur in healthy individuals and after lesions to the central nervous system. These include recruitment of latent synapses, synaptic potentiation, recovery of synaptic function, axonal sprouting, formation of new synaptic connections and the formation of dendritic spines.

Recruitment of latent synapses occurs when synapses which were previously silent or minimally used become more active after a lesion, forming new pathways (Stephenson 1993; Lee & Van Donkelaar 1995; Seil 1997).

Synaptic potentiation occurs when some collaterals of an axon are damaged with resultant redirection of the neurotransmitter substance to the intact terminals. This boosts the function of these terminals as they have more transmitter to release into the synaptic cleft (Annunciato 1995).

Recovery of synaptic function is the result of reabsorption of oedema surrounding the site of a lesion. As the oedema subsides, intact neurons are no longer compressed and begin to function normally again (Annunciato 1995).

Axonal sprouting from intact axons involves the formation of callateral axons which increases the territory of influence of the parent neuron (Seil 1997). Collateral sprouting may also be regenerative in nature. When an axon is damaged or its target cell is destroyed, short sprouts from the axon can develop and form new synapses (Annunciato 1995). The formation of new synaptic connections tends to be one of the slower plastic adaptations (Seil 1997). Finally, an increase in the number of dendritic spines on the post-synaptic cell serves to increase the surface area for reception of incoming signals and therefore increases the efficiency of the connection (Stephenson 1996).

All these plastic adaptations can occur in the damaged nervous systems of patients with neurological disease. In these cases, the therapist manipulates peripheral input to the central nervous system to affect the environment of more central cells in such a way as to engender beneficial neuroplastic adaptation. Without such input, it could be argued that adverse neuroplastic adaptation, for example causing increasing spasticity in hemiplegic limbs, is likely to take place.

Neuroplastic adaptation is also a feature of the healthy nervous system and can be illustrated whenever we learn a new motor skill.

The basis of treatment

In neurology, physiotherapy interventions are based on a problem-solving approach and, as such, require in the therapist an integrated knowledge of neurophysiology, normal movement, normal postural reflex mechanisms, pathology and neuromuscular plasticity. It is from this base that deviations from the normal can be identified and appropriate treatment strategies implemented. For example, a patient with Guillain-Barré syndrome affecting lower motor neurons will, in the recovery stage, benefit from a muscle strengthening regime, as muscle weakness is readily apparent. A factor which must influence our choice of strengthening regime is the knowledge that, in the paralysis stage, adverse neuroplastic adaptation will have occurred in the peripheral nervous system and, by virtue of altered sensory input from this system, there may be plastic adaptations within the central nervous system also. Similar plastic adaptations will have occurred within the muscles. We also know that muscle groups work together in co-ordinated patterns during functional activities. If we therefore wish, for example, to strengthen the abdominal muscles, perhaps the most justifiable approach is one which normalizes neuroplastic adaptation while at the same time incorporating functional patterns of movement. Thus, rather than using isolated abdominal exercises, proprioceptive neuromuscular facilitation techniques using the scapular and pelvic patterns may be used to encourage activities such as rolling over in bed. In this way, we maximize on sensory input to influence neuronal pools in the spinal cord and at higher levels in the central nervous system, i.e. the brainstem, cerebellum, basal ganglia and sensori-motor cortex. In other words, we manipulate the periphery to achieve a more normal central patterning for motor activity.

Adverse neuroplastic adaptation in the central nervous system will also be a feature of hemiplegic patients who are 'locked' into spastic patterns. Technique selection must address this increased tone in order to unmask residual selective movements and facilitate more normal postural reflex mechanisms. A Bobath approach using, for example, central key point mobilizations may achieve both these aims by reducing pathological tone in the trunk, and facilitating weight transference over the base of support. Again this uses manipulation of the peripheral nervous system to influence more normal patterns of neuronal firing in the central nervous system.

In some patients suffering from multiple sclerosis, the excitatory drive to the alpha and gamma motor neurons in the spinal cord is reduced due to lesions within the central nervous system. In such patients, peripheral stimulation may be used to facilitate the anterior horn cells to the hypotonic muscles. An example is an aspect of the Rood approach to treatment which involves tapping the muscle to induce stretch reflexes or brushing over the dermatome of the same root supply as the muscle to facilitate muscle contraction. This sensory bombardment may also induce changes in more central neuronal pools which may influence anterior horn cells via intact but previously underused descending axons, thus strengthening these pathways.

It can readily be seen that the principles of neuroplastic adaptation are central to physiotherapy for neurologically damaged patients. The challenge is to prolong the effects of treatment between physiotherapy sessions so that beneficial adaptation occurs over as much of the 24 hours in each day as possible.

References

Annunciato, N.F. (1995) Plasticity of the nervous system. *Int. Journal of Orofacial Myology*, **xxi**, 53–9.

Bear, M.F., Connors, B.W. & Paradiso, M.A. (1996) *Neuroscience – Exploring the brain*. Williams and Wilkins, Baltimore.

Cockell, D.L., Carnahan, H. & McFadyen, B.J. (1995) A preliminary analysis of reaching, grasping and walking. *Perceptual and Motor Skills*, **81**, 515–19.

Connor, N.P. & Abbs, J.H. (1990) Sensorimotor contributions of the basal ganglia: recent advances. *Physical Therapy*, **70**, (12) 864–73.

Contreras-Vidal, J.L. & Stelmach, G.E. (1995) A neural model of basal ganglia – thalamocortical relations in normal and Parkinsonian movement. *Biological Cybernetics*, **73**, 467–76.

Cote, L. & Crutcher, M.D. (1991) The basal ganglia. In: *Principles of Neural Science* (eds E. Kandel, J.H. Schwartz & T.M. Jessell), 3rd edn, Ch. 42, pp. 647–78. Prentice Hall, London.

Ghez, C. (1991a) The control of movement. In: *Principles of Neural Science* (eds E. Kandel, J.H. Schwartz & T.M. Jessell), 3rd edn, Ch. 35, pp. 533–47. Prentice Hall, London.

Ghez, C. (1991b) Posture. In: *Principles of Neural Science* (eds E. Kandel, J.H. Schwartz & T.M. Jessell), 3rd edn, Ch. 39, pp. 569–607. Prentice Hall, London.

Ghez, C. (1991c) Voluntary movement. In: *Principles of Neural Science* (eds E. Kandel, J.H. Schwartz & T.M. Jessell), 3rd edn, Ch. 40, pp. 609–25. Prentice Hall, London.

Ghez, C. (1991d) The cerebellum. In: *Principles of Neural Science* (eds E. Kandel, J.H. Schwartz & T.M. Jessell), 3rd edn, Ch. 41, pp. 626–46. Prentice Hall, London.

Goldman, S. & Plum, F. (1997) Compensatory regeneration of the damaged adult brain: neuroplasticity in a clinical perspective. *Brain Plasticity, Advances in Neurology*, **73**, 97–107.

Gordon, J. (1991) Spinal Mechanisms of Motor Coordination. In: *Principles of Neural Science* (eds E. Kandel, J.H. Schwartz & T.M. Jessell), 3rd edn, Ch. 38, pp. 581–95. Prentice Hall, London.

Gordon, J. & Ghez, C. (1991) Muscle receptors and spinal reflexes: the stretch reflex. In: *Principles of Neural Science* (eds E. Kandel, J.H. Schwartz & T.M. Jessell), 3rd edn, Ch. 37, pp. 564–58. Prentice Hall, London.

Kidd, G., Lawes, N. & Musa, I. (1992) *Understanding Neuromuscular Plasticity*. Edward Arnold, London.

Lee, R.G. & Van Donkelaar, P. (1995) Mechanisms

underlying functional recovery following stroke. *Canadian Journal of Neurological Sciences*, **22** (4) 257–63.

Martin, J.H. & Jessell, T.M. (1991) Anatomy of the somatic sensory system. In: *Principles of Neural Science* (eds E. Kandel, J.H. Schwartz & T.M. Jessell), 3rd edn, Ch. 25, pp. 351–66. Prentice Hall, London.

Rauschecker, J.P. (1997) Mechanisms of compensatory plasticity in the cerebral cortex. *Brain Plasticity, Advances in Neurology*, **37**, 137–45.

Raymond, J.L., Lisberger, S.G. & Mauk, M.D. (1996) The cerebellum: a neuronal learning machine? *Science*, **272**, 1126–31.

Role, L.W. & Kelly, J.P. (1991) The brain stem: cranial nerve nuclei and the monaminergic systems. In: *Principles of Neural Science* (eds E. Kandel, J.H. Schwartz & T.M. Jessell), 3rd edn, Ch. 44, pp. 683–99. Prentice Hall, London.

Seil, F.J. (1997) Recovery and repair issues after stroke from the scientific perspective. *Current Opinion in Neurology*, **10**, 49–51.

Shumway-Cook, A. & Woolacott, M. (1995) *Motor Control: Theory and Practical Applications*. Williams and Wilkins, Baltimore.

Stephenson, R. (1993) A review of neuroplasticity: some implications for physiotherapy in the treatment of lesions of the brain. *Physiotherapy*, **93** (10), 699–703.

Stephenson, R. (1996) Therapeutic consistency following brain lesions. *Professional Nurse*, **11** (11), 738–40.

Young, P. & Young, P.H. (1997) *Basic Clinical Neuroanatomy*. Williams and Wilkins, Baltimore.

Chapter 19
PROPRIOCEPTIVE NEUROMUSCULAR FACILITATION (PNF)

P. J. Waddington

This technique was developed by Herman Kabat and his work was continued and expanded by Margaret Knott. Herman Kabat was interested in the treatment of 'patients with paralysis' and he stressed the importance of central excitation. The strength of a muscle contraction is directly proportional to the number of activated motor units, which obey the 'all or none' law. The functioning of these is dependent on the degree of excitation of the motor neurons. Thus the basic aim of the method is to stimulate the maximum number of motor units into activity and to hypertrophy all the remaining muscle fibres.

The basic technique

The importance of the proprioceptors, in particular the muscle spindles, was recognized as a key factor in facilitating the contraction of muscles. It was also recognized that to hypertrophy and increase the power of muscles it is necessary to make them work maximally in accordance with the basic principles of progressive resistance exercises.

Stretch

The patterns of movement associated with this technique were evolved from the basic idea of stretching (not overstretching) muscles to stimulate the activity of the muscle spindles, i.e. the patterns evolved from the concept of stretch. The position of stretch, the lengthened position of the muscles, is the starting position of each pattern and this *stretch stimulus* is maintained throughout the movement. An additional advantage of the position of stretch is that any contraction of a muscle on stretch will result in movement and not just in 'taking up' the slack. A simple analogy is that when a child pulls the string to which his toy duck is attached, the duck will not move until the string is taut. This follows Beevor's axiom: 'The brain knows not of muscles but of movement'. This axiom supports the basic idea of working in functional, mass movement patterns rather than trying to activate individual muscles.

Later this concept was extended to the *stretch reflex* which is obtained by an additional stretch superimposed on the muscles in the stretch stimulus position, usually at the outer range of the pattern. All the components of a pattern, particularly the rotary component, must be stretched simultaneously. It must be stressed that it is not excessive additional force, applied by the therapist, which elicits a stretch reflex but the skill with which she applies the stretch to the whole pattern. The reflex contraction of muscles and the movement brought about in this way can be used to initiate voluntary movement. The patient is instructed to make his effort to move to coincide with the reflex movement brought about by the therapist. The stretch reflex can also be used to aid the response of a weak muscle and to establish rhythmic contractions. A stretch reflex may also be used to obtain a lengthening reaction of hypertonic muscles:

(1) By stimulating a contraction of the opposing muscle group, the hypertonic muscles (the antagonists) will reciprocally lengthen.

(2) By reflexly stimulating a contraction of the hypertonic group. This contraction will be followed by a relaxation phase or lengthening reaction of the same muscle group (cf., the muscle twitch).

Patterns of movement

Patterns of movement are movements in a straight line, in a diagonal direction with a rotary component acting as the holding or stabilizing group, i.e. each pattern has three dimensions. For the patterns of the arms and legs these are flexion or extension, abduction or adduction and rotation (Fig. 19.1). These diagonal movements also apply to the head and trunk.

The exact position of the diagonal is critical because muscles are stronger in pattern (in the groove) than out of pattern and the whole basis of the technique is to facilitate the contraction of muscles. The diagonal is in line with the oblique trunk muscles, e.g. the arm must only

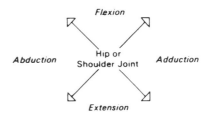

Fig. 19.1 Diagram showing the basic movement diagonals.

be an arm's width from the ear in the flexion, abduction and lateral rotation position; if the eyes and head are turned towards the hand in that position this will place the head and neck in the extension pattern with rotation to that side.

Patterns are named according to the direction of movement and therefore the finishing, not the starting, position. In completing the pattern the muscle contracts through full range from its lengthened to its shortened position.

Timing

The timing of the co-ordinated sequence of movements which form a pattern can be varied. In *normal timing* rotation initiates the movement, giving stability and direction to the pattern. Following this, movement will take place at the distal pivots (joints), e.g. fingers and wrist, and then at the proximal pivots, e.g. shoulder. Movement at the distal pivots must be completed before movement at the proximal pivots is completed. Changes in normal timing can be made to emphasize the contraction of a particular muscle group, i.e. *timing for emphasis*. This will be discussed later.

The grip

The therapist's grip is the key to facilitation. It provides four vital features:

(1) Stretch – the correct grip enables the therapist to stretch all the components of a pattern simultaneously

(2) Exteroception – the grip must be such that it gives sensory stimulation to the skin in the direction of movement, i.e. the therapist's hands must not be on two surfaces at once

(3) Resistance – the grip must be such that the therapist is able to exert maximum resistance throughout the full range of movement

(4) Traction or approximation – the grip must be such that the therapist is able to exert either traction or approximation to the part as and when indicated.

This grip has been called by the author the '*lumbrical grip*' because it is essential for the therapist's hand on the patient's hand or foot to be flexed at the metacarpophalangeal joints and extended, but not rigidly so, at the interphalangeal joints. The more skilled the operator becomes, the more selective and critical she is of her grip in the light of the patient's response.

Maximal resistance

The amount of resistance given by the therapist must be enough to demand from the patient his maximum effort. If the patient cannot lift the limb against gravity it will be necessary for the therapist to assist the movement. PNF can be used to exercise muscles the strength of which relates to any point on the Oxford Scale (Chapter 11).

As with progressive resistance exercises using either weights or springs, the therapist decides on the relationship between the number of repetitions and the amount of resistance. She may decide that the patient needs to repeat the movement many times, in which case the resistance will be reduced accordingly; con-

versely, the number of repetitions can be reduced and the resistance increased proportionately. The speed of the movement may also be controlled by varying the resistance.

The achievement and assessment of maximal resistance is related to the type of muscle work. For an *isotonic muscle contraction* the guide to maximal resistance is that the patient is able to perform a smooth, steady movement through full range; thus the amount of resistance may vary through different parts of the range.

For an *isometric muscle contraction*, where the rotary component (the holding or stabilizing group) is the dominant component, maximal resistance is developed slowly, i.e. the therapist gradually increases the resistance until the patient is making his maximum effort, taking care never to break the patient's hold.

Irradiation/overflow

Maximal resistance may be used to cause irradiation or overflow from stronger patterns to weaker patterns, or from stronger groups of muscles within a pattern to a weaker group within the same pattern (Chapter 23). This phenomenon is familiar to all therapists when strong, resisted dorsiflexion of the ankle is used to facilitate a contraction of the quadriceps. These two groups of muscles work functionally together in the walking pattern of the forward moving leg, i.e. flexion, adduction, with lateral rotation of the hip, extension of the knee and dorsiflexion of the ankle. No part of the body moves independently of other parts of the body. This re-inforcement of activity in one area by activity elsewhere is the basis for the use of the overflow principle.

Another example of re-inforcement frequently used is to obtain a contraction of the abdominal muscles by flexing the neck against resistance, the resistance in most cases provided by gravity as the patient is positioned in lying. If the neck flexors are strong and are made to work against maximal resistance, the abdominal muscles will contract more strongly. Irradiation only occurs from strong muscles to weaker ones. Therefore, when planning a PNF programme, the therapist always starts with the patient's strongest patterns. The concept of re-inforcement utilizes many of the primitive mass flexion and extension reflexes and the postural and righting reflexes.

When patients have spasticity, problems arise with the use of the irradiation principle, which requires the patient's maximal voluntary effort. When patients with spasticity are asked to work against maximal resistance, *associated reactions* may occur. These appear to be movements but are in fact changes of tone and posture due to abnormalities in the central nervous system, i.e. they are pathological and should not be elicited. In individuals with normal tone *associated movements* occur, e.g. swinging the arms when walking, or gritting the teeth when making a great effort to unscrew a jar. These are normal activities and form part of the integrated action of the body.

It could be argued following the definition of maximal resistance for an isotonic muscle contraction, that when associated reactions occur, i.e. abnormal movements, the therapist is applying too much resistance.

The correct use of the concept of maximal resistance requires great skill and accurate assessment and observation.

Voice

To add to the total sensory input the therapist uses her voice to stimulate the patient's voluntary effort. The words of command are also vital in synchronizing the patient's voluntary effort with the stretch administered by the therapist. The action is preceded by the word '*now*' and this is followed by the command '*pull*' or '*push*'.

Joint structures

The proprioceptors in the joints are stimulated by the traction (a force tending to separate joint surfaces) or the approximation (a force tending to compress joint surfaces) applied by the therapist during the movement pattern. Traction is applied when the movement is occurring against gravity, and approximation when the movement is occurring in the direction of the gravitational pull. Approximation may be used to activate postural reflexes.

Eyes

The patient is encouraged, when possible, to follow the movement with his eyes. Thus, by summation of sensory input, the patient's natural movement patterns are facilitated; maximal resistance is used to strengthen muscles and the therapist's skills are augmented by the patient's maximum voluntary effort.

In the next section the basic normal patterns of movement, using normal timing, will be described, together with the therapist's stance and grip. It must be noted that the patterns alone do not constitute PNF. The basic principles must be applied to the patterns and then used in conjunction with additional techniques which may be classified as being either strengthening or relaxation techniques (obtaining a lengthening reaction of antagonists which are preventing movement into the agonist pattern). These techniques will be described in Chapter 23.

Chapter 20
PNF ARM PATTERNS

P. J. Waddington

It is obvious that, to apply this method of treatment, the therapist must know the patterns and techniques in detail, but it is less obvious that the basis for success is the positioning and stance of the therapist: her balance, the use of her body weight and, as stressed before, the grip. For the patient to move in a diagonal direction smoothly against resistance, the therapist must be able to move smoothly herself using her body weight and not just her upper limbs when applying resistance.

The basic position for the therapist to take up is lunge, with the forward foot pointing in the line of the movement diagonal and with the forward knee bent to give flexibility. The rear foot is placed at right angles to the front foot to give stability (Fig. 20.1).

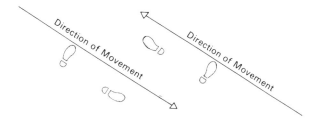

Fig. 20.1 Diagram showing basic foot position in relationship to the movement diagonal.

The therapist must be positioned so that she can use her body weight to apply resistance and traction or approximation throughout the whole movement. She should be close enough to the part being exercised so that her back remains straight to ensure that the weight taken through her arms when applying resistance to gravity-assisted movements is transmitted to the floor without strain. All manually resisted exercise requires effort, but the work can be reduced and the dangers of strain can become negligible if the correct techniques are carefully learned and applied.

Grips and positions are described for the patient's right side. In the photographs which accompany each pattern, note the therapist's position. The patient should be positioned near to the side of the plinth to enable the therapist to obtain stretch on the flexion/adduction patterns by taking the limb over the side of the plinth, and to ensure that she is well balanced and does not over-reach.

Arm patterns

In PNF the term elevation is not used when referring to movements of the arm. Patterns in which the arm is raised above the head are called flexion patterns. Patterns are named according to the direction of movement, i.e. the finishing position. There are two diagonals of movement in line with the oblique trunk muscles and four basic arm patterns (Fig. 20.2).

In the basic arm patterns the elbow remains straight throughout. However, each basic arm pattern may be adapted so that either elbow flexion or elbow extension takes place, for example:

- Flexion/abduction/lateral rotation
- Flexion/abduction/lateral rotation with elbow flexion

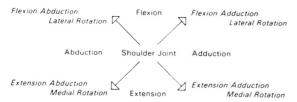

Fig. 20.2 Diagram showing the shoulder movement in the four basic arm patterns.

- Flexion/abduction/lateral rotation with elbow extension.

Thus there are in effect twelve arm patterns, based on movements of the glenohumeral joint. It is obvious that movements of the shoulder girdle will accompany those of the upper limb. The movement patterns of the scapula will be described later (Chapter 22).

It is usual for the patient to be supine although the patterns for the upper limb may be performed with the patient in sitting.

When learning these patterns the patient may be taken through the movement passively. When resistance, i.e. maximal resistance, is applied, the therapist must be guided as to the amount of resistance she gives by the fact that the patient always remains in the 'groove', i.e. does not deviate from the pattern. Once the movement has been learned resistance may be increased.

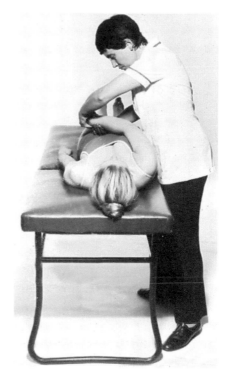

Fig. 20.3 Starting position for the flexion/abduction/lateral rotation pattern of the arm.

Flexion/abduction/lateral rotation

Starting position (Fig. 20.3)

PATIENT Extension/adduction/medial rotation of the shoulder with pronation of the forearm, flexion and ulnar deviation of the wrist, flexion of the fingers and flexion and opposition of the thumb.

THERAPIST

Stance The therapist stands in lunge looking towards the patient's feet with her weight on the forward right leg and parallel with the proposed line of movement at the level of the patient's upper arm. During the movement the therapist transfers her weight from the forward right foot to the left foot and rotates so that she can watch the patient's hand throughout the movement.

Grip The therapist grasps the patient's

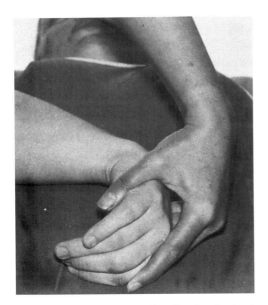

Fig. 20.4 Grip – starting position for the flexion/abduction/lateral rotation pattern of the arm.

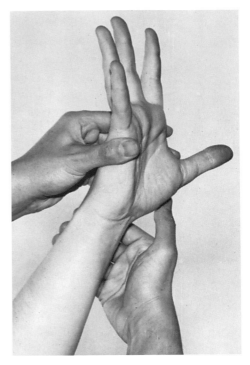

Fig. 20.5 Grip – part way through the flexion/abduction/lateral rotation pattern of the arm.

right hand with her left (Fig. 20.4). Note that because of the flexion of the metacarpophalangeal joints only her fingers, thumb and thenar eminence are in contact with the dorsum of the patient's hand.

Commands

The therapist prepares the patient with the word '*now*', applies stretch to establish the stretch stimulus and gives the executive word '*push*'. After the movement has started, the therapist places the fingers of her right hand on the extensor surface of the patient's wrist approaching from the radial side (Fig. 20.5). If the wrist and finger movements are slow to develop, extra resistance given by the hand on the wrist will facilitate these movements.

Movement

Extension of the fingers (particularly middle and index) and thumb, extension of the wrist with radial deviation, supination of the fore-

arm, flexion, abduction and lateral rotation at the glenohumeral joint, rotation, elevation and adduction (retraction) of the scapula.

In normal timing, movement is initiated by the rotary component. Movement then occurs at the distal joints, to be followed in succession by the more proximal joints. Rotation continues throughout the pattern.

When the pattern is completed the arm should be about an arm's width from the patient's ear (Fig. 20.6).

Flexion/abduction/lateral rotation with elbow flexion

Starting position

PATIENT As for the basic pattern.

THERAPIST *Stance* and *grip* as for the basic

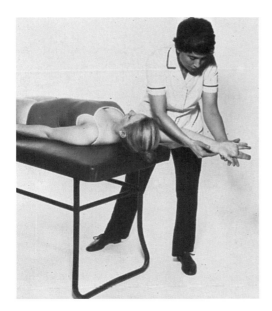

Fig. 20.6 Finishing position of the flexion/abduction/lateral rotation pattern of the arm.

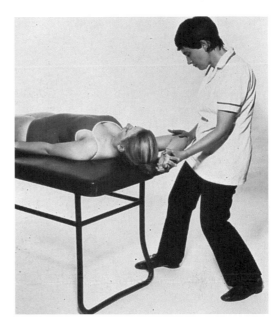

Fig. 20.7 Finishing position for the flexion/abduction/lateral rotation with elbow flexion pattern of the arm.

pattern except that the therapist's right hand is placed over the lateral epicondyle of the humerus to encourage flexion. She may also slip her thumb into the elbow crease.

Movement

As for the basic pattern with the addition of elbow flexion (Fig. 20.7).

Flexion/abduction/lateral rotation with elbow extension

Starting position (Fig. 20.8)

PATIENT As for the basic pattern with the addition of elbow flexion.

THERAPIST

Stance The therapist takes up lunge position near to the patient's head.

Grip She places her right hand over the lateral epicondyle and the point of the elbow

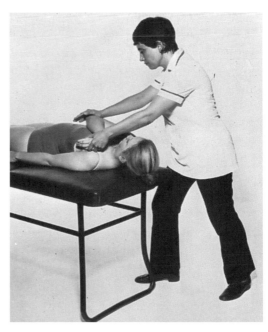

Fig. 20.8 Starting position for the flexion/abduction/lateral rotation with elbow extension of the arm.

to encourage extension, and with the left hand grips the patient's hand as for the basic pattern.

Movement

As for the basic pattern with the addition of elbow extension.

Extension/adduction/medial rotation

Starting position

PATIENT Flexion/abduction/lateral rotation with supination of the forearm, extension of the wrist with radial deviation and extension of the fingers and thumb.

THERAPIST

Stance   The therapist's feet remain in the same place as for the antagonist pattern, i.e. flexion/abduction/lateral rotation, but the lunge stance is reversed: the therapist faces the patient's outstretched hand with her left foot forwards and with the knee flexed. During the movement the therapist transfers her weight from the forward left foot to the right foot.

Grip   The therapist places the palm of her right hand into the palm of the patient's right hand and grasps the palm with the lumbrical grip ensuring that the fingers do not flex and exert pressure on the dorsum of the patient's hand (Fig. 20.9). The therapist places the fingers of her left hand on the flexor surface of the wrist approaching from the radial side. If the movement at the wrist is inadequate, additional resistance at the wrist will stimulate activity.

Commands

The therapist prepares the patient for movement with the word '*now*', applies stretch to establish the stretch stimulus and then instructs the patient to '*grip my hand and pull down*'.

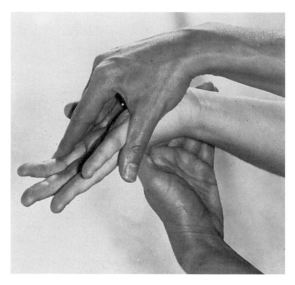

Fig. 20.9 Grip – starting position for the extension/adduction/medial rotation pattern of the arm.

Movement

Flexion of the fingers (with particular emphasis on the index and middle fingers), opposition of the thumb, flexion of the wrist with ulnar deviation, pronation of the forearm, extension, adduction, medial rotation at the glenohumeral joint, depression, abduction of the scapula (Fig. 20.10).

In normal timing movement is initiated by the rotary component. Movement then occurs at the distal joints to be followed in succession by the more proximal joints. Rotation continues throughout the pattern.

Extension/adduction/medial rotation with elbow flexion

Starting position

PATIENT As for the basic pattern.

THERAPIST

Stance   The therapist moves her feet nearer to the patient's hand than for the straight arm pattern.

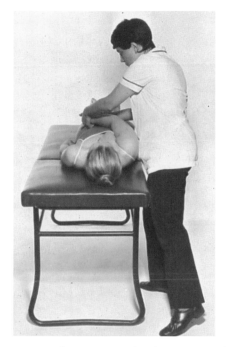

Fig. 20.10 Finishing position for the extension/adduction/medial rotation pattern of the arm.

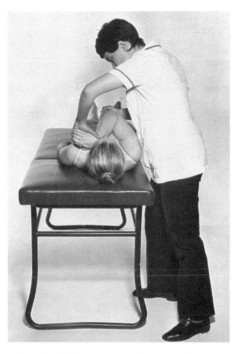

Fig. 20.11 Finishing position for the extension/adduction/medial rotation with elbow flexion pattern of the arm.

Grip This is one of the rare occasions when the grip on the hand does not remain the same for the three similar patterns. The grip is changed so that at the end of the movement the therapist does not find her own arms crossed. The therapist places the palm of her left hand within the patient's outstretched right hand and the fingers of her right hand over the flexor aspect of the patient's elbow to encourage elbow flexion.

Movement

As for the basic pattern with the addition of elbow flexion. Care must be taken to ensure that the arm moves in the diagonal direction as it can easily complete the movement at the patient's side (Fig. 20.11).

Extension/adduction/medial rotation with elbow extension

Starting position (Fig. 20.12)

PATIENT As for the basic pattern with the addition of elbow flexion.

THERAPIST *Stance* and *grip* as for the basic pattern.

Movement

As for the basic pattern with the addition of elbow extension.

In the *flexion/abduction–extension/adduction* diagonal the thumb and radial side of the limb lead throughout the movement. It is in this diagonal, in which opposition of the thumb occurs, that many of the highly skilled movements take place, e.g. writing and threading a needle. The index and middle fingers also work to advantage.

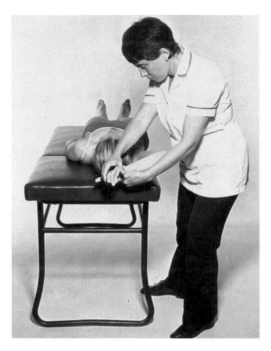

Fig. 20.12 Starting position for the extension/adduction/medial rotation with elbow extension pattern of the arm.

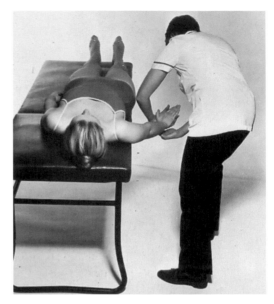

Fig. 20.13 Starting position for the flexion/adduction/lateral rotation pattern of the arm. (In order to show the grip, the arm has been taken too far into abduction.)

Flexion/adduction/lateral rotation

Starting position (Fig. 20.13)

PATIENT   Extension/abduction/medial rotation of the shoulder with pronation of the forearm, extension with ulnar deviation of the wrist, extension of the fingers, extension and abduction of the thumb. The therapist must ensure that the patient is near enough to the side of the plinth to enable the arm to be taken into extension beyond the horizontal. The patient's arm should only be abducted to about an arm's width from the side of the body. It is possible to test for the correct position as muscles are stronger in pattern. Care must be taken to ensure that the patient's fingers are fully extended before the movement begins.

THERAPIST

Stance   The therapist stands at the level of the patient's upper arm in the lunge position facing the patient's feet and with her weight on her forward right foot and parallel with the proposed line of movement. During the movement the therapist transfers her weight from the right to the left foot rotating so that she can continue to watch the patient's hand throughout the movement.

Grip   The therapist grasps the patient's right hand by placing her left palm into the patient's palm approaching from the radial side. She uses the lumbrical grip thus ensuring that she does not touch the extensor surface of the patient's hand. The fingers of her right hand are placed on the flexor surface of the patient's wrist approaching from the ulnar side (Fig. 20.14).

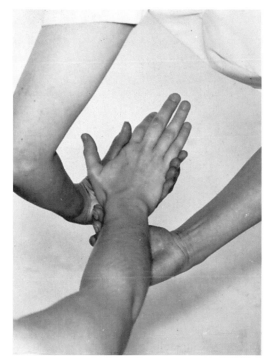

Fig. 20.14 Detail of grip – starting position for the flexion/adduction/lateral rotation pattern of the arm.

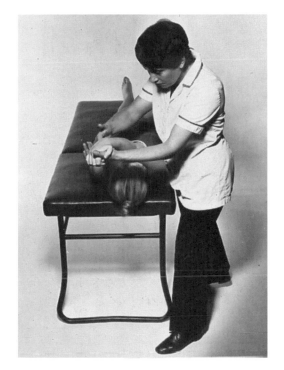

Fig. 20.15 Finishing position for the flexion/adduction/lateral rotation pattern of he arm.

The therapist may delay positioning her right hand until just after the movement has started.

Commands
The therapist prepares the patient for the movement by saying '*now*' and then follows this with the command '*grip my hand, pull up and across your nose*'.

Movement
Flexion of the fingers, particularly the little and ring fingers, adduction and flexion of the thumb, flexion of the wrist towards the radial side, supination of the forearm, flexion, adduction and lateral rotation at the glenohumeral joint, rotation, elevation and abduction (protraction) of the scapula (Fig. 20.15). As in all normal timing the movement is initiated by the rotary component. Movement then occurs at the distal joints to be followed in succession by the more proximal joints until the whole limb is moving.

Flexion/adduction/lateral rotation with elbow flexion

Starting position
PATIENT As for the basic pattern.

THERAPIST *Stance* and *grip* as for the basic pattern. The therapist may move her right hand nearer to the patient's elbow.

Movement
As for the basic pattern with the addition of elbow flexion. This is the eating pattern. It may have been noted when practising the straight arm pattern that the patient has a

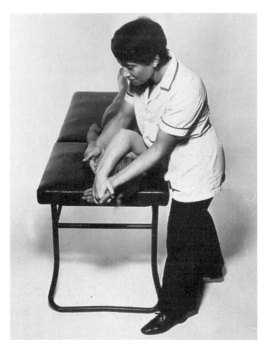

Fig. 20.16 Finishing position for the flexion/adduction/lateral rotation of the elbow flexion pattern of the arm.

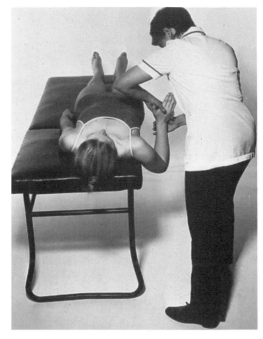

Fig. 20.17 Starting position for the flexion/adduction/lateral rotation with elbow extension pattern of the arm.

tendency to want to flex at the elbow (Fig. 20.16).

Flexion/adduction/lateral rotation with elbow extension

Starting position (Fig. 20.17)
PATIENT As for the basic pattern with the addition of elbow flexion.

THERAPIST *Stance* and *grip* as for the basic pattern.

Movement
As for the basic pattern with the addition of elbow extension. Note this may seem a strange movement at first but a boxer has said that the pattern has the fundamental components of the 'upper cut'.

Extension/abduction/medial rotation

Starting position
PATIENT Flexion/adduction/lateral rotation, supination of the forearm, flexion and radial deviation of the wrist, flexion of the fingers and flexion and adduction of the thumb.

THERAPIST

Stance The therapist stands in the lunge position facing the patient's head at the level of the patient's upper arm with her weight on her forward left foot and parallel with the proposed line of movement. During the movement the therapist transfers her weight from the left to the right foot, rotating so that she can continue to watch the patient's hand.

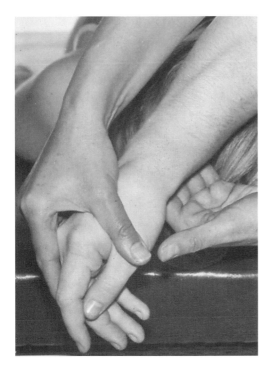

Fig. 20.18 Grip – starting position for the extension/abduction/medial rotation pattern of the arm.

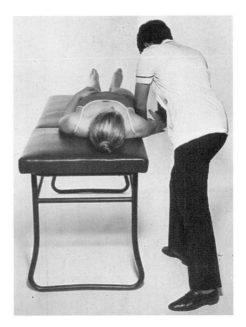

Fig. 20.19 Finishing position for the extension/abduction/medial rotation pattern of the arm.

Grip The therapist, using her right hand and the lumbrical grip, grasps the dorsum of the patient's right hand ensuring that stretch is obtained and that emphasis is given by pressure with her fingers to the exteroceptors on the ulnar side of the patient's hand. After the movement has started the fingers of the therapist's left hand are placed on the extensor surface of the patient's wrist approaching from the flexor aspect and round the ulnar border, i.e. from between the patient's arm and body (Fig. 20.18).

Commands
'*Now*' – '*push*'.

Movement
Extension of the fingers, particularly the little and ring fingers, extension and abduction of the thumb, extension of the wrist towards the ulnar side, pronation of the forearm, extension, abduction and medial rotation of the glenohumeral joint, rotation, depression and adduction of the scapula (Fig. 20.19). As in all normal timing the movement is initiated by the rotary component; movement then occurs at the distal joints to be followed in succession by the more proximal joints until the whole limb is moving.

Extension/abduction/medial rotation with elbow flexion

Starting position
PATIENT As for the basic pattern.

THERAPIST *Stance* and *grip* of the right hand as for the basic pattern but the fingers of the left hand are placed over the point of the elbow approaching from the ulnar side to encourage elbow flexion.

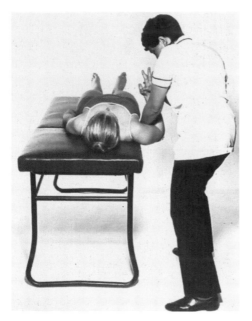

Fig. 20.20 Finishing position for the extension/abduction/medial rotation with elbow flexion pattern of the arm.

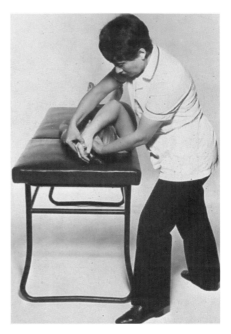

Fig. 20.21 Starting position for the extension/abduction/medial rotation with elbow extension pattern of the arm.

Movement

As for the basic pattern with the addition of elbow flexion. This pattern can be seen in photographs of footballers kicking a ball, particularly when these photographs are 'posed' (Fig. 20.20).

Extension/abduction/medial rotation with elbow extension

Starting position (Fig. 20.21)

PATIENT As for the basic pattern with the addition of elbow flexion.

THERAPIST *Stance* and *grip* as for the basic pattern.

Movement

As for the basic pattern with the addition of elbow extension. This movement occurs in eating when the hand is returning from the mouth.

In the *flexion/adduction – extension/abduction* diagonal the little finger and ulnar side of the limb lead throughout the movement. This is the diagonal of the eating pattern.

Thrust patterns

There are two additional patterns of the upper limb, the *thrust patterns*. One pattern has a flexion, the other an extension component. They are both adduction patterns with elbow extension, in which the rotation occurs in the opposite direction to the basic pattern and flexion of the wrist and fingers is replaced by extension. The addition of these two, to the basic twelve patterns, emphasizes the versatility of movement in the upper limb.

Thrust patterns are powerful movements. They can occur in any position; in prone they are used to support the body on the hands as

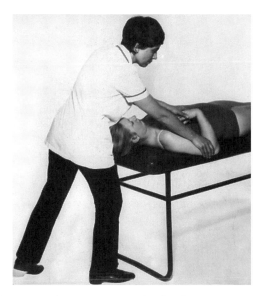

Fig. 20.22 Starting position for the thrust pattern into flexion/adduction.

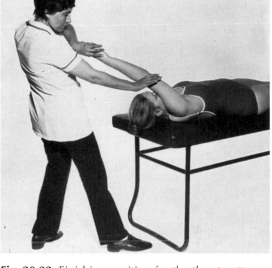

Fig. 20.23 Finishing position for the thrust pattern into flexion/adduction.

in 'press-ups'. The movement also occurs when reaching for an object with an opening hand in preparation for grasping.

Thrust into flexion/adduction

Starting position (Fig. 20.22)

PATIENT   Extension/abduction (an arm's width from the body) with lateral rotation of the shoulder, flexion of the elbow, supination of the forearm, wrist flexion with radial deviation and flexion of the fingers and thumb.

THERAPIST

Stance   The therapist stands at the head of the plinth (as for manual cervical traction) with her right foot forwards in the lunge position.

Grip   She places her left hand over the patient's right hand, grasping the extensor surface, giving pressure with her fingers on the ulnar side of the hand. Her right hand is placed with the thumb abducted over the flexor aspect of the upper arm and into the bend of the elbow. The author prefers this stance and grip but the therapist, if she chooses, may take up her stance as for the basic flexion/adduction/lateral rotation pattern.

Commands

'*Now*' – '*thrust*'. The use of the word thrust appears to have greater impact than push in this situation.

Movement

Protraction of the scapula, flexion, adduction and medial rotation of the glenohumeral joint with elbow extension, wrist extension to the ulnar side, extension of the fingers and thumb (Fig. 20.23). This pattern may be reversed, in which case the therapist slips the fingers of her left hand into the patient's palm from the ulnar side and places her right hand on the point of the elbow.

Thrust into extension/adduction

Starting position

PATIENT Flexion/abduction/medial rotation of the shoulder, elbow flexion (so that the hand is on the shoulder), pronation of the forearm,

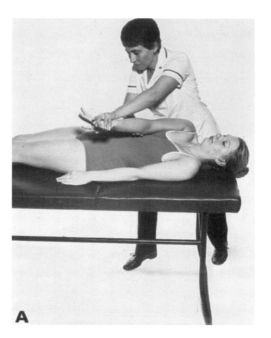

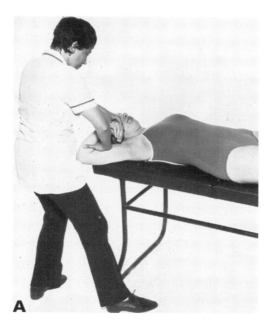

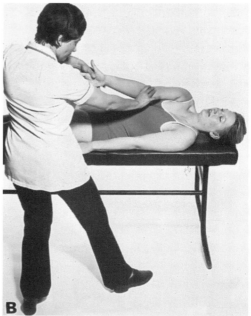

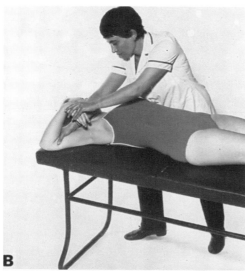

Fig. 20.24 A, Starting position for the thrust pattern into extension/adduction. B, Alternative starting position for the thrust pattern into extension/adduction.

Fig. 20.25 A, Finishing position for the thrust pattern into extension/adduction. B, Alternative finishing position for the thrust pattern into extension/adduction.

wrist flexed towards the ulnar side, flexion of the fingers and thumb.

THERAPIST The therapist may stand in one of two positions, each requiring a different grip:

(1) *Stance* In lunge position as for the basic extension/adduction pattern.
Grip The therapist places her left hand on the extensor surface of the patient's hand obtaining stretch by exerting pressure through her fingers. The therapist's right hand is placed on the upper arm (Fig. 20.24A).

(2) *Stance* The therapist stands in the lunge position with right foot forwards on the patient's left side (i.e. the opposite side to the arm being exercised) facing the patient's head.
Grip The therapist places her left hand over the extensor surface of the patient's hand, obtaining stretch by exerting pressure on the radial side of the hand through her thumb. (This is one of the very few occasions when pressure is exerted through the thumb and not the fingers.) The therapist places her right hand, thumb abducted and extended on the flexor surface of the patient's upper arm (Fig. 20.24B).

Commands
'*Now*' – '*thrust*'.

Movement
Protraction of the scapula, extension, adduction, lateral rotation of the glenohumeral joint, elbow extension, supination, wrist extension to the radial side, extension of the fingers and thumb (Fig. 20.25A and B).

This pattern may be reversed. Reversals are more easily done if the therapist takes up starting position 2. The therapist slips the fingers of her left hand into the patient's palm from the ulnar side and places her right hand over the olecranon process.

Chapter 21
PNF LEG PATTERNS

P. J. Waddington

For the leg, as with the arm, there are two diagonals of movement (Fig. 21.1) in line with the oblique trunk muscles and four basic patterns.

In the basic leg patterns the knee remains straight throughout. However, each basic pattern may be adapted so that either knee flexion or knee extension takes place, for example:

- Flexion/adduction/lateral rotation
- Flexion/adduction/lateral rotation with knee flexion
- Flexion/adduction/lateral rotation with knee extension.

Thus there are twelve leg patterns, based on the hip joint. It should be noted that throughout the movements the heel should lead the way.

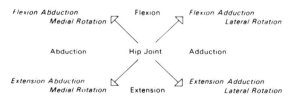

Fig. 21.1 Diagram showing the hip movements in the four basic leg patterns.

It is usual for the patient to be supine on a plinth.

Flexion/adduction/lateral rotation

Starting position (Fig. 21.2)

PATIENT Extension/abduction/medial rotation of the hip, plantarflexion and eversion of the foot and flexion of the toes.

The patient lies at the side of the plinth so that the leg can be taken into full extension over the side without too much abduction which would take it out of pattern.

THERAPIST

Stance The therapist stands in the lunge position in line with the diagonal of movement and with the forward left foot about level with the patient's foot. The therapist's weight is on the right foot so that her body weight can be used to exert traction. Both her knees are flexed.

Grip The therapist holds the patient's heel with her left hand and places her right hand over the dorsum of the patient's foot and uses the 'lumbrical grip'. With her thumb on the lateral border and fingers spread out on the medial border of the foot she exerts pressure through her fingers to give the correct exteroception and stretch (Figs 21.3 and 21.4).

Commands

'*Now*' used as a preparation for action. '*Turn your heel in and pull your foot up.*' The patient

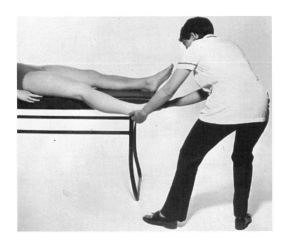

Fig. 21.2 Starting position for the flexion/adduction/lateral rotation pattern of the leg.

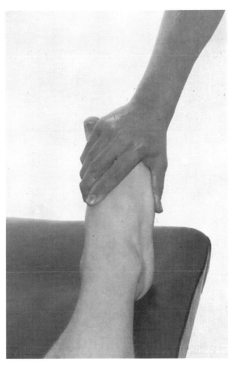

Fig. 21.3 Basic grip for the hand placed on the patient's foot in the flexion/adduction/lateral rotation pattern of the leg.

may respond initially and certainly will later to the simple commands '*now*' – '*pull*'.

Movement

In this pattern the therapist must pivot on her forward left foot taking a forward step with her right foot so that she is able to maintain her grip on the foot of the extended leg.

The position of the therapist's left hand also changes quickly. Once the rotation has started, her left hand is placed on the extensor and adductor aspects of the patient's leg at the level of the knee. The patient's movement is lateral rotation of the hip, inversion and dorsiflexion of the foot and extension of the toes, followed by flexion and abduction at the hip (Fig. 21.5).

In normal timing movement is initiated by the rotary component. Movement then occurs at the distal joints to be followed in succession by the more proximal joints. Rotation continues throughout the pattern. The length of the patient's hamstring muscles will determine the range of movement.

Flexion/adduction/lateral rotation with knee flexion

Starting position

PATIENT As for flexion/adduction/lateral rotation.

THERAPIST

Stance The therapist stands as for the flexion/adduction/lateral rotation pattern.

Grip As for the flexion/adduction/lateral rotation pattern.

Commands

'*Now*' – '*Pull up and bend your knee*'.

Movement

As the patient's knee flexes in this pattern it is not necessary for the therapist to take

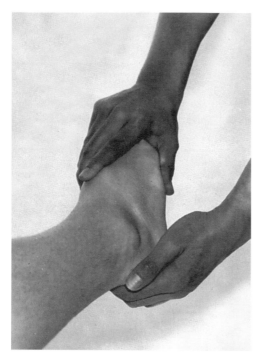

Fig. 21.4 Grip (both hands) – starting position for the flexion/adduction/lateral rotation pattern of the leg.

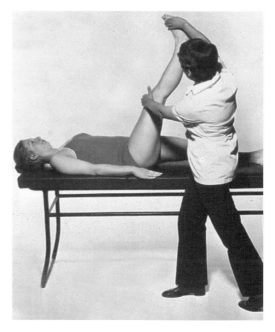

Fig. 21.5 Finishing position for the flexion/adduction/lateral rotational pattern of the leg.

a step; it is sufficient for her to flex the forward left knee and perhaps glide forwards a little. The therapist's weight is transferred from the rear right foot to the forward left foot.

The patient's movement is as for the flexion, adduction, lateral rotation pattern with the addition of knee flexion. The therapist must ensure that knee flexion is active and resisted throughout the pattern by using her right hand, otherwise flexion can be brought about passively by gravity.

It is very easy to allow incorrect medial rotation to occur in this pattern if the knee is allowed to lead and the foot to follow in the movement diagonal. The therapist must ensure that the knee and foot move across diagonally together maintaining a vertical relationship to each other (Fig. 21.6).

Flexion/adduction/lateral rotation with knee extension

Starting position (Fig. 21.7)

PATIENT   As   for   flexion/adduction/lateral rotation but with the knee flexed.

THERAPIST

Stance   The therapist stands adjacent to the patient's flexed knee in the lunge position facing the foot of the plinth, i.e. right foot forwards and knee flexed and her weight through the flexed left leg.

Grip   The therapist grasps the foot with her right hand as before, slightly adapting her grasp to accommodate her changed stance. She places her left hand on the extensor and adductor aspect of the patient's knee. Care must be taken not to overstretch rectus femoris in this position.

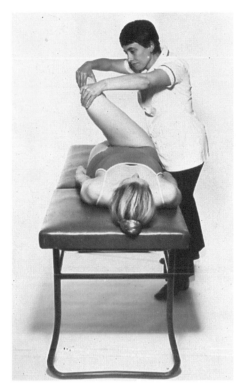

Fig. 21.6 Finishing position for the flexion/adduction/lateral rotation with knee flexion pattern of the leg.

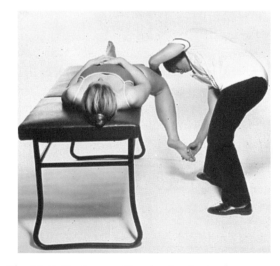

Fig. 21.7 Starting position for the flexion/adduction/lateral rotation with knee extension pattern of the leg.

Commands

'*Now*' – '*turn your heel in and straighten your knee*'.

Movement

As before with the addition of knee extension. To accommodate the adduction movement the therapist, having transferred her weight to the forward right foot, takes a step towards the plinth with her left foot.

Extension/abduction/medial rotation

Starting position

PATIENT   Flexion/adduction/lateral rotation of the hip, dorsiflexion and inversion of the foot, extension of the toes.

THERAPIST

Stance   The therapist faces the head of the plinth in lunge in the line of the basic diagonal. She is near to the patient's hip and with the left foot forwards.

Grip   The therapist places her right hand held slightly in the 'lumbrical position' on the plantar surface of the patient's foot, with the thumb, in line with the palm, lying under the toes in a position to resist flexion. The therapist exerts pressure through her fingers on the medial border of the foot (Fig. 21.8). The therapist stretches her left hand and places the thumb on the lateral surface of the patient's thigh near to the knee with the border of the index finger on the posterior aspect of the thigh. As the patient extends the leg this hand is in a position to catch and control the knee.

Commands

'*Now*' – '*turn your heel out and push your toes down*'. The patient may respond to the simple commands '*now*' – '*push*'.

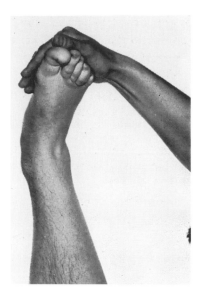

Fig. 21.8 Grip on the foot – starting position for the extension/abduction/medial rotation pattern of the leg.

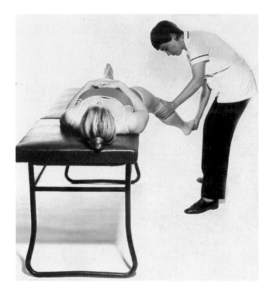

Fig. 21.9 Finishing position for the extension/abduction/medial rotation pattern of the leg.

Movement

Medial rotation of the hip, plantarflexion and eversion of the foot, flexion of the toes and extension and abduction of the hip (Fig. 21.9).

In normal timing movement is initiated by the rotary component. Movement then occurs at the distal joints to be followed in succession by the more proximal joints. Rotation continues throughout the pattern. The therapist transfers her weight from the left to the right foot and flexes her knee.

Extension/abduction/medial rotation with knee flexion

Starting position

PATIENT As for extension/abduction/medial rotation.

THERAPIST *Stance* and *grip* as for extension/abduction/medial rotation except that the left hand is placed slightly more

proximally so that it will not impede knee flexion.

Commands

'Now' – *'turn your heel out, push your toes down and bend your knee'.*

Movement

Medial rotation of the hip, plantarflexion and eversion of the foot, flexion of the toes, knee flexion, extension and abduction of the hip. The therapist, having transferred her weight onto the forward right foot, takes a step to the side with her left foot to allow room for the patient's foot (Fig. 21.10).

Extension/abduction/medial rotation with knee extension

Starting position (Fig. 21.11)

PATIENT Flexion/adduction/lateral rotation of the hip with knee flexion, dorsiflexion and inversion of the foot and extension of the toes. The therapist must ensure that the knee

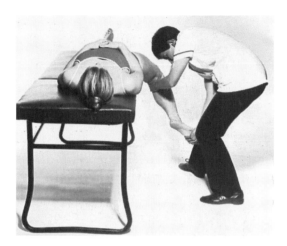

Fig. 21.10 Finishing position for the extension/abduction/medial rotation with knee flexion pattern of the leg.

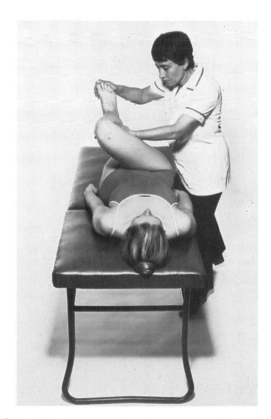

Fig. 21.11 Starting position for the extension/abduction/medial rotation with knee extension pattern of the leg.

and foot are in the line parallel with the side of the plinth and the resting leg, i.e. that the hip is in lateral rotation. It is easy to deviate from this so that the knee and foot are diagonally related to each other. In this position the hip is medially rotated.

THERAPIST

Stance The therapist stands facing the patient in lunge position with her weight on the forward left leg.

Grip As for the extension/abduction/medial rotation pattern.

Commands
'*Now*' – '*push*'.

Movement
Medial rotation of the hip, plantarflexion and eversion of the foot, flexion of the toes, extension of the knee and extension and abduction of the hip.

This pattern and the other mass extension pattern of the leg, i.e. extension/adduction/lateral rotation with knee extension, are the strongest patterns in the body.

Flexion/abduction/medial rotation

Starting position (Fig. 21.12)
PATIENT Extension/adduction/lateral rotation of the hip, plantarflexion and inversion of the foot and flexion of the toes.

To allow the leg to be adducted the other leg must be taken into abduction. In this position the final few degrees of extension cannot be obtained.

THERAPIST

Stance The therapist stands in lunge position at the level of the patient's thigh facing the foot of the plinth and with her right foot forwards.

Grip The therapist places her right hand, using the lumbrical grip, on the dorsum of

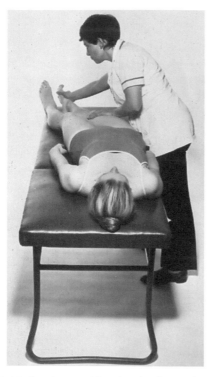

Fig. 21.12 Starting position for the flexion/abduction/medial rotation pattern of the leg.

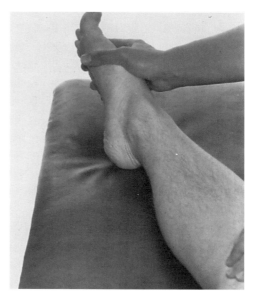

Fig. 21.13 Grip on the foot – starting position for the flexion/abduction/medial rotation pattern of the leg.

the patient's foot and, by exerting pressure through the fingers, she is able to obtain stretch (Fig. 21.13).

The left hand is placed on the upper and outer aspect of the thigh.

Commands

'*Now*' – '*turn your heel out and pull your foot up*'. This may later be reduced to '*now*' – '*pull up*'.

Movement

Medial rotation of the hip, dorsiflexion and eversion of the foot, extension of the toes and flexion and abduction of the hip (Fig. 21.14). In normal timing movement is initiated by the rotary component. Movement then occurs at the distal joints to be followed in succession by

the more proximal joints. Rotation continues throughout the pattern.

To ensure good balance the therapist must transfer her weight to the rear left leg as the movement proceeds.

Flexion/abduction/medial rotation with knee flexion

Starting position

PATIENT   As   for   flexion/abduction/medial rotation.

THERAPIST

Either

Stance and *grip* as for flexion/abduction/medial rotation.

Or Fig. 21.15.

Stance   The therapist stands in the lunge position, right foot forwards, facing the patient on the opposite side of the plinth, i.e. when the patient's right leg is being exercised she stands on the patient's left. The forward

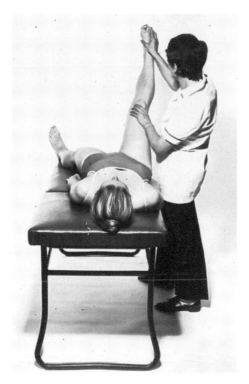

Fig. 21.14 Approaching the finishing position for the flexion/abduction/medial rotation pattern of the leg.

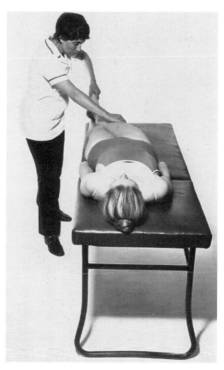

Fig. 21.15 Alternative starting position for the flexion/abduction/medial rotation with knee flexion pattern of the leg.

right foot is placed at about the level of the patient's right ankle and her weight is on the left foot. It is usual when using this method to cross the patient's active leg over the resting leg.

Grip The therapist places her left hand on the dorsum of the patient's foot exerting pressure through her fingers. Her right hand may be placed under the patient's heel with pressure given to the lateral aspect; otherwise it is placed on the lateral aspect of the thigh.

Commands
'*Now*' – '*pull*'.

Movement
Having used both hands on the foot to obtain stretch and thus initiate the movement, the therapist immediately transfers the hand on the right heel onto the patient's knee giving pressure on the lateral aspect. This encourages both flexion of the knee and abduction of the hip. Care must be taken to keep the knee and foot in line with each other parallel to the resting leg, i.e. the leg is carried across as one piece. If this point is not observed the wrong rotation will occur at the hip. The therapist must ensure that the knee flexion is caused by activity of the hamstrings and not passively by gravity. This is achieved by actively resisting the movement.

The patient moves into medial rotation of the hip, dorsiflexion and eversion of the foot, extension of the toes, knee flexion and flexion and abduction of the hip (Fig. 21.16).

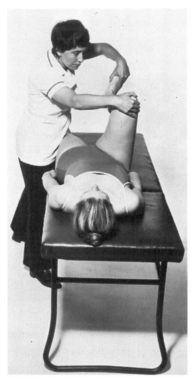

Fig. 21.16 Approaching the finishing position for the flexion/abduction/medial rotation with knee flexion pattern of the leg.

Flexion/abduction/medial rotation with knee extension

Starting position (Fig. 21.17)

PATIENT To enable the patient to flex the knee of the extended and adducted leg in preparation for knee extension, he is moved down the plinth until his knees are level with the foot of the plinth. Both knees can then be flexed. Care must be taken when deciding to use this position as some individuals find that it causes discomfort in the lumbar region even if a pillow is used to support this area. It may be necessary to abandon the normal timing of this pattern and use the timing for emphasis technique (Chapter 23) in the sitting position.

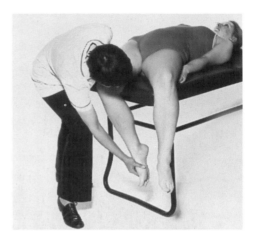

Fig. 21.17 Starting position for the flexion/abduction/medial rotation with knee extension pattern of the leg.

THERAPIST *Stance* and *grip* as for the basic pattern. The therapist will need to flex her forward knee more fully to enable her to reach the foot.

Commands

The basic command is '*now*' – '*pull up and straighten your knee*' although specific instructions, for example '*turn your heel out*', may be necessary.

Movement

Medial rotation of the hip with dorsiflexion and eversion of the foot, extension of the toes, extension of the knee and flexion and abduction of the hip.

Extension/adduction/lateral rotation

Starting position

PATIENT Flexion/abduction/medial rotation of the hip, dorsiflexion and eversion of the foot and extension of the toes. The resting leg must be abducted to allow the moving leg to come to rest in adduction.

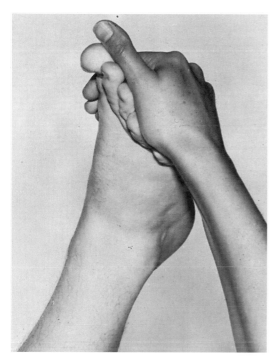

Fig. 21.18 Grip on the foot – starting position for the extension/adduction/lateral rotation pattern of the leg.

THERAPIST

Stance   The therapist stands in line with the movement diagonal opposite to the patient's hip facing the foot of the plinth with her right foot forwards.

Grip   The therapist places her right hand on the plantar surface of the patient's foot with her thumb under the toes and the heel of her hand giving pressure on the outer border of the foot (Fig. 21.18). Her left hand is placed, approaching from above the leg, on the adductor surface of the thigh with the fingers on the flexor surface of the knee.

Commands

'Now' – 'turn' your heel in and push your foot down'. This may be reduced to 'now' – 'push'.

Movement

Lateral rotation of the hip, plantarflexion and inversion of the foot, flexion of the toes and extension and adduction of the hip.

In normal timing movement is initiated by the rotary component. Movement then occurs at the distal joints to be followed in succession by the more proximal joints. Rotation continues throughout the pattern. The therapist transfers her weight from the rear left foot to the forward right foot and bends the right knee.

Extension/adduction/lateral rotation with knee flexion

Starting position

PATIENT   To accommodate the knee flexion the patient is moved towards the foot end of the plinth until the knees conveniently flex with the patient in lying. This position, as in the flexion/abduction/medial rotation with knee extension pattern, may cause discomfort in the lumbar region. In this case it should not be used. The starting position is as for extension/adduction/lateral rotation.

THERAPIST   *Stance*   and *grip* as for extension/adduction/lateral rotation except that the left hand is moved proximally away from the knee.

Commands

'Now' – 'push'. Additional commands such as 'bend your knee' may be used as necessary.

Movement

Lateral rotation of the hip, plantarflexion and inversion of the foot, flexion of the toes, flexion of the knee, extension and adduction of the hip (Fig. 21.19).

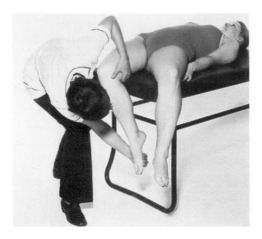

Fig. 21.19 Finishing position for the extension/ adduction/lateral rotation with knee flexion pattern of the leg.

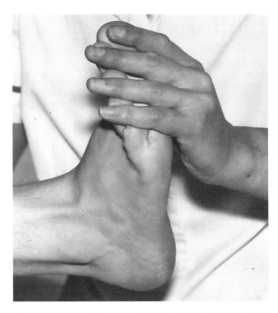

Fig. 21.20 Grip on the foot – alternative starting position for extension/adduction/lateral rotation with knee extension pattern of the leg.

Extension/adduction/lateral rotation with knee extension

Starting position

PATIENT Flexion/abduction/medial rotation of the hip with knee flexion, dorsiflexion and eversion of the foot and extension of the toes.

THERAPIST

Either *Stance* and *grip* as for extension/ adduction/lateral rotation. In this position the therapist is unable to resist a powerful thrust.

Or

Stance The therapist stands in the lunge position, right foot forwards, facing the patient on the opposite side of the plinth, i.e. when the patient's right leg is being exercised she stands on the patient's left. In this position she can use her body weight more effectively to give resistance.

Grip The therapist places her left hand on the plantar surface of the patient's foot so that her fingers are exerting pressure on the patient's toes (Fig. 21.20). The right hand with the thumb abducted is placed on the posterior and medial surfaces of the patient's thigh. Initial contact is made with the index finger on the posterior surface and with the thumb on the medial surface. As the movement is executed the thigh 'falls' into the therapist's outstretched hand.

Commands

'*Now*' – '*push*'.

Movement

Lateral rotation of the hip, plantarflexion and inversion of the foot, flexion of the toes, extension of the knee and extension and adduction of the hip. The patient's moving leg crosses the resting leg.

This is the second 'thrust' or 'mass extension' pattern of the lower limb.

Chapter 22
PNF HEAD AND NECK, SCAPULAR, AND TRUNK PATTERNS

P. J. Waddington

Head and neck patterns

As with the limb patterns, each head and neck pattern has three components resulting in a diagonal movement. These are rotation either to the right or left, most of which takes place at the atlanto-axial joint and either flexion or extension at two levels, i.e. at the atlanto-occipital joint only, a nodding movement of the head on the neck, and the second a large movement involving in addition the whole of the cervical vertebrae.

Care must be taken to ensure that rotation occurs throughout the whole movement. If full rotation is allowed to occur too soon, extension and flexion will be limited and the movement will not be in a diagonal direction. This diagonal is in line with the oblique muscles of the trunk. The therapist may ask the patient to look at the hand in the extension/adduction/medial rotation position to give the inner range position of the flexed and rotated head and neck and may ask the patient to look at the hand in the flexion/abduction/lateral rotation position to give the inner range position of the extended

and rotated head and neck. The chin will be seen to move in a straight line in a diagonal direction.

Extension with rotation to the right

Starting position (Fig. 22.1)

PATIENT Supine with the shoulders level with the end of the plinth. Flexion of the head with rotation to the left.

THERAPIST

Stance   The therapist stands at the head end of the plinth in the lunge position with the right leg forwards.

Grip   The therapist places the thumb of her right hand on the lateral surface of the right half of the mandible. The rest of the hand and fingers are kept well away from contact with the patient.

The left hand is placed, thumb abducted with fingers down, on the occiput. The temptation to put this hand near to the nape of the neck must be resisted as the wrist will be placed in an uncomfortable position when the patient moves into extension.

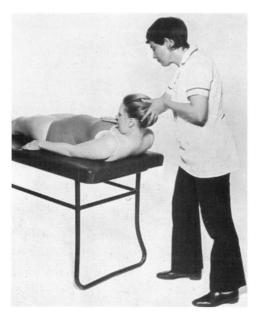

Fig. 22.1 Neck patterns – starting position for extension with rotation to the right.

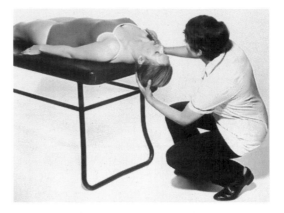

Fig. 22.2 Neck patterns – finishing for extension with rotation to the right.

Commands

'*Now*' – '*push and look to the right*'.

Movement

Extension of the head and neck with rotation to the right (Fig. 22.2).

Flexion with rotation to the right

Starting position (Fig. 22.3)

PATIENT Lying with the shoulders level with the edge of the plinth. Extension of the head and neck with rotation to the left.

THERAPIST

Stance   As for extension with rotation to the right, but with the left foot forward.

Grip   The therapist may choose to use either hand on the chin and vice versa on the occiput but it is convenient to use the left hand on the mandible so that the slow reversal technique (Chapter 23) may be used.

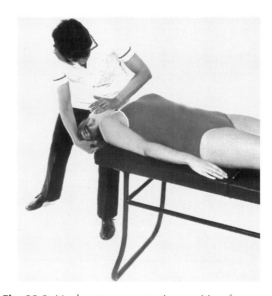

Fig. 22.3 Neck patterns – starting position for flexion with rotation to the right.

The little and ring fingers of the left hand are placed on the inferior border of the right half of the mandible. If more fingers are used there is a tendency to press on the patient's larynx and cause discomfort.

The right hand is on the occiput as for extension with rotation to the left.

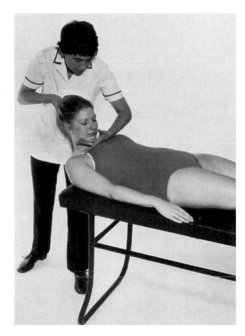

Fig. 22.4 Neck patterns – finishing position for flexion with rotation to the right.

Commands

'*Now*' – '*pull your chin up towards your breast pocket*'.

Movement

Flexion of the head and neck with rotation to the right (Fig. 22.4).

Head and neck patterns can usefully be done with the patient in forearm support prone lying either on the plinth or on the mat. It may also be found to be of value to use the extensor patterns with the patient in the sitting position. This will assist the patient to gain a good position of the head and thus will favourably affect posture in general.

Using the timing for emphasis technique (Chapter 23) and the head and neck as the 'handle', the strong neck muscles can be used to obtain a contraction of the abdominal muscles (flexion with rotation) and the erector spinae (extension with rotation).

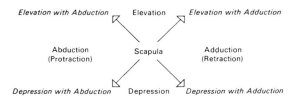

Fig. 22.5 Diagram showing the diagonal movements of the scapula.

Shoulder girdle or scapular patterns

Each scapular pattern has three components: either elevation or depression, either abduction (protraction) or adduction (retraction) and rotation round the chest wall (Fig. 22.5).

It will be noted that the terms abduction and adduction are used instead of the more usual protraction and retraction. This is quite logical as the protracted scapula has been moved away from the central axis of the body, i.e. into abduction; and the retracted scapula has been moved towards the central axis, i.e. into adduction.

Elevation with abduction

Starting position

PATIENT The patient is placed either on the plinth or on the mat in side lying with hips and knees flexed sufficiently to give stability. Care must be taken not to allow the patient to assume a semi-prone position.

THERAPIST

Stance The therapist stands or kneels behind the patient in line with the movement diagonal, i.e. near to the patient's hips.

Grip The therapist places her left hand on the point of the patient's shoulder and exerts stretch by pulling the shoulder into depression and adduction, i.e. towards the left hip. She may use her right hand to support her left hand or to control the patient's arm.

Commands

'Now' – 'pull up towards your nose'.

Movement

Elevation and abduction of the scapula with rotation round the chest wall. This movement is associated with the flexion/adduction/lateral rotation pattern of the arm.

Depression with abduction

Starting position

PATIENT As for elevation with abduction.

THERAPIST

Stance The therapist stands or kneels behind the patient in line with the movement diagonal, i.e. near to the patient's head.

Grip As for elevation with abduction except that the pressure is such that it stimulates the movement required. The therapist exerts stretch by pulling the shoulder into elevation and adduction, i.e. towards the nape of the patient's neck.

Commands

'Now' – 'pull down towards your left hip'.

Movement

Depression and abduction of the scapula with rotation round the chest wall. This movement is associated with the extension/adduction/medial rotation pattern of the arm

Note for both abduction patterns of the scapula the therapist positions herself behind the patient.

Elevation with adduction

Starting position

PATIENT As for elevation with abduction.

THERAPIST

Stance The therapist stands or kneels in front of the patient in line with the move-

ment diagonal, i.e. near to the patient's hip.

Grip The therapist places both hands usually left on top of right on the scapula with her fingers round the medial border. She exerts stretch by pulling the shoulder into depression and abduction, i.e. toward's the patient's left hip.

Commands

'Now' – 'pull up towards the back of your neck'.

Movement

Elevation and adduction of the scapula with rotation round the chest wall. This movement is associated with the flexion/abduction/lateral rotation pattern of the arm.

Depression with adduction

Starting position

PATIENT As for elevation with abduction.

THERAPIST

Stance The therapist stands or kneels in front of the patient in line with the movement diagonal, i.e. near to the patient's head.

Grip As for elevation with adduction except that the pressure is such that it stimulates the movement required. The therapist exerts stretch by pulling the shoulder into elevation and abduction, i.e. towards the patient's nose.

Commands

'Now' – 'pull down towards your left hip'.

Movement

Depression and adduction of the scapula with rotation round the chest wall. This movement is associated with the extension/abduction/medial rotation pattern of the arm.

Scapular patterns are important in two specific areas of rehabilitation:

(1) Correct movement of the scapula is vital for normal functioning of the upper limb
(2) Strong movements of the scapula working in pattern may be used to facilitate rolling activities on mats

Pelvic girdle patterns

There are four movements of the pelvis in line with and exercising the oblique abdominal muscles.

Pelvic girdle patterns are usually done in side lying on the mat, where the patient feels more secure and where they can be used as a means of teaching rolling.

The therapist kneels at one end of the diagonal line of movement behind the patient. She grasps the iliac crest, using this as a 'handle' to obtain stretch and give resistance to the forward movements of the pelvis. For the backwards movements of the pelvis the therapist presses with the heel of one hand supported by the other hand on the ischial tuberosity.

Trunk patterns

Using the head and neck and arms

Flexion with rotation (chopping)

Starting position for rotation to the right

PATIENT The patient is in lying. His right arm is placed in the position of flexion/adduction/lateral rotation. He grasps his right wrist with his left hand. His forearm is supinated.

The patient is instructed to look at his right hand thus assuming the head and neck

position of extension with rotation to the left.

THERAPIST

Stance The therapist is on the patient's right at the side of the plinth in the lunge position with her left foot forwards facing the patient's head, as for the extension/abduction/medial rotation pattern of the arm.

Grip The therapist uses her right hand to grasp the patient's right hand as for the extension/abduction/medial rotation pattern of the arm. She places her left hand, as if she were pushing, over the near part of the patient's forehead.

Commands

'*Now*' – '*push*'.

Movement

The head and neck move into flexion with rotation to the right. The right arm moves into extension/abduction/medial rotation of the shoulder, pronation of the forearm, extension of the wrist and fingers with abduction of the thumb and the left arm moves in a supporting role. The trunk is flexed and rotated to the right (Fig. 22.6).

The timing for emphasis technique (Chapter 23) may be used here to strengthen the abdominal muscles with the head and neck and the arms used as the 'handle' held in inner range and using the lumbar spine as the 'pivot'. For the average individual very little resistance will prove to be maximal.

Extension with rotation (lifting)

Starting position for rotation to the right

PATIENT The patient is supine with his shoulders level with the top of the plinth. His right arm is placed in the position of extension/adduction/medial rotation. He grasps his

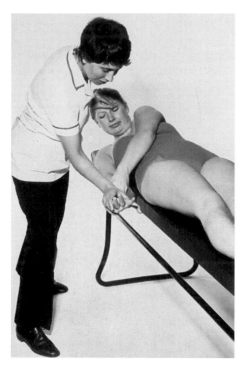

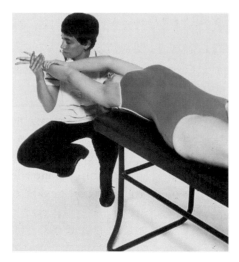

Fig. 22.7 Finishing position for 'lifting' to the right.

Fig. 22.6 Finishing position for 'chopping' to the right.

of the patient's head, fingers towards the nape of his neck.

Commands
'Keep looking at your hand', 'now' – 'push'.

Movement
The head and neck move into extension with rotation to the right. The right arm moves into flexion/abduction/lateral rotation of the shoulder, supination of the forearm, extension of the wrist, fingers and thumb. The left arm moves in a supporting role. The trunk is extended and rotated to the right (Fig. 22.7).

right wrist with his left hand with supinated forearm. The patient is instructed to look at his right hand, thus assuming the head and neck position of flexion with rotation to the left.

THERAPIST
Stance The therapist is on the patient's right at the side of the plinth in the lunge position with her right foot forwards facing the patient's feet. She should be as near to the patient's head as possible while still able to reach his right hand with her right hand. Her reach will be increased by flexing her right knee.

Grip The therapist grasps the patient's right hand with her right hand. On this occasion the thumb and not the fingers will be in a position to resist the rotation of the upper limb. She places her left hand on the crown

Using the legs

The basic patterns of the legs are used as a means of obtaining trunk movement. In these patterns both legs move simultaneously keeping together throughout the movement. Thus they move in asymmetrical patterns; for example, for the left leg to remain with the right leg throughout the flexion/adduction/lateral rotation pattern, it will have to move into flexion/abduction/medial rotation.

Flexion with rotation (straight knees)

Starting position for rotation to the left

PATIENT The patient is in supine close to his right-hand side of the plinth.

The right leg is in extension, abduction, medial rotation of the hip, plantarflexion and eversion of the foot and flexion of the toes. The left leg is in extension, adduction, lateral rotation of the hip, plantarflexion and inversion of the foot and flexion of the toes.

THERAPIST

Stance The therapist stands facing the patient on his right side in the lunge position in a diagonal direction with her left foot forwards and slightly proximal to the level of the patient's feet.

Grip The therapist places her right hand on the dorsum of both of the patient's feet and her left hand and forearm are placed on the anterior aspect of the patient's thigh near to the knees. If the patient has difficulty in lifting his legs the therapist may place her left forearm underneath the patient's knees supporting his legs while the hand is in contact with the lateral surface of the patient's left thigh.

Commands

'*Now*' – '*turn your heels away from me – pull up*'. The patient may need to be reminded to dorsiflex the feet.

Movement

The legs move as one. The right leg into flexion/adduction/lateral rotation of the hip, dorsiflexion and inversion of the foot with extension of the toes. The left leg moves into flexion/abduction/medial rotation of the hip, dorsiflexion and inversion of the foot with extension of the toes. This is followed by flexion of the trunk with rotation to the left.

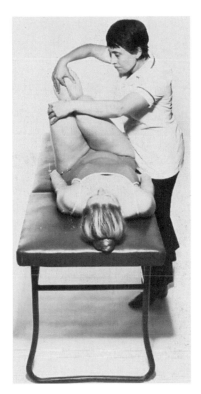

Fig. 22.8 Finishing position for the double leg, hip and knee flexion pattern.

This is a very difficult exercise and with the average patient it will be noted that the pull of psoas major and iliacus will have an adverse effect on the lumbar spine and pelvic tilt, causing extension of the lumbar spine.

The same pattern but with knee flexion will be found to be strong enough for the vast majority of patients (Fig. 22.8). The timing for emphasis technique (Chapter 23) is of value here. The legs, with flexed knees, form the 'handle' and the lumbar spine is the 'pivot'. A series of repeated contractions done in this way is valuable for strengthening the abdominal muscles.

The pattern starting with the knees flexed and finishing with the knees in extension may also be used, but again the therapist and patient may experience the same problems with the lumbar spine and pelvic tilt as in the straight leg pattern.

Extension with rotation (straight knees)

This is a valuable pattern for facilitating back extension.

Starting position for rotation to the right

PATIENT The patient is in supine close to his right-hand side of the plinth. The right leg is in flexion/adduction/lateral rotation of the hip, dorsiflexion and inversion of the foot and extension of the toes. The left leg is in flexion/abduction/medial rotation of the hip, dorsiflexion and eversion of the foot and extension of the toes.

The therapist may have to assist the patient into the starting position.

THERAPIST

Stance The therapist stands on the patient's right at the side of the plinth, in the lunge position with her left foot forward facing the patient's head. The therapist must stand close to the patient with her elbows tucked into her body so that the force of the patient's effort is transmitted as directly as possible, through her straight back, to the floor.

Grip The therapist places her right hand on the plantar surface of the patient's feet with her thumb as far as possible under his toes in a position to resist flexion. The therapist places the left forearm under the patient's legs at above the level of his knees.

Commands

'Now' – 'turn your heels towards me and push down'.

Movement

The legs move as one, the right leg into extension, abduction, medial rotation of the hip with plantarflexion and eversion of the foot and

flexion of the toes and the left leg into extension, adduction and lateral rotation of the hip with plantarflexion and inversion of the foot and flexion of the toes.

Knee extension

This is probably the strongest movement available to an individual, i.e. thrusting with both legs. The therapist must be able to control the patient and care must be exercised in selecting suitable patients. It may be used when one leg is reasonably strong and the other weak. The therapist uses 'overflow' from the stronger leg to facilitate activity in the weaker. It may also be used to gain general extension in the very weak patient.

The pattern and positioning are the same as for the straight knee pattern except that the patient starts with his knees flexed.

Knee flexion

This pattern may be used to facilitate back extension. The pattern and positioning are the same as for the straight knee pattern except that the patient finishes the movement with flexed knees.

Side flexion (quadratus lumborum pattern using the legs)

Side flexion of the trunk to produce a 'hip hitching' movement is valuable but sometimes difficult to teach a patient. It can be achieved easily by applying PNF principles.

Starting position for left side flexion (Fig. 22.9)

PATIENT The patient is placed in lying on a plinth with his heels minimally over the end of the plinth.

THERAPIST

Stance The therapist stands at the foot

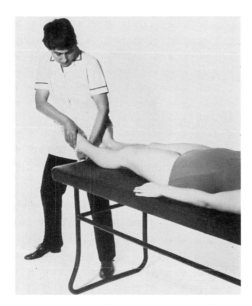

Fig. 22.9 Starting position for trunk side flexion to the left.

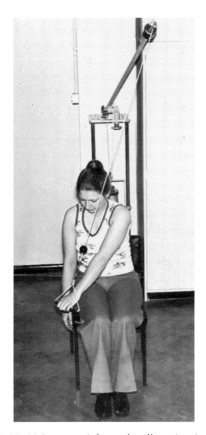

Fig. 22.10 Using a weight and pulley circuit to resist the extension/adduction/medial rotation pattern of the arm.

of the plinth in the lunge position with her left foot forwards. She places the patient's right foot onto her left hip giving enough pressure to keep his leg straight in that position.

Grip The therapist places her left hand under the patient's left heel and her right hand on the dorsum of his foot near to the ankle. She then pulls down with both hands in the direction of the long axis of the leg. Care must be taken to pull equally with both hands. Too much pressure with the right hand will force the foot into plantarflexion. This should be avoided.

Commands

'*Now*' – '*pull up*'.

Movement

The patient side flexes by hitching his hip and in effect 'shortening' his left leg.

A quick gentle stretch will initiate the stretch reflex and result in contraction and movement. The therapist must be careful to allow the movement to take place as such a contraction is weak. The maximal resistance principle together with repeated contractions (Chapter 23) may be used as a strengthening technique.

Other considerations

PNF principles can be applied to exercises for the respiratory muscles, the muscles of the face and jaw, and, by using a wooden tongue depressor, exercises can be given to the tongue and the buccinator muscles.

Stimulation round the face and mouth can be very valuable as these areas are well supplied with sensory receptors.

Mechanical loading

Progressive resistance exercises using pulley and weight circuits form a part of many treatment programmes. When viewed from the neurophysiological standpoint exercises done against mechanical resistance cannot be considered to be as effective as those done against manual resistance. The features associated with the expert grip of the therapist are absent:

(1) Precise exteroceptive stimulation
(2) Stretch stimulus
(3) Graduated resistance ensuring the patient's maximum effort through full range

However, a pulley and weight circuit may form a useful part of an intensive treatment programme. It is valuable in increasing the patient's exercise tolerance and the therapist can supervise a small group of patients. This may have the beneficial effect of reducing the patient's dependence on the therapist, which can develop in a one-to-one situation.

It is possible to arrange such circuits so that the patient is working in pattern by positioning him so that the rope is in the line of the diagonal on completion of the movement. All patterns may be done in this way (Fig. 22.10).

The main aim of a mechanically resisted programme when used in conjunction with manually resisted exercises is to improve the patient's endurance. It is therefore advisable to give low resistance so that a high number of repetitions is necessary for maximum effort.

Chapter 23
PNF TECHNIQUES

P. J. Waddington

In therapeutic exercise co-ordinated patterns of movement facilitated by the correct sensory input must be augmented by specific techniques of emphasis.

Basically these fall into the two fundamental categories, muscle strengthening and joint mobilizing techniques. Although it is theoretically and practically convenient to conceive the problems presented by patients in this way, therapists are well aware that the two are indivisible although certain techniques are much more effective in strengthening muscles and others in increasing the range of movement.

Strengthening techniques

There are two main techniques which may be used for strengthening: *repeated contractions* and *slow reversals*.

Repeated contractions

There are three variations of this technique: normal timing, timing for emphasis and combining isotonic and isometric muscle work.

Normal timing
Normal timing is probably the simplest of all the techniques once the patterns have been learned. It consists of repeating any chosen pattern several times through full range against maximum resistance ensuring smooth movement at all times. As with other methods of applying progressive resistance exercises, the therapist may determine the relationship between the amount of resistance and the number of repetitions.

The therapist selects the pattern or patterns in which the muscle to be strengthened works to advantage and the patient moves through full range. Once the pattern has been completed, i.e. the muscles are in their shortened range, the therapist passively returns the limb to the lengthened position ready for the next repetition.

The firing of motor units is prolonged due to bombardment of the motor neurons by many impulses (summation). This prolongation of the response is called 'after discharge'.

Timing for emphasis (pivoting)
Timing for emphasis is a technique in which the irradiation/overflow principle is used to facilitate the contraction of a weak group of muscles.

The patient's strong muscles, maximally contracting, facilitate the contraction of a weaker group through recruitment. This 'overflow' principle can be used from one limb to another or from the head or limbs to the trunk or vice versa. The therapist must analyse the patient's strengths and weaknesses as overflow is only effective from strong to weak muscles. Timing for emphasis is the method by which this overflow principle is applied to the muscles within a single pattern. For example, a weak deltoid muscle may be strengthened by exercising it in two patterns, i.e. flexion/abduction with lateral rotation and extension/abduction with medial rotation. The fundamental feature of timing for emphasis is that the other muscles in the pattern are made to contract maximally to facilitate the contraction of the weak muscle, while movement is allowed only in one joint or in the case of the elbow, movement is also allowed in the radioulnar joints.

It is natural for an individual to make every effort to complete a movement.

A pattern used in this manner is described as having three parts: *pivot*, *handle* and *stabilizing*.

Pivot

The pivot is the joint in which movement is taking place. This movement is brought about by the weak muscles.

Handle

The handle is the part the therapist is holding, distal to the pivot. The strong muscles in this part of the pattern are contracting in inner range.

Stabilizing part

This is the part of the pattern proximal to the pivot controlled by strong muscles. The muscles here are usually contracting in middle range. There are two methods by which this can be achieved:

(1)   The therapist may prevent the patient from moving in any part of the pattern except over the pivot, i.e. the patient is prevented from further contracting iso-

tonically by the resistance applied by the therapist.

(2)   The therapist takes the part passively to the strongest point in the range. The patient is then encouraged to 'hold' at that point, i.e. to perform an isometric contraction and then movement is allowed at the pivot.

The wrist flexors may be used as another example. Flexion of the wrist towards the radial side takes place in the flexion/adduction/lateral rotation pattern with elbow flexion and supination. The pattern is allowed to proceed or the limb is taken to a point in the range where the proximal components are in middle range and the distal components, the flexors of the fingers, are contracting in inner range. Further movement ceases except in the wrist joint where movement is allowed and the range completed. The therapist, while maintaining the position of the rest of the pattern, returns the wrist to the extended position and the patient is encouraged to repeat the movement. Thus the normal timing sequence has been changed to emphasize the contraction of the weak component, i.e. the wrist flexors – especially flexor carpi radialis. This group is then subjected to a form of repeated contractions facilitated by the other strong muscles in the pattern working maximally.

In this example the flexors, adductors and lateral rotators of the glenohumeral joint, the flexors of the elbow and supinators form the *stabilizing part*, the wrist joint is the *pivot* and the flexors of the fingers and adductor of the thumb constitute the *handle*. The therapist's grip is that used in the basic pattern.

When learning and exploring the possibilities of this technique the therapist may choose to analyse the movements and muscles involved in two ways:

(1) By taking each pattern the therapist may allow movement to occur in successive pivots, i.e. glenohumeral, elbow, wrist, etc., or hip, knee, ankle, etc. For example: flexion/adduction/lateral rotation with knee extension; grip as for basic pattern (Table 23.1).

(2) The therapist may prefer to analyse the movement and muscle work occurring at each joint in all four patterns before moving on to the next joint. For example: A, the wrist (Fig. 23.1); B, the thumb (Fig. 23.2).

Table 23.1

Pivot	Starting position	Movement	Muscles subjected to repeated contraction

Hip	Supine lying
	   Hip flexed and adducted in the part of the range selected for strengthening – this is frequently middle or inner range.
	   Knee flexed in middle range (care must be taken to ensure that the patient is actively contracting his hamstring muscles).
	   Ankle and foot dorsiflexed, inverted, toes extended in inner range.
		Flexion adduction, lateral rotation	Hip flexors – psoas major, iliacus, rectus femoris (acting over the hip); hip adductors and lateral rotators – adductor brevis, adductor longus, gracilis, pectineus and the small lateral rotator muscles

Knee	Either supine lying or sitting over the side of the plinth.
	   Hip flexed and adducted in middle range.
	   Knee flexed in preparation for extension in the part of the range selected for strengthening.
	   Ankle and foot dorsiflexed, inverted, toes extended in inner range
		Extension of the knee	Vastus medialis and rectus femoris (medial component)

Ankle and talocalcaneonavicular joint	Any starting position although supine lying is frequently convenient.
	   Hip flexed and adducted in middle range.
	   Knee, the therapist has to decide whether she requires flexion or extension – she must consider two major factors: the length of and/or tone of gastrocnemius and, that the functional combination of movements in walking is dorsiflexion with knee extension.
	   Ankle and foot plantarflexed and everted in preparation for movement, toes extended
		Dorsiflexion and inversion	Tibilais anterior

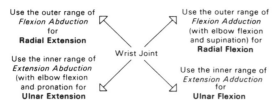

Fig. 23.1 Diagrammatic representation of the movements occurring at the wrist in the four basic arm patterns; giving the range in which the best results may be obtained when using the timing for emphasis technique.

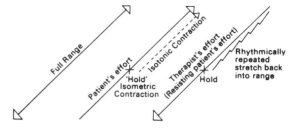

Fig. 23.3 Diagrammatic representation of the strengthening technique combining isotonic and isometric muscle work.

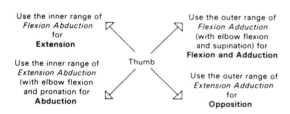

Fig. 23.2 Diagrammatic representation of the movements occurring at the thumb in the four basic arm patterns; giving the range in which the best results may be obtained when using the timing for emphasis technique.

Combining isotonic and isometric muscle work (Fig. 23.3)

This method is designed to strengthen a muscle in a specific part of the range and is of particular value in strengthening a muscle following an increase in the range of movement, e.g. when treating a frozen shoulder.

The therapist's aim is to facilitate the isotonic contraction of muscles which have not been active for some time in this shortened range.

Take the limb either passively or actively to a strong part of the range adjacent to the range selected for strengthening. The patient is then instructed to '*hold*' and a maximal isometric contraction of the agonists is developed at this point where the muscles are strong. The patient is then instructed to '*push*' or '*pull*', i.e. to endeavour to complete full range – the muscles working isotonically.

The therapist then rhythmically and repeatedly rotates the limb a short distance into the antagonist pattern; each time giving the contracting muscle a gentle stretch to stimulate further muscle contraction.

This method also aids the relaxation or lengthening reaction of the antagonist group (reciprocal innervation) by facilitation of the contraction of the agonists, thus assisting in maintaining the increased range previously gained.

Slow reversal

In this technique the contraction of the strong muscles in the antagonist pattern is used to facilitate the contraction of the weaker muscles of the agonist group. The basis for the slow reversal technique is Sherrington's principle of successive induction. Sherrington noted that immediately the flexor reflex had been elicited the excitability of the extensor reflex was increased.

When the therapist is applying the slow reversal technique she uses the maximal contraction of the stronger antagonist group to facilitate the contraction of the weaker agonist group. For example, to strengthen deltoid in the flexion/abduction/lateral rotation pattern the patient is instructed to complete the extension/adduction/medial rotation pattern. The therapist ensures that the patient is working maximally. On completion of the movement the therapist, smoothly and without pause, changes her grip and the patient moves into the flexion/abduction/lateral rotation pattern. The sequence is then repeated several times.

Relaxation/lengthening techniques

There are two methods by which the therapist may endeavour to obtain a lengthening reaction of the antagonist group, hypertonus of which is preventing the patient from moving further into the agonist pattern: working the hypertonic group and working the reciprocal group.

Working the hypertonic group

The therapist elicits a maximal contraction of the antagonist group, ensuring that the maximum number of motor units is contracting simultaneously. Following the contraction the muscle will relax and the therapist takes advantage of the relaxation to move the part further into the agonist range. The more motor units the therapist can facilitate to contract together, the better the result, as all these motor units will also relax simultaneously.

There are two techniques which take advantage of this physiological fact: *contract relax* and *hold relax*. The fundamental difference between these techniques is the type of muscle contraction. Contract relax uses an iso-

tonic contraction of the antagonists and hold relax, as the name implies, uses an isometric contraction.

Contract relax

For contract relax the therapist takes the part passively or resists the active movement of the part to the point where further movement into the agonist pattern is limited by tension in the antagonist group. She then changes her grip to that used for the antagonist pattern and instructs the patient to '*pull*' or '*push*'. By her resistance the therapist only allows the patient to move a short way into rotation, preventing movement from occurring in the other components of the pattern. When the therapist is sure that the patient is working maximally she instructs him to '*relax*' and then she gradually relaxes her resistance while maintaining her grip. Time is then allowed for relaxation to occur. The therapist then changes her grip carefully and moves the part gently further into the agonist pattern. The process can be repeated at the point where resistance to further movement is experienced.

Hold relax

As for contract relax, for hold relax the therapist takes the limb to the point where further movement into the agonist pattern is prevented by tension in the antagonists. This movement may be passive or active. The therapist smoothly changes to the grip for the antagonist pattern and instructs the patient to '*hold*' slowly; by concentrating on the rotary component, the therapist builds up the resistance until the patient is contracting his muscles maximally. The therapist must never break or overcome the patient's maximal isometric contraction. The patient is instructed to '*relax*' and the sequence is completed as for the contract relax technique.

Advantages and disadvantages

Hold relax is frequently the technique of choice. The slow build up and isometric contraction ensures that there is no joint movement and when the problem is one of pain the lack of movement will ensure that the patient is relatively pain-free. Pain is counter productive as it will increase the unwanted hypertonus.

The other advantage of hold relax is that when treating a particularly strong patient the therapist maintains control of the situation. If she were to allow movement the patient might be able to overcome her resistance.

The advantage of contract relax is that in some situations the patient may find it difficult to perform an isometric contraction.

Working the reciprocal group (to the hypertonic group)

Contraction of a muscle is accompanied by relaxation of the antagonist group.

Slow reversal – hold relax

The method for the hold relax technique is used until the point when the patient is told to relax, i.e. the patient is taken actively or passively to the point where limitation occurs, he is then instructed to contract in the direction of tightness, and this is followed by relaxation. The therapist then changes her grip to the reverse pattern. The patient moves further into the previously restricted range (isotonic contraction) against maximal resistance. This technique thus uses both approaches to obtaining the lengthening reaction. This method is particularly valuable when the agonist group of muscles is strong.

Reciprocal lengthening reaction

Although it is not included as a PNF technique, the therapist can obtain a reciprocal lengthening reaction of a group of muscles in spasm (the antagonists) by causing the agonist group to contract isometrically against maximal resistance at the point of limitation.

This method is particularly successful when trying to increase the range of movement at the knee joint, when further flexion is prevented by the failure of the quadriceps to lengthen due to spasm. The therapist gains relaxation by causing the hamstrings to contract maximally. Overflow may be used by maximally resisting the contraction of the hamstring group of the uninjured leg. The patient is positioned in sitting over the side of the plinth and the therapist sits on the floor. The therapist gives resistance to the hamstrings by grasping the plantar surfaces of the patient's feet, thus activating the gastrocnemius (a knee flexor) and the other plantarflexors as well.

Additional techniques

Rhythmic stabilization

Rhythmic stabilization is based on isometric muscle work where there is a simultaneous isometric contraction of all muscles controlling the joint. The result is called co-contraction. Rhythmic stabilization can be used either to gain relaxation or increase strength.

Relaxation

The part is taken to the point where limitation occurs. The therapist gives the command '*hold*'. Emphasizing the rotary component of the pattern the therapist alternates her pressure and thus alternates the resistance between the agonist and antagonist patterns. Gradually the resistance is increased until the patient is working maximally. The therapist must not break the hold. The final '*hold*' is in the pattern antagonistic to the tightness. The patient is then asked to contract isotonically by moving through as much range as possible.

Strength

The muscle to be strengthened is facilitated to contract maximally in the strongest part of the range. At that point the resistance is alternated, building up a maximal co-contraction. The final hold is on the side of the muscle to be strengthened and then the patient is instructed to move further into the desired range.

It may take up to 15 minutes after the treatment for the strengthening technique to exhibit its maximum effect. An additional effect of rhythmic stabilization will be to increase the circulation.

Rhythm technique

The rhythm technique is applied to the limbs when the patient has difficulty in initiating movement, particularly for patients with Parkinsonism. It is very beneficial when used in conjunction with trunk rotation (as advocated by Mrs Bobath), as relaxation gained centrally affects the peripheral muscles.

The therapist applies the technique to each limb and each pattern in turn. The therapist takes hold of the patient with a usual grip for the selected pattern. When using this technique with the upper limbs the therapist may find it an advantage to grasp the patient with only the hand which holds the patient's hand, as the two-handed grip tends to impede the rhythmic movement. She begins by passively taking the limb through full range. This is repeated several times until a good rhythm of moderate speed is established. The patient is then instructed to join in gently and assist the movement. Gradually the patient is encouraged to increase his effort, ensuring that the tone is not in-

creased. The therapist then repeats the method in the antagonist pattern.

Stretch reflex

The stretch reflex may be used in several ways:

(1) The stretch reflex can be used with the 're-peated contraction' technique when the extra stretch gives added rhythm to the movement.

(2) When the patient cannot move voluntarily a series of stretch reflexes, each followed by the responsive muscle contraction and movement, may be used, resulting in a series of repeated contractions. This has value as the patient gets the feeling of movement. He can then try to 'join in'.

(3) The stretch reflex can be used to obtain a lengthening reaction:
   (a) By obtaining a contraction of the agonist group the antagonist group will reciprocally relax.
   (b) A series of contractions of the antagonist (tight) group caused by the therapist applying quick and controlled stretch will result in relaxation or lengthening of the muscle. The therapist gradually takes the limb further into the desired range.

When using stretch reflex the therapist must be sensitive to the resultant movement which is brought about by a relatively weak contraction, and allow it to occur. Any appreciable resistance will prevent movement.

Chapter 24
FUNCTIONAL ACTIVITIES ON MATS

P. J. Waddington

Functional activities on mats are designed to improve progressively the patient's independence. It is as important to teach the helpless patient to turn in bed as it is to teach re-education of walking to another. The progression of mat activities is based on the main theme of the normal development sequence, i.e. rolling from supine to prone and from prone to supine, getting to prone kneeling, then to standing and eventually to gait training. Such activities as teaching the patient to get up from the floor into the sitting position are also included. These activities are based on the normal patterns of movement but each activity will include more than one pattern.

The basic techniques of PNF are applicable to this work. In the actual treatment of a patient, balance activities (Chapter 25), also done for the most part on mats, cannot be divorced from functional activities on mats. As a general rule it is advsiable to:

(1) *Help* the patient *to take up* a position, e.g. prone kneeling, and *teach* him *to retain* that position (power and balance). A patient cannot be expected to attempt with confidence to achieve a position if he

believes that he will fall down again once he has gained it.
(2) *Teach* the patient *to take up* the position.
(3) *Teach* the patient *to move* in the position, e.g. crawl.

Ideally there should be a mat area in the department, the size of which will depend on the number of patients treated at any one time. Each patient will require a mat at least 1800 × 1740 cm (low mat). Mats raised from the floor on a platform 46 cm high (high mat), i.e. the height of the seat of the average wheelchair, have many advantages, particularly when getting a patient onto and off the mat. Patients can also easily be progressed from mat activities to sitting balance on the side of the mat. Ideally a department should have both high and low mats side by side.

The therapist should ensure that people using mats remove their shoes to keep the mats clean.

The basic principles of maximum resistance and the selection of strong patterns to overflow to weaker muscles and movements are the basis of teaching the patient to achieve a specific function. However, it is implicit in these principles that the patient must be allowed to move smoothly through the available range. Therefore, where spasticity is a factor in preventing normal movement, inhibition should always precede and accompany movement, which must be at a less voluntary level as voluntary effort will have the effect of potentially increasing tone.

The descriptions and illustrations in this section give the main movements and resistance points which may be used by the therapist. It must be remembered that many more combinations of patterns and techniques, for example repeated contractions, may be used by the therapist based on her assessment of each patient's specific needs.

As with balance, it is important for the therapist to observe normal functional movement in others as most of these activities take place at a subconscious level. The individual knows that he has rolled over, that he has gone from lying to prone kneeling or to standing, but cannot afterwards describe his movements in detail. This, the therapist must know when faced with the problems of rehabilitation. When conscious control is exerted it is unlikely that the normal individual will achieve such a flowing co-ordinated movement.

In each section below the main patterns of movement involved in the functional activity are given.

Rolling

From side lying

If the patient is weak, side lying is a good starting position, for very little effort by the patient will result in movement as he is assisted by gravity in either direction. The facilitation of trunk rotation is important when re-educating functional activities. The therapist must position herself in the line of movement, i.e. on the diagonal, as it is very easy to get out of pattern and thus make the patient's task more difficult. To aid accuracy of pattern and to give some stability to side lying as a starting position, the patient's knees are flexed.

Scapular patterns

Abduction patterns, particularly the depression/abduction pattern, will cause the model to roll forwards towards the prone position.

Adduction patterns, particularly the elevation/adduction pattern, will cause the model to roll backwards towards the supine position.

Pelvic patterns

The patterns are based on the line and contraction of the oblique abdominal muscle, i.e. from the crest of the ilium and inguinal ligament to the lower ribs of the opposite side. Movement occurs in two directions:

(1) Flexion of the trunk with rotation – rolling forwards. The therapist grasps the patient's iliac crest near to, and including, the anterior superior iliac spine. Using her body weight by leaning backwards she applies a stretch stimulus. On the command 'now – pull' the patient moves the pelvis forwards.

(2) Extension of the trunk with rotation – rolling backwards. The therapist, using her body weight, gives forward pressure to the patient's pelvis (over gluteus maximus). On the command 'now – push' the patient moves the pelvis backwards.

This rotation of the pelvis resulting in an arc of movement can be observed in many of the functional activities on mats and in sideways transfer activities, e.g. from chair to bed (Fig. 24.1).

The other basic arc of movement, i.e. in a forwards and backwards or straight movement,

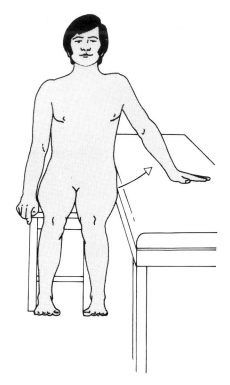

Fig. 24.1 The basic arc of movement used in sideways transfers.

can be *observed in* many of the mat and transfer activities, e.g. backwards into a chair drawn up facing the bed (Fig. 24.2).

Scapular and pelvic patterns

A combination of the depression/abduction, scapular pattern and the flexion with rotation, pelvic pattern may be used to teach forward rolling into the prone position.

A combination of the elevation/adduction scapular pattern and the extension with rotation, pelvic pattern may be used to teach rolling into the supine position.

As the patient's function improves he can be gradually moved further into either the supine or the prone position, thus increasing the range of movement and resistance by gravity. Manual resistance will also be graded to allow for smooth movement throughout the available range.

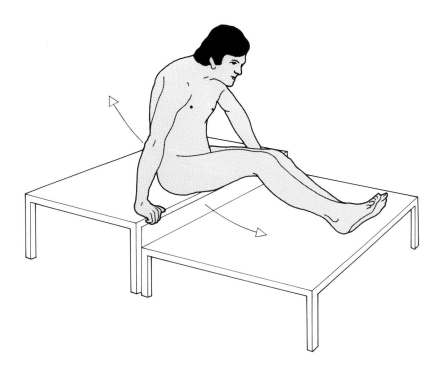

Fig. 24.2 The basic arc of movement used in forwards and backwards transfers.

From supine to prone lying

Most normal individuals when rolling from supine to prone use a combination of head and neck, arm and leg patterns. It will be noted that in the majority of instances the head is raised and rotated towards the direction of movement fractionally before the arm and/or leg is moved. Occasionally the normal individual may use mass extension pivoting on the head and heels to initiate a roll. This potentially pathological method should not be encouraged.

The following movements will assist the patient to roll.

Head and neck
Flexion with rotation in the direction of movement.

Arm
The following methods of using the right arm will cause the patient to roll to the left:

(1) Flexion/adduction pattern. The patient reaches across his face. He grasps the top edge of the mat or head of the bed and pulls.
(2) Extension/adduction pattern. The patient reaches across his body. He grasps the side edge of the mat or bed and pulls (Fig. 24.3).
(3) Extension/abduction/elbow extension pattern. The patient places his hand on the mat at waist level and pushes.

The following methods of using the right arm will cause the patient to roll to the right:

(1) Flexion/abduction pattern. The patient reaches for the top edge of the mat or bed. He grasps and pulls.
(2) Extension/abduction pattern. The patient reaches for the side edge of the mat or bed. He grasps and pulls.

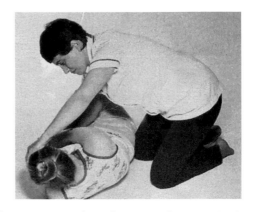

Fig. 24.3 Using the right arm in the extension/adduction position to assist rolling to the left, starting in the supine position. The therapist may resist the movement using the head and arm.

Leg
The following methods of using the right leg will assist the patient to roll to the left:

(1) The flexion/adduction knee flexion pattern.
(2) The extension/abduction/with knee extension pattern. The patient flexes his hip and knee and places his foot on the mat lateral to the mid-line. He thrusts, extending both the hip and the knee.

The following methods of using the right leg will assist the patient to roll to the right:

(1) Flexion/abduction pattern either with a straight leg or a flexed knee. The patient should create enough momentum to help his trunk to rotate.
(2) Extension/adduction pattern with either a straight leg or extending knee. The patient flexes at the hip and knee (when used) and places the limb in an adducted position. He then pushes with his leg or thrusts his foot into the mat or bed and rolls over.

From prone lying to supine

Head

By extending the head and turning it to the right the patient is assisted in rolling to the left.

Arm

By placing the right arm in the following positions with the hand flat on the mat or bed and thrusting, the patient will be assisted in rolling to the left:

(1) Flexion/abduction with the elbow flexed sufficiently to allow the palm to be placed on the mat or bed.
(2) Extension/abduction with sufficient elbow flexion to allow the palm to be placed on the mat or bed.

By placing the right arm in the position of flexion/adduction with sufficient elbow flexion to allow the palm of the hand to be placed on the mat or bed and thrusting, the patient will be assisted in rolling to the right (Fig. 24.4).

Leg

By raising the right leg backwards, i.e. into the inner range of the extension/adduction pattern, the patient will be assisted in rolling to the left.

Bridging

The term bridging denotes pelvic raising from the crook lying position. This activity is useful as a preparation for transfers and also for the patient who has to pull clothing over the hips when in lying. Some patients may find crook lying to be a good position from which to initiate rolling.

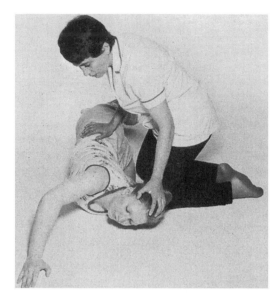

Fig. 24.4 Using the right arm in the flexion/adduction position to assist in rolling to the right starting in the prone position. The therapist may resist the movement using the head and pelvis.

Before attempting to bridge, the patient must be assisted to maintain the starting position by 'rhythmic stabilization' or 'tapping'. The therapist positions herself in standing, facing the patient, with her feet astride his raised knees. She then flexes her hips and knees until she can control the patient's knees with her own knees. It is difficult, in this position, to block the patient's feet as well. If this is necessary a sandbag may be used. The therapist must take care not to strain her back when assisting a patient to bridge.

The therapist places her thumbs inside the waistband of the patient's trousers at the level of the seam. This position enables her either to resist the patient's bridging activities by pressing on the anterior superior iliac spine, or to assist him to lift his hips by taking a firm grip of the trousers and through them to control the pelvis. As the aim is to achieve movement, assistance may be necessary initially but the patient

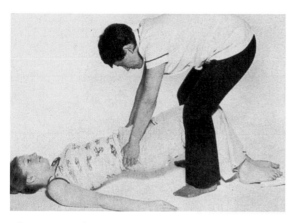

Fig. 24.5 Bridging.

should be encouraged to work maximally (Fig. 24.5).

Bridging may be done either sideways with rotation or straight by simply lifting the buttocks straight off the mat. When asking the patient to do the former, the therapist exerts pressure on one anterior superior iliac spine and instructs the patient to raise that hip. The patient may then return to the starting position or, while in the bridging position, raise first one hip and then the other, thus rotating the pelvis. The therapist gives alternating pressure first on one side and then on the other. For the straight raise pressure is exerted on both hips simultaneously.

Crook lying is a useful position in which to strengthen the trunk rotators and the hip abductors and adductors.

Trunk rotators
(1) The therapist, with her hands in position on the patient's knees, opposite to the proposed direction of movement, instructs the patient to roll the knees towards the mat, first in one direction and then in the other. Resistance is given to the movement, ensuring that the patient is working maximally.

(2) With the patient in the bridging position, i.e. pelvis raised, the therapist uses the rhythmic stabilization technique working on the rotators. The therapist's hands are placed one over the anterior superior iliac spine and the other on the opposite buttock. The hands are thus in a position to exert pressure in a rotatory direction. They then alternate.

Hip abductors and adductors
The therapist places each of her hands on the lateral aspect of the appropriate knee. She then resists the movement of abduction with lateral rotation. She then places her hands on the medial aspect of the abducted knees and resists adduction with medial rotation (to mid-line).

Creeping

The term creeping denotes either forward or backward progression in either prone lying or forearm support prone lying.

The more primitive form of creeping is an ipsilateral (amphibian) movement of the head, trunk, arm and leg. Later this may develop into the more mature contralateral movement.

Starting position
As the individual's mode of progression matures, he will gradually raise his head more and assume the forearm support prone lying position.

In preparation for this activity, the patient may be placed in the forearm support prone lying position. The patient rolls into prone lying and the therapist stands astride his thorax facing towards his head. To raise the patient onto his right elbow the therapist places her left hand under the patient's shoulder girdle (clavicle) and lifts his shoulder off the mat. With her right hand she positions the patient's arm ensuring that his elbow is directly below the point of the shoulder. Any deviation from this exact position will cause instability. To retain the elbow in the correct position, the therapist fixes it with her right foot. The same method is used to position the patient's left elbow.

Rhythmic stabilization using the head and/or shoulder or tapping on the shoulders may be used to teach the patient to maintain the position.

The patient is then taught to get into this position unaided.

Movement
Creeping forwards
The therapist takes up a position behind the patient, grasps the feet and resists the forward movement of the leg as it flexes and abducts with lateral rotation. The patient is then instructed to move the arm into flexion/abduction and to turn his head towards the moving limbs.

Progress is made by alternate total flexion on one side and then on the other.

Creeping backwards
Reverse movements cause the individual to progress backwards.

Other activities
The forearm support position is useful to enable the patient to learn early control of the head. The rhythmic stabilization technique may be used. Repeated contraction and slow reversal techniques, working in the neck flexion and extension patterns, can be successfully done in this position as a means of strengthening weak muscles.

Where the neck muscles are strong they may be used in accordance with the overflow principle to strengthen weaker back extensor and abdominal muscles.

Crawling

It is not necessary, particularly with adult patients, always to progress through creeping to crawling. Crawling can be attempted as the first mode of progression. To achieve crawling the patient is taken through several stages.

Starting position
Forearm support prone lying
See above.

Forearm support prone kneeling
The patient takes up the forearm support prone lying position. The therapist stands astride him at hip level facing the patient's head. Bending at the hips and knees, she inserts her thumbs into the waistband of the patient's trousers and grasps the pelvis. She then lifts and raises his pelvis well clear of the mat. The patient's knees are either positioned under the raised hips or the hips are taken slightly backwards over the knees. The patient's knees are abducted a little to ensure a stable position. The therapist's knees which are on either side of the pelvis can, if necessary, control the patient's buttocks.

The patient then learns to balance in this position.

Prone kneeling
From the forearm support prone kneeling position the patient is raised into prone kneeling. The therapist raises the patient's right shoulder by placing her left hand over the clavicle from behind and uses her right hand to support the patient's right elbow as she lowers his weight onto his out-stretched hand. If the patient cannot fully extend the wrist and fingers some adjustment can be made, for example, the hand may be placed on a sandbag. This enables the patient to place weight through the upper limb and to establish the

positive support reaction (protective extension reaction). In some situations the patient may find it helpful to take his weight through his knuckles. This has the effect of elongating the arm, thus causing the elbow to flex and giving a better position for weight bearing and a thrust.

To free her hands to position the patient's left arm the therapist may have to support his right elbow with her knee.

In this description the right arm has been positioned first; in practice if the patient has one arm which functions better than the other, that arm will be positioned first or the therapist may raise both shoulders simultaneously by placing her hands one over each clavicle and lifting.

The patient then learns to balance in the position.

Teaching the patient to achieve the starting position

There are two basic ways for an individual to achieve prone kneeling.

Through side sitting

From prone lying the patient raises his head, places one or both hands flat on the floor beneath his shoulder(s) and thrusts. Simultaneously he rotates his trunk and pushes himself into side sitting. When one hand is used the patient rotates towards and sits to that side.

From the supine position the patient raises his head, rotating it towards the stronger side. Almost simultaneously he raises the opposite shoulder (depression/abduction), rotates his trunk and raises himself up to rest on his forearm. The knees are flexed and the pelvis rotated in the same direction. The patient then pushes on his forearm and hand until he has achieved side sitting supported by the extended upper limb. With one or both hands on the mat

he thrusts on his hands and knees and raises his pelvis sideways in an arc of movement.

To train the patient to do this the therapist places the patient in the prone kneeling position and kneels at one side of him. If the patient has weakness down one side the therapist will kneel at the stronger side.

The therapist grasps the patient's waistband and pulls his pelvis slightly towards herself. The patient is then instructed to '*pull up*' and applying the maximal resistance principle, the therapist allows him to regain the prone kneeling position (Fig. 24.6).

The therapist gradually moves herself into the kneel sitting position, so that each time the patient will be pulled further towards the side sitting position and he will have to raise his pelvis through a larger arc of movement to return to prone kneeling. Finally, the patient raises his own pelvis from side sitting on the mat.

The advantage of the therapist working from the stronger side will now be obvious, i.e. the patient is able to use the stronger (under-

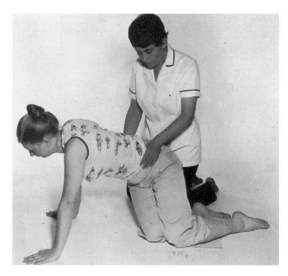

Fig. 24.6 Teaching the patient to achieve prone kneeling from side sitting.

neath) arm and leg to thrust himself from the floor. The therapist may decide that it is to the patient's advantage to teach him to do the movement from both sides.

Movement backwards from prone lying

Prior to which the patient places his hands under his shoulders. He will either extend his neck in midline or extend and rotate the head to one side as he thrusts backwards with his arms and bends his hips and knees.

In practice it will be noted that it is usually the younger people, or those with good power in both arms, who use this method.

To emphasize the movement the therapist gives resistance with one hand to the extensors and rotators of the neck by placing one hand on the head opposite to the direction of movement and the other hand over the opposite scapula.

In preparation for crawling the patient learns to balance both in the basic prone kneeling position and with alternate arm and leg forwards.

Movement

Crawling forwards

The therapist positions herself in kneeling behind the patient and grasps both his feet by the dorsum only.

To crawl forwards and to the right the therapist raises the patient's right leg into extension/adduction with lateral rotation. On the command '*pull*' the patient flexes, abducts and medially rotates the leg. The therapist then raises the left leg into extension/abduction with medial rotation and on the command '*pull*' the patient flexes, adducts and laterally rotates the leg.

This method is adapted to enable the patient to crawl forwards towards the left.

The patient either automatically adopts contralateral movements of the arms or is instructed to do so.

In the early stages of crawling infants keep their knees in abduction. This method of crawling may be adopted for a patient with poor balance.

Crawling backwards

The therapist positions herself as before, kneeling behind the patient, and grasps both feet ensuring that pressure is exerted on the plantar surface of the feet only.

To crawl backwards towards the right the therapist pushes the right leg into flexion/adduction with lateral rotation and on the command '*push*' the patient thrusts the leg into extension/abduction with medial rotation. The therapist then resists the thrust of the left leg into extension/adduction with lateral rotation. This method should be adapted for crawling backwards to the left.

The patient either automatically adopts or is instructed to make contralateral movements with the arms.

These resisted movements of the legs as described can be used as resisted exercises by applying either the repeated contraction or slow reversal techniques.

Kneeling

Kneeling is a more difficult position to maintain, as the centre of gravity is raised, the base is smaller and the line of gravity falls near to the edge of the base. Developmentally the child achieves standing and walking before he learns to kneel and walk on his knees. However, it is usually through this position that the adult achieves standing or raises himself from the floor into sitting on a chair or bed. Walking on the knees is a necessary activity in some cases.

Starting position

(1) The patient may be helped into kneeling from prone kneeling by the therapist who takes up a position of kneel sitting facing the prone kneeling patient. The patient places his hands one at a time on the therapist's shoulders, who then raises herself into the kneeling position, moving towards the patient until they are both kneeling facing each other, with the patient supporting himself with his hands on the therapist's shoulders and the therapist supporting the patient at waist level.

(2) The patient may get himself into kneeling by crawling up to the wallbars and 'walking' up the bars with his hands, moving his knees towards the bars as necessary.

The patient is then taught to balance in the position by the therapist, using the head, shoulders and hips as stabilizing points.

Teaching the patient to achieve the position

Kneeling is achieved from side sitting, i.e. sideways with rotation, or from kneel sitting, a straight thrust.

From side sitting

The patient is positioned in kneeling either facing the wallbars which he grasps, or facing a high mat which he uses to support himself with his arms. The therapist kneels at one side and grasping the patient by the waistband (iliac crest) rotates his pelvis towards herself. The patient is then instructed to '*pull up*' and against resistance he is allowed to return to kneeling. Gradually the therapist pulls the patient further towards the side sitting position and each time he returns to the starting position until he can raise himself from the floor. The patient can learn to raise himself into the kneeling position from side sitting by pushing

on his supporting hand and underneath leg. Obviously, if the patient is weak down one side he will find it easier if he sits towards the stronger side so that he will be supported by the stronger arm, which he can then use to push himself into kneeling.

From kneel sitting

The patient sits back onto his heels from prone kneeling and places his hands on his thighs. By thrusting with his hands and extending his neck and hips he can raise himself into the kneeling position. The therapist can assist by giving direction to the movement by placing one hand on the front of the patient's head and the other on one of his shoulders. She may find it necessary to help the patient to extend his hips by grasping his iliac crests or waistband.

Movement

The patient may be taught to walk on his knees against resistance; he can walk forwards or backwards, towards the right or left, or sideways in a similar manner to resisted crawling. The therapist gives resistance either at the head and shoulder or on the iliac crests.

The therapist may find it useful to give the patient shortened axillary or elbow crutches and teach balance and knee walking on these.

From the floor to sitting on a chair/bed

Sideways with rotation

This activity is achieved through half kneeling. The patient takes up the kneeling position with his stronger side against the support. The support should be large and very stable (high mat or low plinth) so that the patient will feel secure. As he gains in ability and confidence he can be taught to get into an armchair or even onto a stool, but the latter is unstable and only has a small area on which to place his buttocks. In most instances it is unsafe and unnecessary for a patient to use a stool.

From the kneeling position the patient puts his near hand onto the high mat and, taking weight through this hand he raises the ipsilateral (inside) knee and places the foot on the floor. The therapist may need to assist him to do this. The patient is taught to balance in half kneeling using the head, shoulder, hips, raised knee and foot as pivots for rhythmic stabilization.

It will be noted that in this position the patient's buttocks are level with the support. To raise himself into the sitting position it is only necessary for him to pivot on the supporting hand, thrust with the raised leg and rotate the pelvis towards the support (Fig. 24.7).

To assist the patient the therapist takes up a position behind him and places her nearside knee onto the high mat, ensuring that the foot that remains on the floor and the supporting knee are in the line of movement to be taken by the patient's pelvis. She then grasps the waistband of the patient's trousers. The patient and the therapist synchronize their efforts and the patient achieves the sitting position.

This sideways movement is the basis for transfers either from sitting through standing or direct from sitting to sitting.

The reverse movement may be used to enable the patient to return to the floor. Some patients prefer to rotate the trunk through a greater range so that they can place both hands on the bed or chair arms. They then flex their knees and rotate the pelvis. At the completion of the movement the patient is kneeling facing the support rather than sideways to it.

Straight anteroposterior movement

This method may be preferred by patients who have good power in both arms.

As a preparatory exercise the patient takes up the position of long sitting on the mat and grasps a pair of blocks which are placed one on either side at hip level. The therapist kneels at the patient's feet and grasps them over the dorsum in such a way that she can lift them off the mat (Fig. 24.8). The patient is instructed to raise his hips off the mat by thrusting on the

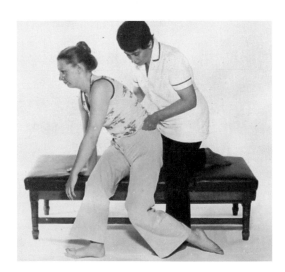

Fig. 24.7 Assisted/resisted movement from half kneeling to sitting.

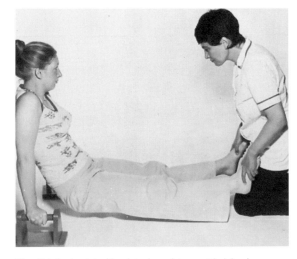

Fig. 24.8 Assisted/resisted rocking with blocks.

blocks and the therapist raises his feet. The patient retains this position and starts to move his hips backwards and forwards. As the hips move backwards his head moves forwards, i.e. flexes, and vice versa. This rocking takes the hips through an anteroposterior arc of movement. That is, as the hips move backwards they are raised further from the mat, sufficient to clear a low obstacle. When resisting the forwards movement of the patient the therapist should change her grip so that she is giving pressure over the plantar surface of the feet.

To get from the floor using this method it may be necessary, certainly at first, for the movement to take place in two stages: stage one onto a low platform or firm cushion, stage two up onto the high mat or chair. The patient sits with his back to the bed or chair, places his hands onto the support and, using the same movement as previously practised, thrusts with his arms, raises his hips clear of the mat and carries them backwards onto the support (Fig. 24.2).

Kneeling to standing

The patient takes up the half kneeling position:

(1) Facing and supporting himself on the wallbars. The therapist stands behind the patient and places one hand on the hip of the forward leg and the other on the opposite shoulder.

(2) Facing the therapist and supporting himself by placing his hands onto her shoulders. The therapist grasps the patient's waistband.

The raised knee and foot should be placed to one side, i.e. in the flexion/abduction position. (It is quite difficult for a normal individual to stand from half kneeling if the foot is placed directly in front of the body.)

Using the principle of maximum resistance the therapist allows the patient to stand. Standing unaided is difficult or impossible for many patients. Before attempting to get the patient to stand either directly from the floor or through sitting the therapist must ensure that he can balance in the position.

Chapter 25
BALANCE

P. J. Waddington

Balance and posture are interrelated. Depending on the base and the position of the centre and line of gravity a body is either balanced – in equilibrium – or not. Posture is the word used to describe any position of the human body. Some positions or postures require more muscle work to maintain than others, but whatever the position, balance must be maintained otherwise the force of gravity will impose a change of posture.

The maintenance of balance is dependent on the one hand upon the integration of sensory input from exteroceptors, proprioceptors and the special senses – the eyes and the vestibular apparatus – and on the other hand on an integrated motor system and the basic postural reflexes. In the normal individual, balance is maintained almost completely at a subconscious level. In retraining a patient's balance this fact must be considered and the patient trained to react to stimuli rather than to make a conscious, voluntary effort to maintain equilibrium. At times voluntary control will have to be exercised, but this causes the patient to be at a great disadvantage.

Balance, therefore, is the basis of all static or dynamic postures and should be considered when planning any exercise or rehabilitation programme. Its re-education should not be confined to patients with neurological conditions, as balance is frequently impaired following fractures, soft tissue lesions and surgical procedures involving the lower limb.

Balance reactions can also be used to facilitate the contraction of selected muscle groups and as part of a muscle strengthening programme.

There are two approaches to balance, both of which are necessary for normal function: static balance and dynamic balance.

Static balance

The static balance approach is based on PNF principles and techniques.

Static balance is the rigid stability of one part of the body on another and is based on isometric and co-contraction of muscle. The rhythmic stabilization technique and the irradiation principle are used to develop a contraction of postural muscles. These techniques may be used in any position. They are frequently combined with compression to stimulate postural reflexes.

As a general principle balance is developed progressively by moving from the most stable to the least stable position, for example from forearm support prone lying to standing with sticks.

Stability and control of the head should be established first as these are vital in all positions. Strong neck muscles can then be used to reinforce muscle contraction elsewhere.

Assessment of the patient's muscle strength will guide the therapist in the application of the irradiation principle. Note that the possibilities of associated reactions and an undesirable increase in tone must always be considered. However, this method is useful with patients who are hypotonic or ataxic.

Application

As indicated above, positions for the retraining of balance are selected on the basis of progression from the easy to the more difficult.

Positions
Forearm support prone lying
Forearm support prone kneeling
Prone kneeling
Reach grasp kneeling
Half kneeling
Sitting
Walk standing
Standing

Although in the normal development of the child standing is achieved before kneeling, for the adult, kneeling, and certainly reach grasp kneeling are frequently easier to maintain than standing. If required as a progression, shortened crutches may be used for support in kneeling.

In standing and walk standing the patient may be progressed from using parallel bars, through the range of walking aids to standing unaided.

Resistance is applied to all the components needed to maintain a particular position. Selection is made from the following:

- Head
- Shoulders
- Pelvis
- Knees
- Toes for gripping the floor

- Hands for gripping a support or a walking aid.

A slow increase of alternating resistance is used to build up a co-contraction, i.e. rhythmic stabilization. The direction of the resistance will vary with the point selected, for example:

(1) The pelvis
  - Forwards and backwards
  - Laterally
  - Diagonally
  - Rotation
(2) The knee
  - Forwards and backwards

A combination of stabilizing points may be used to advantage, e.g. the shoulder and the pelvis, the head and the pelvis, the pelvis and the knee.

In some situations the principles of maximal resistance are used to stimulate a unilateral isometric contraction instead of a co-contraction; this is of particular value when working to obtain extension of the cervical spine in forearm support prone lying.

Dynamic balance

This approach is based upon Bobath principles and techniques.

The body, unless it is fully supported and relaxed, is in a constant state of adjustment to maintain its posture and its equilibrium. The forces tending to upset this balance may vary in strength from the infinitesimal to sufficient to completely upset the individual's equilibrium so that he falls to the ground. Consequently, the body's reactions to maintain its equilibrium will vary in degree. For example, the amount of adjustment will be greater and more obvious when an individual slips on an ice-covered road than when he raises his hand to his mouth. The normal individual will find the former a difficult if not impossible exercise in regaining balance but he will not even be aware of the adjustments he makes when eating. However, raising the hand to the mouth will prove a severe test of balance for a paraplegic patient early in his rehabilitation, while he is still learning to compensate for the loss of sensory input from below the lesion.

At the level of minor adjustments, the muscles may be working either isometrically or isotonically but when larger adjustments are necessary the type of muscle work will become definitely isotonic. If one had to try to clarify this it is easier to work with the concept of static balance as being isometric, and dynamic balance as being isotonic contraction.

It is convenient to think of these balance reactions as occurring in two ways:

(1) An adjustment in tone to maintain a position.
(2) An adjustment in posture to maintain or regain balance. This can involve either movements designed to keep the individual in more or less the same place, or those in which the base is moved.

Maintenance of position

This method, unlike rhythmic stabilization, allows for a little movement.

The patient is instructed to maintain the position, for example, prone kneeling, kneeling, sitting or standing against the therapist's tapping technique. This technique simply consists of tapping the patient's shoulders or thorax at shoulder level, first in one direction and then in the other. The tap should be strong enough to cause the patient to adjust his muscle tone but not strong enough to make him change his position. For example, when he is standing, a tap on the patient's back causing the body to move slightly forwards will cause the calf

muscles to contract, a tap in the opposite direction will cause a contraction of the anterior tibial muscles. This is obviously an oversimplification as changes in muscle tone will occur elsewhere, particularly in the feet.

Maintaining or regaining balance

It has been said that our whole life consists of constantly regaining our balance. We are never static. One view of walking is that it is simply a transferring of weight forwards and that the leg moves to regain balance.

Balance reactions are immediate and reliable and are not learned at a voluntary level. Therefore, the therapist does not instruct the patient in how to react but puts him into such a situation that he has to react to maintain or regain his balance. It is usually a wise precaution to explain to the patient that you are going to work on balance, otherwise he may get very frustrated as most patients expect to be told what to do in the form of a definite task or exercise. Further instruction would destroy the patient's ability to react spontaneously.

The therapist must know the normal balance reactions, so that she will be able to recognize the abnormal and also so that she can facilitate normal reactions where they are absent.

An interesting point to note is the change of tone in a limb before it actually moves. The student can easily try this for herself. In the prone kneeling position do not move but think about lifting one hand from the ground and note the change of pressure and of tone. Without this preparation movement would not be possible.

The use of a moving support is valuable in some positions to facilitate movement and in others can be related to balance maintenance in such common situations as riding in a bus or car or on a bicycle or ship.

There are three basic types of movable support:

(1) *A balance board*, which can vary in size from the usual balance wobble board (Chapter 2) to a polished piece of wood 2000 mm long and 610 mm wide with a rocker at either end

(2) *A roll*, which can be made of a cardboard tube, as used in carpets, is padded and covered with plastic

(3) *Large inflated balls* of varying size and type (Chapter 7).

Lying

This position is not usually associated with problems of balance but if the therapist wishes to stimulate movement, particularly trunk movement, the patient can be placed in lying on a polished balance board. The therapist controls the board from one end and tilts it so that the patient has to react to remain on the board. From the age of 6 months a child will try to stay on the board. The disadvantage is that it is difficult for the therapist to control both the board and the patient.

Rolling a patient on a mat may be used as a method for reducing tone. A pathological pattern and the accompanying hypertonus is a complete entity. General reduction in tone as a preparation for movement starts with efforts to produce symmetry and trunk rotation. Trunk rotation is lost in patients with Parkinson's disease and trunk rolling can be used followed by the rhythm technique (Chapter 23). Following the reduction in tone, active balance reactions occur. These movements, in themselves, tend to reduce tone still further. Even where hypertonus is not a problem balance reactions in lying may be used as a form of exercise. There are several ways of producing trunk rotation passively but to activate the patient the

following methods will form a basis for stimulating activity.

The patient is placed in lying with the therapist kneel sitting so that the patient's head is resting on her knees. The patient's arms, when possible, are placed in the flexion/abduction/lateral rotation position which is a reflex inhibitory pattern, i.e. a position opposite to the basic pathological pattern of spasticity. This position in itself will tend to reduce tone as a preparation for movement. The therapist places her hands high on the patient's scapulae and rolls him first to one side and then to the other. Once the patient begins to show some movement more time is spent with him in the side lying position. The therapist slightly adjusts the patient's position, constantly putting him off balance so that he has to move either his trunk or the upper leg to regain his equilibrium (Fig. 25.1).

This method can prove impossible if the patient is too heavy to move from the supine position. When this is so, side lying can be used as a starting position to activate balance

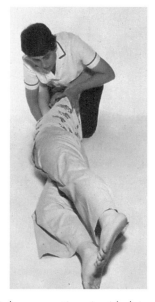

Fig. 25.1 Balance reactions in side lying.

reactions. Also side lying is useful as the labyrinthine reflexes are not stimulated in that position, and if care is taken to ensure that the head and neck are aligned neither are the asymmetrical tonic neck reflexes.

Prone kneeling (normal reactions)
The patient takes up the prone kneeling position. The therapist raises one of his limbs to elicit balance reactions. When the arm is used it should be kept laterally rotated and the thumb extended. There are three basic types of reaction (Figs. 25.2 and 25.3):

(1)   When a normal limb is raised and moved slowly, without the help of the patient, it will feel light and easy to move and the body will adapt itself easily to maintain its balance.

The next two types of reaction occur when enough force is applied to endanger the patient's equilibrium. Each person, depending on his physical strength and possibly his personality, will have an automatic preference for one or the other.

(2)   The patient tries to maintain his position by developing a co-contraction, i.e. static balance. This is usually adequate up to a certain point, at which the patient can no longer resist and he collapses onto the mat.

(3)   The patient moves another limb to maintain his equilibrium. If the therapist moves one limb into abduction the patient will raise his contralateral limb (Fig. 25.2). If she adducts the limb the patient will raise the ipsilateral limb (Fig. 25.3).

Some people will crawl about following the limb that is being moved. This really does not come under the narrow heading of balance reactions. Patients who do this are obviously

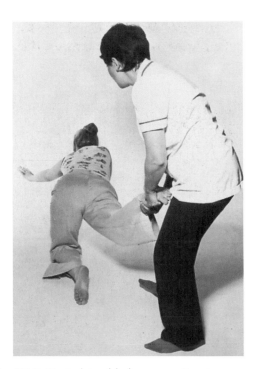

Fig. 25.2 Contralateral balance reaction in prone kneeling.

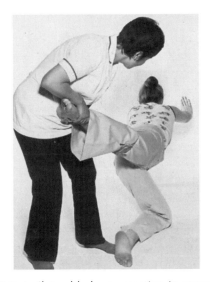

Fig. 25.3 Ipsilateral balance reaction in prone kneeling.

quite safe in prone kneeling. If the therapist wishes to use these equilibrium reactions as a form of exercise for such patients she may have to give him a further explanation of what is required.

Kneeling (normal reactions)

(1) Weight transference forwards – the therapist kneels in front of the patient and displaces his weight forwards holding him at waist level. The patient reacts by abducting the arms and extending the fingers and thumb, flexing the knees and plantar-flexing at the ankle (Fig. 25.4).

(2) Weight transference laterally – again the arms abduct and the fingers extend. The non-weight bearing leg is abducted (Fig. 25.5).

Standing (normal reactions)

The therapist, standing behind the patient, can hold the patient at the pelvis (thumbs inserted into waistband or belt), shoulders, knees or head. Obviously the patient feels safer if held at the pelvis and in practice this is usually done as the majority of patients are apprehensive. Again

a judgement has to be made as the patient must not feel too secure.

These balance reactions may be done with either the patient standing on a mat or on the floor. Many nervous patients prefer to stand on the mat, although a thick mat forms a less secure base and may be selected by the therapist for that reason, i.e. to elicit a reaction.

The therapist may decide to cause a patient either to take weight on an affected leg or to move it.

(1) Weight transference backwards – causes dorsi-flexion at the ankle. Further disturbance will cause the patient to take a step backwards. If he is prevented from doing this by the therapist placing a foot at the back of his heels, the patient will bend forward from the waist and hips raising the arms forwards simultaneously. Some people may prefer this reaction in any situation.

(2) Weight transference forwards – will cause the patient to stand on his toes. If this is

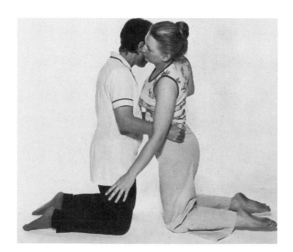

Fig. 25.4 Balance reaction in kneeling – weight transferred forwards.

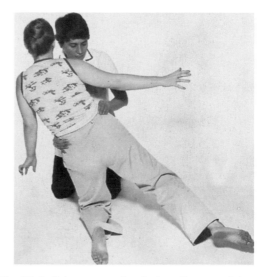

Fig. 25.5 Balance reaction in kneeling – weight transferred laterally.

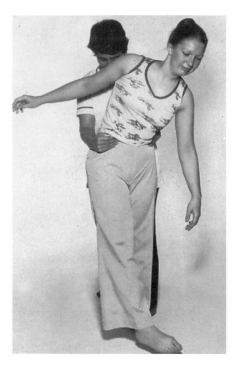

Fig. 25.6 Balance reaction in standing – weight transferred laterally.

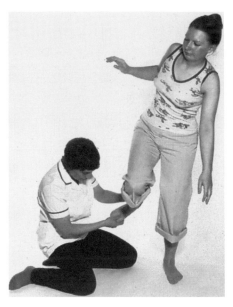

Fig. 25.7 Balance reaction – standing on one foot.

the reaction required, the therapist would be better standing facing the patient. Further transference of weight forwards will cause the patient to step.

(3) Weight transference laterally – the therapist transfers the patient's weight onto one foot, the patient either abducts the non-weight bearing leg or crosses it in front of the weight bearing leg (Fig. 25.6). The first reaction may be followed by the second. If the weight is then transferred in the opposite direction the leg will return to the starting position. This alternating weight transfer may be done rhythmically causing the moving leg to react repeatedly.

Standing on one foot (normal reactions)
The therapist asks the patient to stand on one foot. She grasps the raised leg taking the foot

in one hand, using the other to grasp the posterior aspect of the leg just below the knee. It is usually preferable to keep the patient's knee flexed.

Reactions:

(1) Slight movement of the raised leg by the therapist will result in considerable activity of the standing foot which will remain stationary (Fig. 25.7).

(2) Further movement of the raised leg by the therapist will cause the patient to move, either by doing a heel–toe pivot or by hopping. Again the normal person will have his own preferred reaction.

Sitting
The patient sits so that the feet are unsupported.

(1) Weight transference backwards – the therapist may stand either behind or in front of the patient, grasping the pelvis.

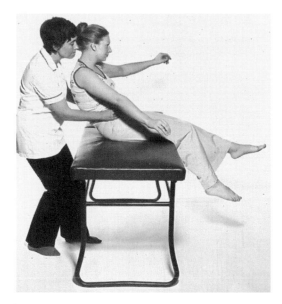

Fig. 25.8 Balance reaction in sitting – weight transferred backwards.

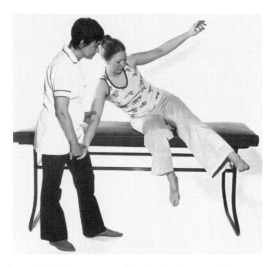

Fig. 25.9 Balance reaction in sitting – weight transferred laterally.

The patient reacts by extending the knees (Fig. 25.8).

(2) Weight transference forwards – the therapist stands facing the patient and grasps the pelvis. The patient reacts by further flexion of the knees.

(3) Weight transference laterally – the patient's weight may be transferred by moving either the arm or the leg. The weight is transferred laterally initially (Fig. 25.9). Once the patient's balance reactions are facilitated many movements can be elicited by further movements of the limb. These movements involve a considerable amount of effort on the patient's part to maintain his balance. Some individuals react by resisting the therapist and so develop a co-contraction.

Note: A knowledge of normal balance reactions enables the therapist to use these not only in the retraining of balance and thus confidence in the patient, but also as a means of eliciting a contraction in exercising specific muscle groups.

Protective extension reaction of the arms

If balance reactions fail, protective extension (saving reactions) of the arms is one of the most important reactions. In patients with central nervous system damage it may be necessary to facilitate this reaction either in infants and children who have never developed it or in adults where it has been disturbed. Again these techniques may be used as a means of eliciting a muscle contraction.

Such discussion moves into the area of normal development and the treatment of specific conditions which are outside the scope of this book.

It may be useful to indicate some of the ways in which this reaction may be elicited.

(1) The patient is placed in the sitting position.
    (a) The therapist holds the unaffected arm and transfers the patient's

weight sideways towards the affected side.

(b) The therapist holds the affected arm by *either* using one of her hands to keep the patient's wrist and fingers extended and her thumb abducted, and the other hand to control the elbow, *or* using both hands to maintain the extended wrist and fingers and the abducted thumb. Some of the patient's weight is then transferred through the affected arm. The therapist may then use a pull–push technique in the long axis of the limb to facilitate the protective extension reaction.

(2) The patient is placed in the prone kneeling position. The therapist raises either one or both of the patient's arms by grasping at the shoulder, and releases her grasp.

(3) The patient is standing. The therapist stands facing the patient and grasps the hands, palm-to-palm, keeping the wrists extended and when possible the thumbs abducted. The patient's arms are raised into the reach position and the therapist gently pulls the patient towards herself so transferring his weight forwards. The push–pull technique through the longitudinal axis of the arm may again be used to elicit a response.

The reactions of some patients who have made an almost complete recovery may be speeded up by pushing them forwards onto a plinth or wall. The therapist may keep control of the patient by retaining her hold of one arm.

Chapter 26
GAIT

P. J. Waddington

The problems presented by the patient who is unable to walk, but has the potential to do so, and by the patient with abnormal gait, are manifold. The assessment of each patient must be the basis for satisfactory treatment. The therapist who looks at the problem from more than one standpoint will have a better chance of solving it.

Walking is a complex combination of balance and co-ordinated muscle contraction based on normal tone and power and on sensory input. Too much time can be spent in instructing the patient to perform specific movements at a conscious voluntary level. Walking is a reflex activity which takes place at a subconscious level. It is obvious that the patient who is being instructed in the use of a walking aid will have to know what is expected of him, but the aim is to produce a conditioned reflex so that the aid becomes part of his normal walking pattern.

When possible, walking should be trained as a reaction to sensory input based on normal muscle tone, and the use of specific instructions about localized movement should be reduced to a minimum. With some patients the difficulty facing the therapist is to decide at what point the effort at attempting to train a normal gait pattern should be abandoned and the patient and the therapist should accept an abnormal pattern and/or the introduction of an appliance or a walking aid, i.e. to consider walking merely as a means by which the patient can have some degree of independence in moving from place to place.

Standing balance is an essential prerequisite to walking. Time spent in gaining this before walking is attempted is vital as the patient who is unsure of his balance will be tense and afraid to move.

Walking aids feature in most gait training programmes (Chapter 10) as:

(1) A progression from parallel bars to the minimum necessary to enable patients who have been immobile for a period to develop their full potential.
(2) A temporary measure, for example for patients with lower limb injuries who have to be non-weight bearing or partial weight bearing for a limited period.
(3) A permanent aid for patients with no possibility of improvement.

The usual type of stick or crutch has been found to have an undesirable effect on some patients with cerebral palsy. The position in which sticks are usually held emphasizes the spastic pattern. In such cases the use of poles about half as long again as normal sticks may be used to help the patient's balance. To grip the poles, which he is encouraged to keep well out to the side, the patient's arms will be laterally rotated and the forearms supinated

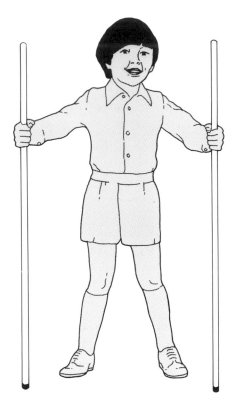

Fig. 26.1 Standing – using poles to aid balance.

(Fig. 26.1). The therapist can control the poles from the top when standing behind the patient.

Gait training is not complete until the patient can walk forwards, backwards, sideways and in a diagonal direction. To be fully independent the patient also needs to be able to negotiate stairs, slopes, uneven surfaces and other people moving or standing in close proximity.

Resisted walking

The therapist selects the walking aid which will enable the patient to concentrate his maximum effort on walking. The parallel bars are frequently used in the early stages of training.

Resisted walking may be selected with one of two aims:

(1) As a means whereby the therapist can give as much sensory information as possible while allowing the patient to move smoothly through the walking pattern which in itself establishes his sensory image of walking.

(2) As a means of increasing joint range, particularly at the knee and ankle, when it is limited following injury. The therapist encourages the patient, usually within the parallel bars, to work against a high degree of resistance thus exaggerating the walking pattern and the power of contraction of the muscles bringing about the movement.

Method

The therapist ensures that the patient has adequate balance.

She also ensures that he is in control of the walking aid and using it effectively. The patient's grip is tested and reinforced. The therapist grasps the patient's fingers with one hand and his thumb with the other. She then exerts resistance to the grip until the patient is working maximally. The grip must not be broken. Frequently when patients first use a crutch or stick they fail to exert enough downward pressure. In some instances they simply lift the aid off the floor. This downward pressure and stability can be facilitated by the therapist tapping the stick about halfway down, first from one side and then from the other in quick succession. Alternatively she may place her hand over the patient's and try to lift the aid off the floor. The command will be '*Don't let me move it*'.

The therapist stands in front of the patient if he is to walk forwards (Fig. 26.2) or behind him if he is to walk backwards. She places her hands on his iliac crests with either forward or backward pressure as necessary to give extero-

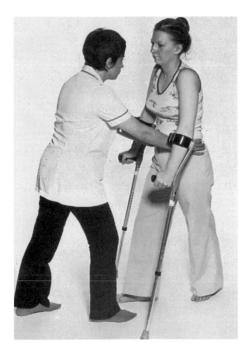

Fig. 26.2 Resisted walking.

ceptive stimulation for the direction of movement and in preparation for resisting walking.
The therapist may find it useful to slip her
thumbs into the waistband of the patient's
trousers, through which, if necessary, she can
control the pelvis.

As the patient walks, the therapist exerts
firm pressure downwards at every step on 'heel
strike' to facilitate the postural reflexes. She
then ensures that the patient transfers his
weight into the now standing leg simultaneously resisting or assisting the progression of
the moving leg. On 'heel strike' of the other leg,
downward pressure is again given and the cycle
repeated.

When resisted walking is being used to
increase range of movement at a particular
joint, emphasis is placed on resisting the
forward movement. The patient may appear to
be moving in slow motion and feel that he is
walking uphill.

Facilitating normal gait through trunk rotation

Trunk rotation is the foundation of correct
walking and when this is absent an abnormal
pattern results. Trunk rotation is lost in patients
with rigidity, e.g. with Parkinsonism, and in
patients who hold themselves stiff usually
through fear and lack of confidence in their
ability to walk following injury. It is not
unusual when young children are learning to
march to see one, who perhaps is a little unco-
ordinated, making a great effort, the result
being ipsilateral instead of contralateral movements of both the arms and the legs.

Method

Trunk rotation can be imposed on the patient
when he is walking by the therapist who either
rotates the trunk directly by using the pelvis or
shoulder girdle, or indirectly through the arms.
It is usual only to use these techniques when the
patient is walking forwards.

Both these methods when first used by the
therapist may pose a rather difficult problem of
co-ordination.

Directly

The therapist stands behind the patient. In the
early stages of using this technique it is advisable to establish with the patient which leg he
is going to move forwards initially, because
the therapist needs to be in position before the
patient starts to walk as she has to change her
manual contacts quickly. The patient takes
the first step with his right leg:

(1) The pelvis – the therapist places her right
    hand over the anterior superior iliac spine
    and her left on the posterior aspect of the
    iliac crest. As the patient moves his right
    leg forwards she pulls backwards with her
    right hand and pushes forwards with her

left hand. This has the effect of rotating the trunk to the right and the left arm swings forwards. She reverses the position of her hands and the pulling and pushing movements with each step.

(2) The shoulders – the therapist places her right hand on the front of the patient's right shoulder and her left hand on the back of the patient's left shoulder. As the patient moves his right leg forwards she pulls backwards with her right hand and pushes forwards with her left hand. As with the pelvic control this has the effect of rotating the patient's trunk to the right and the left arm swings forwards. She reverses the position of her hands and the pulling and pushing movements with each step.

The therapist's selection of either the pelvis or shoulders as a point of control will depend on the patient's response and the relative height of the patient and the therapist.

Indirectly
The therapist obtains a pair of wooden sticks or poles of similar length and stands in front of the patient facing him. She holds one end of each stick ands the patient holds the other end. They both allow their arms to hang loosely at their sides. Having established with the patient the leg with which he will take his first step, e.g. the right, she prepares to step backwards simultaneously with her left leg. The therapist instructs the patient to start walking; she walks backwards keeping in step and at the same time moving the patient's arms contralaterally through the sticks. Vigorous, large range movement of the arms imposes trunk rotation. If necessary the therapist, through the sticks, can help the patient to keep his balance.

INDEX